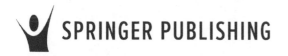 **SPRINGER PUBLISHING**

T0074888

GET THE MOST FROM YOUR BOOK

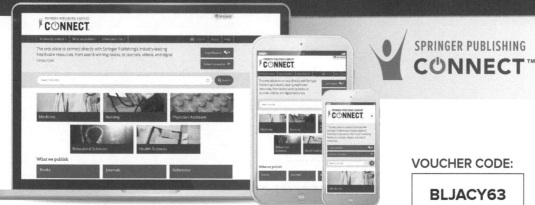

SPRINGER PUBLISHING
CONNECT™

VOUCHER CODE:

BLJACY63

Online Access

Your print purchase of *The Social Work Field Placement, Second Edition*, includes **online access via Springer Publishing Connect**™ to increase accessibility, portability, and searchability.

Insert the code at https://connect.springerpub.com/content/book/978-0-8261-3753-1 today!

Having trouble? Contact our customer service department at cs@springerpub.com

Instructor Resource Access for Adopters

Let us do some of the heavy lifting to create an engaging classroom experience with a variety of instructor resources included in most textbooks SUCH AS:

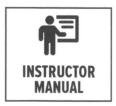

INSTRUCTOR MANUAL

POWERPOINTS

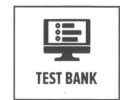

TEST BANK

Visit **https://connect.springerpub.com/** and look for the **"Show Supplementary"** button on your **book homepage** to see what is available to instructors! First time using Springer Publishing Connect?

Email **textbook@springerpub.com** to create an account and start unlocking valuable resources.

The Social Work
Field Placement

John Poulin, PhD, MSW, is a professor emeritus and adjunct professor at Widener University's Center for Social Work Education in Chester, Pennsylvania, currently teaching the foundation field seminar in Widener's online MSW program. In 2016, he retired from Widener University, where he taught generalist practice, research, and policy courses for 32 years. Dr. Poulin received a BA from the University of Southern Maine, an MSW from the University of Michigan, and a PhD from the University of Chicago's School of Social Service Administration. As a former director of Widener's BSW program, he founded its MSW program and served as the dean and director for 13 years. He also served for 10 years as the executive director of Social Work Consultation Services (SWCS), an innovative community-based field placement agency developed by the school of social work in collaboration with local community human services organizations. SWCS provides a wide range of free social work services to low-income community residents as well as free capacity-building services to underresourced community-based human services organizations. SWCS has served as a field placement site for hundreds of BSW and MSW students. Dr. Poulin has published numerous journal articles and book chapters and three editions of a generalist social work practice textbook. He also has to his credit many national and international conference presentations.

Selina Matis, PhD, LCSW, LICSW, is a lifelong resident of southwestern Pennsylvania. She received her doctoral degree in social work from Widener University. Additionally, she has an MSW, a BS in elementary education, and an MS in school psychology, all from California University of Pennsylvania. Dr. Matis is a full-time practice education associate faculty member at Capella University in the MSW program. Clinically, she has worked primarily in the mental health arena supporting children and their families in a variety of settings. She has specialized in treating trauma across the lifespan. She currently runs a private practice providing counseling, consultation, and supervision services. Educationally, Dr. Matis has taught at both the BSW and MSW levels in a variety of subject areas including practice education, clinical practice, research, policy, human behavior in the social environment, child welfare, and program evaluation. She has experience supporting students through the social work practice internships in a variety of ways as well, including as a practice coordinator, practice faculty liaison, and MSW supervisor. Dr. Matis has been published and presented on a variety of topics including resilience, self-care and burnout, ethics, trauma-informed social work, working with families, helping students succeed, and the social work competencies. She has two current social work textbooks in print—*Social Work Practice* and *The Social Work Field Placement.*

Heather Witt, PhD, LMSW, MEd, is a licensed social worker and assistant professor of social work at Boise State University. She received her PhD and MSW from Widener University in Chester, Pennsylvania. As a clinical social worker, she worked with children, adolescents, adults, and older adults providing individual, group, family, and relationship therapy. This work focused on a variety of issues including sexual trauma, infertility, depression, anxiety, and sexual functioning difficulties. Additionally, Dr. Witt provided psychoeducational sex education groups for families. Dr. Witt also has experience in administration in community health and nonprofit education settings, which informs her approach to policy and macro-level social work practice. Her current research focus is on human rights and policy practice, with a focus on social justice related to human sexuality. Her past scholarship topics include infertility; body image, eating disorders; gender differences; humility; trauma-informed approaches in the classroom; and cross-cultural research on body image, fear of intimacy, psychological well-being, and sexual anxiety. She recently published a chapter in *The Routledge Handbook on Social Work Ethics and Values.*

The Social Work Field Placement

Second Edition

A Competency-Based Approach

John Poulin, PhD, MSW
Selina Matis, PhD, LCSW, LICSW
Heather Witt, PhD, LMSW, MEd

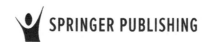 SPRINGER PUBLISHING

Springer Publishing Company, LLC
11 West 42nd Street, New York, NY 100036
www.springerpub.com
connect.springerpub.com

Acquisitions Editor: Rhonda Dearborn
Compositor: Transforma

ISBN: 978-0-8261-3752-4
ebook ISBN: 978-0-8261-3753-1
DOI: 10.1891/9780826137531

SUPPLEMENTS:

 A robust set of instructor resources designed to supplement this text is located at http://connect.springerpub.com/content/book/978-0-8261-3753-1. Qualifying instructors may request access by emailing textbook@springerpub.com.

Instructor Materials:
Instructor Manual: 978-0-8261-3754-8
Instructor PowerPoints: 978-0-8261-3758-6

Student Materials:
Student Resources: 978-0-8261-3755-5

23 24 25 26 27 / 5 4 3 2 1

Library of Congress Cataloging-in-Publication Data

Names: Poulin, John E., author. | Matis, Selina, author. | Witt, Heather, author.
Title: The social work field placement : a competency-based approach / John Poulin, PhD, MSW, Selina Matis, PhD, LCSW, Heather Witt, PhD, MEd, LCSW.
Description: 2 Edition. | New York, NY : Springer Publishing Company, [2023] | Revised edition of The social work field placement, [2019] | Includes bibliographical references and index. | Summary: "This book is designed to help BSW and MSW students enrolled in foundation field placements and field seminars structure their field placement learning around the nine Council on Social Work Education (CSWE) profession social work competencies defined in the 2022 Educational Policy and Accreditation Standards (EPAS). Our goal is to ensure that foundation field placement students integrate course learning related to the social work competencies with their field placement learning experiences in a purposeful, reflective, and integrated manner. It focuses the field experience and learning opportunities on the social work competencies. Each chapter is directly linked to a professional competency with substantive content on the competency, field reflection questions, critical thinking questions, a detailed case example illustrating one or more competencies with discussion questions, and electronic competency resource links to websites and videos"– Provided by publisher.
Identifiers: LCCN 2022049392 | ISBN 9780826137524 (paperback) | ISBN 9780826137531 (ebook)
Subjects: LCSH: Social work education. | Social service–Fieldwork.
Classification: LCC HV11 .P66 2023 | DDC 361.3071/55–dc23/eng/20221013
LC record available at https://lccn.loc.gov/2022049392

Contact sales@springerpub.com to receive discount rates on bulk purchases.

John Poulin: https://orcid.org/0000-0003-2165-8242

Publisher's Note: **New and used products purchased from third-party sellers are not guaranteed for quality, authenticity, or access to any included digital components.**

Printed in the United States of America by Gasch Printing.

For my family and friends whose support means the world to me. Thank you!
—SM

This book is dedicated to the social workers, social work students, and others who are fighting for the rights of women, LGBTQIA+ individuals, immigrants, refugees, and all other oppressed, targeted, and excluded people in the United States and throughout the world. Social workers combat social and economic injustice daily and are on the front lines in the struggle for equality and social justice in these troubling times.
—HW & JP

Contents

PART II: DEVELOPING YOUR PROFESSIONAL COMPETENCIES

6. Demonstrating Ethical and Professional Behavior   *101*

7. Advancing Human Rights and Social Justice in Your Field Placement   *121*

Contributors

Marina Barnett, DSW, MSW, is currently an associate professor in Widener University's Center for Social Work Education. Dr. Barnett teaches social welfare policy, organizational practice and grant writing, and community organization at the BSW, MSW, and PhD levels. Dr. Barnett has served in the Philadelphia and Chester communities as a consultant to numerous community-based organizations and government offices. Her research interests include geographic information system (GIS) mapping of community assets and using community empowerment approaches to train community residents to understand and conduct research in their own communities.

Stephen E. Kauffman, PhD, is a professor at Widener University's Center for Social Work Education, where he has taught community practice, program evaluation, research, and policy since 1991. He received his PhD from Bryn Mawr College and his MSW from Washington University in St. Louis. His research and practice have focused on citizen participation and community and organizational responses to global problems, such as environmental decay, poverty (in all its dimensions), and education.

With this focus, major research projects have included program evaluations of U.S. Department of Justice (DOJ) violence prevention programs, U.S. Department of Health and Human Services housing programs, 21st Century Community Learning Centers school performance studies, lead abatement, and teenage pregnancy prevention. The programs (and evaluations) have received funding from the DOJ, U.S. Department of Housing and Urban Development, the state of Pennsylvania, and several private foundations. He has also examined the relationship between universities and their surrounding environments.

He is currently developing a comprehensive assessment tool for examining trauma-informed care in organizations. He has published in *Social Work, Journal of Social Work Education, Journal of Community Practice, Journal of Baccalaureate Social Work,* and elsewhere. He also has coauthored one book.

Preface

GOAL OF THE BOOK

This book is designed to help BSW and MSW students enrolled in foundation field placements and field seminars structure their field placement learning around the nine Council on Social Work Education (CSWE) professional social work competencies defined in the 2022 Educational Policy and Accreditation Standards (EPAS). Our goal is to ensure that foundation field placement students integrate course learning related to the social work competencies with their field placement learning experiences in a purposeful, reflective, and integrated manner.

In our opinion, social work field education is facing three related challenges in relation to the mandated professional competencies and students' field placement experiences. The first is the disconnect between social work education's emphasis on the competencies and the practice of social work in the field. Unlike social work education, agency-based social work practice is not organized around the CSWE competencies. Thus, social work field placement students are faced with two competing pressures: their social work programs' focus on professional competencies development and their field placements' focus on the tasks and skills related to the delivery of services and adherence to the agency's model of practice. This book helps structure students' field learning to ensure that competency development is addressed throughout the field experience. It focuses the field experience and learning opportunities on the social work competencies. Each chapter is directly linked to a professional competency with substantive content on the competency, field reflection questions, critical thinking questions, a detailed case example illustrating one or more competencies with discussion questions, and electronic competency resource links to websites and videos.

A second challenge is that most field instructors are not well versed on competency-based education and the 2022 EPAS' emphasis on professional competencies. This leads to a lack of direct emphasis in student supervision related to the students' competency development. It is natural for supervisors to focus their supervision on the students' field tasks, work with clients, use of self, and administrative issues. However, including or framing supervision around the nine professional competencies does not happen organically with most field instructors. This book addresses this challenge by providing students with a toolbox that includes a competency field log intended to ensure that their field supervision includes discussions of their experiences and progress on each of the nine professional competencies. The Student Materials also contains an instrument to assess their field supervision as a way to increase the students' and field instructors' awareness of the administrative, educational, and supportive components of supervision to help ensure that all three are covered in the supervisory processes. As noted earlier, students' competency development around the educational component is often not addressed in field supervision. The Supervisory Relationship Inventory and the Competency Reflection Logs provided in the Student Materials help ensure that the students' experiences and progress related to the professional social work competencies are directly addressed in their field supervision. As an additional supplement to the field instructors' training and education on the 2022 EPAS, purchase of the print book includes digital access for use on most mobile devices and computers.

A third challenge facing field education in social work is that the EPAS 2022 mandates that at least one assessment measure be based on demonstration of the competency in real or simulated practice situations. Students' field placements meet the "real" practice situation criteria and are often used for one of the required outcome measures for each competency. Typically, the field instructor is tasked with completing the student's evaluation, which is tied in some way to the professional competencies. The challenge is obtaining meaningful data on competency assessment. This becomes problematic when competency development has not been incorporated into the ongoing supervisory process. When this happens, supervisors do not have the data needed to make accurate and valid assessments. The evaluation tends to be based on overall impressions without supporting data. This, in our opinion, raises serious questions about the validity of the data used for one of the mandated two measures.

This book helps address this challenge. The competency field log used to help structure field learning and supervision centered on competency development is also an excellent tool for a competency-based assessment conducted by the field instructors. The competency field log documents the students' experiences, affective reactions, and critical thinking on each competency throughout the field placement. It becomes the data on which the field instructors can base their assessment in completing the schools' field assessment tool. When used this way, the field instructor has the students' documentation and reflections from their field experiences related to each competency to help in evaluating student progress. This helps ensure that the field instructor's evaluation is data driven and not just based on an overall impression. We believe that the use of the competency log will help field instructors differentiate the students on each competency-based on actual experiences related to each competency. This will not happen if experiences related to each competency during the internship are not processed and discussed in supervision during the field placement and if a record of those experiences is not part of the students' field evaluation.

Thus, the goal of this book is threefold. First, it helps structure students' field learning on the social work competencies. Second, it helps educate social work field instructors on the social work competencies mandated by CSWE. Third, it helps provide valid data to social work programs on their students' mastery of the nine social work competencies if they use the student field evaluation by their field instructors as one of their required two program outcome measures.

DISTINGUISHING FEATURES/LEARNING TOOLS

In this book, we cover topics students need for successful field experiences and tie these topics to the professional social work competencies. To accomplish this, we have incorporated several distinguishing features and learning tools. One such feature is the use of Field Reflection Questions in each chapter. These questions engage students with the chapter content by asking about their field placements. How does the specific content relate to or apply to the student's field placement experience?

Another key feature is that each chapter has multiple critical thinking questions to help students think about the chapter content and its application to their field placement. The chapter critical thinking questions in Part II of the book focus on the specific competency covered in the chapter. Our critical thinking questions help students begin to understand how they might apply the chapter content and/or the professional social work competencies in their field placement.

Each chapter also has a detailed case example that illustrates the chapter competency and other professional competencies. These case examples bring to life the application of social work competencies in actual case situations. The case examples provide students with an opportunity to reflect on a case situation and describe how they would respond. Each case example is designed to engage the students' critical thinking and decision-making skills in relation to the identified social work competency.

As another key feature of the book, each chapter has suggested Learning Activities for the student that are related to the chapter content and/or the chapter competency. We believe that the Learning Activities will help students become proactive in structuring their field placement experiences to ensure that they have learning opportunities related to all nine of the professional social work competencies.

Other key features of this book are the Student Materials (available by accessing Springer Publishing Connect™ via the instructions on the opening page of this book, and clicking on the drop down Show Supplementary, Student Materials), the QR codes included throughout the book, and the numerous website and video links located at the end of each chapter. The materials provide students with electronic access to all the tools discussed in the book. These tools, especially the Competency Reflection Logs and Supervisory Relationship Inventory, will help students have a successful competency-focused field placement experience. The Student Materials also has several micro- and mezzo-level assessment tools that will aid students in their social work practice experiences. The Student Materials, the QR codes, and website and video links provide students with a wealth of supplemental resources to enhance their field placement learning opportunities.

This book has several instructor resources. PowerPoint presentations for each chapter cover the key points in each chapter and provide a structured guide for presenting the chapter content to the students. There also are additional case examples for each chapter as well as small group discussion assignments. Finally, there are case assignments and grading rubrics for each competency. All the assignments are applicable for use in site-based, hybrid, and online course formats. **Qualified instructors can access these materials by sending an email to textbook@springerpub.com.**

CHANGES AND ADDITIONS TO THE SECOND EDITION

Changes and additions to this version of the book include:

1. Updating the entire book with the 2022 Educational Policy and Accreditation Standards (EPAS).

2. Expanding the content on anti-racism, diversity, equity, and inclusion (ADEI) throughout the book.

3. Adding a new chapter on understanding the student's field placement agency and community. The aim of this new chapter is to help students successfully negotiate their field placement agency and to understand the community served by the agency. This additional content on organizational functioning and the community context of the field placement experience is based upon the recognition that understanding how organizations function internally and externally is a critical component to having a productive field placement experience. The chapter guides students in an exploration of their field placement agency's vision, mission, and goals as well as its organizational auspices and structure. It also helps students' development of understanding their agency's organizational culture and the need to be sensitive to the informal organizational culture or ways of doing things as well as its formal policies and procedures. The chapter also covers information on defining community and retrieving descriptive demographic information on their field placement community and/or population. Finally, the chapter describes approaches to identifying and locating community resources.

4. Adding student Learning Activities to every chapter. The Learning Activities provide examples of field placement tasks and projects that are aimed at developing learning opportunities related to the chapter topics and competencies. The aim here is to help ensure that students are proactive in creating learning opportunities that cover the full range of the professional social work competencies.

5. Including a pre- and posttest competency self-assessment instrument to the chapter on documenting your professional competencies. The tool focuses on the skill dimension of the competencies and contains an expanded list of

behavioral indicators for each competency. The self-assessment tool will help students identify areas of strength as well as areas that need development. It also can be used to help document their competency development.

6. Adding information on developing a performance improvement plan to the chapter on supervision. A sample performance improvement plan has also been added to the chapter. This information will help students struggling in their field placement make a plan to improve their performance and have a successful field placement experience.

7. A separate chapter on research-informed practice. The aim of this chapter is to help students incorporate research into their social work practice. The chapter describes critical thinking skills and their application, critiquing existing research, and incorporating the use of evidence-based practice. The chapter expands the coverage of research-informed practice from the previous edition of the book.

8. A separate chapter on applied research. Chapter 16 focuses on program evaluation and practice evaluation, the two types of applied research that students will most likely encounter in the field placements. The chapter covers the practice-informed research component of Competency 4 and the practice evaluation competency (Competency 9). The aim of the chapter is to provide students with the skills and knowledge to conduct formative and summative program evaluations as well as informal and formal evaluations of their social work practice with clients and constituencies. The chapter expands the coverage of program evaluation from the previous edition.

9. Adding content on cultural competence from the National Committee on Racial and Ethnic Diversity to Chapter 8. The section on forms of oppression has been moved to Chapter 7, where it fits better with our discussion of human rights and social justice. Information on cultural safety has been infused into the diversity chapter as well.

10. Infusing additional information about human rights in the field of social work, including information on rights-based approaches to social work practice. Content on forms of oppression has been expanded and justice-informed practice models has been added to Chapter 7.

11. Adding new content infusing recent research on policy practice for social workers as well as new information on recent policy changes that impact social welfare with special attention to social policy priorities established by the NASW.

Available Resources

 A robust set of instructor resources designed to supplement this text is located at http://connect.springerpub.com/content/book/978-0-8261-3753-1. Qualifying instructors may request access by emailing textbook@springerpub.com.

INSTRUCTOR RESOURCES

- **Instructor Manual** containing competency-based case summary assignments, grading rubrics, and small group exercises
- **Lecture PowerPoints**

STUDENT RESOURCES

- **Student Materials** including self-assessment tools

Maximizing Your Field Placement Learning Experience

The Social Work Field Placement

Jan is a first-year MSW student with a field placement in a public child welfare agency. She is assigned to a unit that provides case management services for adolescents in foster care, their birth parents, and their foster parents. In her internship, Jan monitors clients' service plans, provides supportive counseling for adolescents, helps link clients to other services and resources, and advocates for clients who need help from various systems and organizations.

Jan is pleased with her field placement because she is getting experience in working with individual clients and families. However, she is concerned about the services being provided to one of her families. The family clearly needs parenting classes, but they are not eligible because of program requirements about prior participation. Jan feels that not providing parenting programming is an ethical concern and a violation of the National Association of Social Workers (NASW) Code of Ethics regarding services to clients. Although Jan feels that she is facing an ethical dilemma, she is unsure what she can do to change the rules or get the families the needed services.

Jan decides to talk to Mary, her field instructor, about her concerns. Mary helps Jan realize that generalist social work practice includes macro practice activities as well as her micro activities with the children and their families. Together they formulate a plan in which Jan advocates for her clients' participation in the parenting program and for a change in the program requirements. Both activities enable Jan to address her ethical concerns and to develop her competence as a generalist social worker.

Why was it important for Jan to talk with her field instructor about how she was feeling? How should field students handle ethical concerns that occur at their placement?

LEARNING OBJECTIVES

By the end of this chapter, you will be able to:

- Describe the process of field education.

- Identify and define the roles of the field coordinator, field faculty liaison, field supervisor, task supervisor, and intern.

LEARNING OBJECTIVES

- Describe the NASW safety guidelines.
- Identify five steps in de-escalating an angry/hostile client.
- Identify the value base of the profession and its ethical principles.
- Apply frameworks for ethical decision-making.

WELCOME TO FIELD PLACEMENT

You are about to embark on the adventure that is field education, social work's signature pedagogy. Many professions require internships of sorts, but field work is unique to social work and has a long-standing history tied to the profession's early days.

During your field experience, you will have the opportunity to integrate your course content and experiences and apply that understanding to your social work practice. The hours you spent reading, studying, in lectures, and completing assignments have all sought to prepare you for this point. All senior BSW students and first-year MSW students are required by the Council on Social Work Education's (CSWE) Commission on Accreditation (COA) to have a generalist field placement that consists of at least 400 hours of supervised generalist social work practice opportunities to demonstrate social work competencies in field settings with individuals, families, groups, organizations, and communities (CSWE, 2022).

Field Reflection Questions

What are your expectations of your field experience?

What do you hope to gain during your placement experience?

THE FIELD PLACEMENT PROCESS

There are several stages in the field placement process. The first step in the field process is one that you have most likely already completed—the field placement assignment. As you will begin your field placement and your accompanying field course you will need to develop a learning plan, sometimes referred to as learning contract, with your field supervisor. Your institution will have a format for this document. The purpose of this plan is to develop mutually agreed-upon goals and related activities that will guide your learning and mastery of the professional competencies. It ensures that you receive the learning opportunities that are required to meet the CSWE (2022) Educational Policy and Accreditation

Standards (https://www.cswe.org/getmedia/94471c42-13b8-493b-9041-b30f48533d64/2022-EPAS.pdf). The learning contract and the professional social work competencies are discussed in detail in Chapter 3.

Throughout the semester, you will be meeting weekly with your field course, and there will be required assignments and discussions to explore and reflect upon the learning that is occurring in your field placement. You will have evaluations to be completed at the midpoint and the end of the semester. There will also be a site visit by your field faculty liaison who will review your placement progress with you and your field supervisor.

EXPECTATIONS AND REALITY

It is important to be clear about what your field placement it is and is not. Your field placement is:

- an educational opportunity in a real-world setting to engage with individuals, families, groups, organizations, and communities

- a time to incorporate all that you have learned in your social work courses in a supervised setting

- a time to grow your social work self

Your field placement is not:

- the same as a full-time job (although it may look a lot like a typical job position, the focus of field should be on the educational experience you are having)

- simply a required number of hours that you must complete at an agency (the time you spend in the field must be meaningful and directed toward meeting the goals that you have outlined in your learning plan)

> **Field Reflection Question**
>
> Can you identify two areas of growth you hope to focus on in your field experience?

STAGES OF INTERNSHIP

As you set out to begin your social work field placement it is helpful to know that there are stages in an internship. Though you may be very excited to dive in and begin working with clients, it is normal if that does not happen on day 1. Typically, there is an orientation period when you learn about the organization followed by a shadowing period when you observe your supervisor or a social work staff member. After you have been able to observe other staff working with clients, you will be able to start working with clients with the staff present to support you. During this co-facilitation phase you work with the client directly with the support of a more seasoned clinician by your side. In the final stage you move to independent practice with your clients, sometimes even maintaining your own caseload of clients under the supervision of your field instructor.

ROLES AND RESPONSIBILITIES

You will be working with many people during your field experience, some more directly than others, but everyone is working together to help you succeed and develop into the best social worker you can be. It is important to be clear on the roles of each person you will be working with during your field placement so that you understand how they are available to support you. But first let us review your role as a field placement student.

SOCIAL WORK INTERN

As a student, in what is probably your first social work field placement, your primary responsibility is to adopt a learner role. You are there to learn the practice of social work. This is done through gaining social work practice experiences at your placement, reflecting upon your experiences, and discussing your experiences with your field instructor. Be open to learning. *You are not expected to know everything.* You are expected to ask questions and adopt a position of not knowing. This is often hard for students who want to do well and show their field instructors and professional colleagues that they are competent and capable. Nevertheless, adopting the learner role is critical to a successful field placement and professional growth. Relax and accept that you are not expected to know everything. You are there to learn about social work practice. Ask questions, reflect upon your experiences with your field instructor, and be open to constructive feedback.

FIELD COORDINATOR

This person is an employee of the institution where you are enrolled, and their primary responsibility is to coordinate placements for social work students. The field coordinator works year-round to identify potential placements and cultivate relationships with agencies that host social work students. The field coordinator will help you throughout the preplacement setup process.

FIELD FACULTY LIAISON

This person is also an employee of the institution. Their primary responsibility is to support your learning throughout the semester. You will most likely be meeting with your field faculty liaison weekly in class (or online) to provide updates regarding your placement. Any institutional assignments or requirements (e.g., learning plan and evaluations) will be submitted to your liaison. Visits to your field site will also be conducted by your liaison. In almost all cases, this person is the direct connection between what is happening in your field placement and the institution. If there is a problem in field, your faculty liaison is there to support you and mediate if necessary. Ultimately, your faculty liaison is an advocate for you and your educational experience in the field.

FIELD INSTRUCTOR/SUPERVISOR

This person is the social worker who will support you throughout your placement. You will meet with your field instructor every week for supervision (more about this in Chapter 4). Your field instructor is most likely an employee of the agency where you are completing your field placement; however, in some instances that is not the case. When the field instructor is not an employee of the agency, you will also have a task supervisor who is an employee.

TASK SUPERVISOR

This person is responsible for overseeing your day-to-day tasks while you are at your field placement. Not all placements require a task supervisor. Some reasons that you may have a task supervisor include that the task supervisor does not have a social work degree or that the field instructor's job responsibilities require that this person is not on-site to the degree necessary to support you.

SOCIAL WORK PEERS

Your fellow classmates who are going through the field process with you are an excellent resource and source of support during your own field experience. When you meet during your field seminar classes, your peers can often offer insights and suggestions that may provide a fresh perspective on issues you are facing in the field. Do not underestimate the value of having this network of fellow social workers!

PROFESSIONAL EXPECTATIONS

In field, you should always present yourself as a professional. Being a professional is a multidimensional task that envelops all aspects of what you do in the field. There are a variety of ways that you can demonstrate that you are a professional. Arriving on time and being prepared is a simple way to demonstrate professional commitment. If you are sick and cannot make it to the agency, it is your responsibility to reach out to your field supervisor and let them know. Dependability is an important aspect of professionalism.

Acting with integrity and follow-through is another important aspect of the professional expectations that come along with field. If you are asked to complete a task during your field placement, do your best to complete it. With that being said, if you are unsure of what you are to do or have a question, it is absolutely okay to ask your field supervisor. Remember, field work is a learning experience; no one expects you to have all the answers on day 1. This is a process whereby you will be able to grow over time.

Professionalism can also be demonstrated through how you present yourself. Is your dress appropriate for the setting you are in? Depending on where you are placed, there is a wide range of acceptable attire for social workers. No matter how formal or casual the attire, your attire should be clean, neat, and respectable. Although ripped jeans and cropped tops may be in style, they may not be appropriate when working in the field. If you have questions regarding what professional attire is appropriate in your placement, ask your field supervisor.

How you dress is one way that you present yourself; another way is through your verbal and nonverbal communication. In the field, you are going to be meeting and interacting with many individuals. It is important to make good first impressions, and one way to do that is by using good communication skills. When meeting individuals, remember the power of making a good first impression by offering a greeting and making eye contact. Engage in conversations with those who are with you and pay attention. Turn off or silence your cell phone when in meetings or when you are with clients.

PROFESSIONAL SOCIALIZATION

One key aspect to social work education is professional socialization. Professional socialization refers to the process by which an individual becomes a member of a select profession. Your socialization to the social work profession began when you took your first social work course. Throughout your education you have been learning not only how to engage in the practice of social work but also what is expected of you as a social worker. The social work profession has high standards for members of the professions. As the old adage says, with great power comes great responsibility. As social workers we have a great power in our ability to serve and shape the lives of those with whom we work. As a result, there is great responsibility on us to uphold the values of this profession and to always practice ethically. The burden of ethical responsibility always falls upon us as the professional (not onto the client).

In field education, your professional socialization is taken a step further. As you engage in this signature pedagogy of our profession, you are given the opportunity to practice as a social worker under the direct supervision of another social work professional. Through this process you can take concepts from your coursework and apply them in a real-world setting. You are also able to benefit from the practice wisdom of your field supervisor. During this time, you further develop your professional self as an upcoming independent social worker. Developing your professional self is a key piece of your field placement experience.

Another aspect of professional socialization is the commitment to the profession of social work (Freund et al., 2017). One way that social workers are required to demonstrate a commitment to the profession is to adhere to the NASW *Code of Ethics* (2021; www.socialworkers .org/About/Ethics/Code-of-Ethics/Code-of-Ethics-English).

SOCIAL WORK VALUES AND ETHICS

The practice of social work is based on a number of value positions and principles that guide the work with clients irrespective of the approach used, the presenting client problem, the client population, or the setting in which services are provided. These values and principles apply to all forms of social work practice.

CORE SOCIAL WORK VALUES

Social work is a value-based profession (Reamer, 1990). What we mean by that is that values are at the heart of the work we do as social workers. They guide the actions we take and our evaluations of what is "good" (DuBois & Miley, 2014). Social work has a rich tradition of principles and beliefs. The heart of these is reflected in the NASW's (2021) *Code of Ethics*, which identifies core social work values, associated ethical principles, and ethical standards. The core professional values are the following: service to others, social justice, dignity and worth of the person, and importance of human relationships, integrity, and competence. These values and their associated ethical principles all play a critical role in generalist social work practice. It is important that you are familiar with the core values of our profession because they are the foundation for our practice.

Service

The first ethical principle is that "social workers' primary goal is to help people in need and to address social problems" (NASW, 2021, Ethical Principles, para. 1).

Service to others is placed above self-interest. Volunteering to serve others and address social problems is a commitment that all social workers are charged with accepting. Social work is a service profession dedicated to providing help to individuals, families, and groups in need, and to improving community and social conditions. The focus is on helping others directly by enhancing their capacities to resolve problems and indirectly by linking clients with resources, improving service delivery systems, and developing social programs and policies.

Social Justice

The second ethical principle is that social workers fight for social injustice. Social justice has long been valued in social work. Concern with social justice and inequality in the profession goes back to the advocacy efforts of Jane Addams and the settlement house movement of the early 1900s. The *Code of Ethics* states that challenging social injustice is an ethical principle of the profession.

Social workers traditionally work with people who are victims of discrimination and prejudice. Many of our clients are unemployed or underemployed, have limited access to resources, received inadequate education and training, and are among the most disadvantaged members of society. They often face prejudicial attitudes and are identified as lesser persons (DuBois & Miley, 2014). Social injustice is manifested in discrimination based on race, gender, social class, sexual orientation, age, and disability. Prejudicial attitudes provide justification for social structures that provide fewer prospects—fewer opportunities, fewer possibilities, and fewer resources—for those persons with lower status (DuBois & Miley, 2014).

Social workers' commitment to social justice is based on concern about the negative effects of discrimination and prejudice on disadvantaged populations. We often work with clients who have been denied basic rights and opportunities. We are called on to challenge social injustice and to increase the opportunities, possibilities, and resources of our clients. We have an ethical responsibility to address the social, physical, and economic needs of our clients as well as their psychological needs. The social work competencies expand the concept of social justice to include racial, economic, and environmental justice (CSWE, 2022).

Dignity and Worth of the Person

The third ethical principle is that "social workers respect the inherent dignity and worth of the person" (NASW, 2021, Ethical Principles, para. 3). This entails treating our clients in a caring and respectful fashion and being mindful of individual differences and cultural and ethnic diversity. The underlying assumption of this value is that all human beings have intrinsic worth, irrespective of their past or present behavior, beliefs, lifestyle, race, or status in life (Hepworth et al., 2017).

As a social worker, you are expected to treat your clients with respect and dignity. They deserve respect by virtue of their humanness. This does not mean that you must agree with your clients' life choices or decisions. It *does* mean that you should strive to affirm their dignity and self-worth. Not doing so can have profound negative effects on the helping process, and doing nothing could potentially cause harm.

Closely associated with respect for the individual is a nonjudgmental attitude. As a social worker, you must not place blame on the client through either your attitude or your behavior. Focus on understanding your clients and their difficulties and on helping them find solutions or alternative ways of behaving. If you blame them for their difficulties and assign pejorative labels, most will become defensive and unwilling to trust you. The more you understand the life experiences of your clients, no matter how personally distressing their behaviors or beliefs may be, the more likely it is that you will be able to accept them as human beings (Hepworth et al., 2017).

Many of our clients' behaviors conflict with our personal values and beliefs. Often, there will be a clash of values between you and your clients. These differences should be viewed as a normal part of generalist social work practice. Expect them and accept them. There are going to be differences; in fact, there are going to be major differences. If you focus on your values and assign blame to clients for adopting behaviors or attitudes with which you disagree, you will not be able to help them.

Importance of Human Relationships

The fourth ethical principle is that social workers value the centrality and importance of relationships. The *Code of Ethics* states that "social workers seek to strengthen relationships among people in a purposeful effort to promote, restore, maintain, and enhance the well-being of individuals, families, social groups, organizations, and communities" (NASW, 2021, p. 5). Focusing on the relationship issues of clients is common in generalist social work. Many clients need help in improving their human relationships and interpersonal interactions.

Integrity

The fifth ethical principle is that "social workers behave in a trustworthy manner" (NASW, 2021, Ethical Principles, para. 5). You have probably heard the sentiment that honesty is the best policy; in the social work profession, we value honesty very much. Social workers should demonstrate integrity at all times through honesty, sincerity, and responsibility. This is the key to developing trust and a positive helping relationship. Be open and honest. It is okay to admit that you do not

Field Reflection Questions

How can you demonstrate the six core values of social work during your field placement?

Which values and ethical principles are most challenging for you?

know or are unsure about something. If that happens, let your clients know that you will find out, and then follow through and get back to your clients with the information.

Competence

The sixth ethical principle is that "social workers practice within their areas of competence and develop and enhance their professional expertise" (NASW, 2021, Ethical Principles, para. 6). Social workers are to practice within their areas of training and seek ongoing supervision, education, and support on a regular basis. As a social work intern, your primary learning objective for your field placement is to become a competent generalist social worker. This is done by demonstrating proficiency through your practice experiences as they relate to the nine professional competencies defined by the CSWE (2022). The development of competence is a lifelong undertaking that involves critical thinking, reflection, and ongoing professional development.

ETHICAL STANDARDS

The core social work values and ethical principles embody the ideals to which all social workers should aspire. The *Code of Ethics* sets specific standards and explains how the core values and principles influence the actions of professional social workers. The standards spell out social workers' ethical responsibilities to clients, to colleagues, in practice settings, as professionals, to the social work profession, and to the broader society (NASW, 2021). They are detailed, comprehensive guidelines for social work professionals. Each area of responsibility includes several subareas. For example, ethical responsibilities to clients cover 16 subareas, such as commitment to clients, self-determination, informed consent, and competence. A detailed discussion of each ethical standard in the six areas of professional behavior areas may be found in the *Code of Ethics* (NASW, 2021).

As a social work intern, it is important that you become very familiar with the areas of professional responsibility. A thorough knowledge of the NASW *Code of Ethics* early in your field placement experience will help ensure that you engage in ethical practice and help you avoid unethical behavior. It is your responsibility as a professional social worker to be familiar with the *Code of Ethics* and follow it in your professional practice.

Ethical Dilemmas

Social workers frequently have ethical obligations to several parties at the same time. For example, we have ethical obligations to both our clients and our employing organizations. This creates the potential for conflict, or ethical dilemmas. An ethical dilemma occurs when one or more social work values are in conflict.

In these situations, you are forced to choose between two competing values or undesirable courses of action. Because we have ethical responsibilities to our clients, our colleagues, our practice settings, the profession, and the broader society, value conflicts and ethical dilemmas occur often within and between the six areas of professional responsibilities.

Resolving ethical dilemmas is never easy or straightforward. Rarely is there a clear-cut right or wrong choice. The choice is between two seeming "rights"; the task is to determine which "right" is more so given the circumstances.

The first step in addressing ethical dilemmas is to refer to the *Code of Ethics* for clarification of the standards of practice. The *Code*, however, does not offer bases for choosing between two or more conflicting standards. A number of guidelines have been developed to help individuals resolve ethical dilemmas. A hierarchy of value assumptions is the basis for decision-making; the hierarchy developed by Reamer (1990) is shown in the following list.

ETHICAL GUIDELINES

1. The rights to life, health, well-being, and necessities of life are superordinate and take precedence over rights to confidentiality and opportunities for additive "goods" such as wealth, education, and recreation.

2. An individual's basic right to well-being takes precedence over another person's right to privacy, freedom, or self-determination.

3. People's right to self-determination takes precedence over their right to basic well-being, provided they are competent to make informed and voluntary decisions with consideration of relevant knowledge and so long as the consequences of their decisions do not threaten the well-being of others.

4. People's rights to well-being may override laws, policies, and arrangements of organizations.

The first guideline proposes that a person's right to health and well-being takes precedence over the right of confidentiality. If you had to choose between protecting a person's health and well-being and violating a client's confidentiality, you would choose health and well-being. For example, the right of neglected and abused children to protection takes precedence over their parents' rights to confidentiality.

The second guideline proposes that a person's right to health and well-being takes precedence over another person's right to privacy, freedom, or self-determination. When you must choose between protecting a person's freedom and protecting another person from harm, the choice is to protect the person from harm. For example, if a client reveals plans to seek physical revenge on their former spouse, you should warn the former spouse.

The third guideline states that a person's right to self-determination takes precedence over their own right to well-being. That is, an individual's self-determination supersedes that person's well-being. The principle promotes freedom to choose and possibly fail or make mistakes. It protects the right of people to carry out actions that do not appear to be in their own best interests, if they are competent to make informed and voluntary decisions. However, the first guideline takes precedence if the individual's decision might result in death or serious harm. For example, you must take action to protect a client who is at risk of committing suicide.

The final guideline proposes that the right to well-being may override agency policies and procedural rules. Social workers are obligated to follow the policies and procedures of social work agencies, voluntary associations, and organizations. When agency policy has a negative effect on a client's well-being, however, violating the policy or procedure may be justified.

The guidelines described earlier—or any other guidelines—will not always provide clear-cut courses of action. They will, however, help you prioritize values to help clarify your thinking about an ethical issue. Resolving ethical dilemmas almost always entails making value judgments and subjective interpretations. For example, the third guideline states that a person's right to self-determination takes precedence over their right to basic well-being, provided that person is competent to make an informed decision. A social worker may have to apply this guideline to a person who is mentally ill and homeless, who prefers to remain on the street, and who has little or no interest in participating in a treatment program. Does this person have the right to refuse treatment as well as the right to live wherever they want? The complicating factor in this situation is determining the person's competence and the degree of physical or mental harm that is likely to ensue. Can a person who is mentally ill, delusional, and exhibiting psychotic behavior make informed decisions? At what point does refusing shelter or treatment create a serious risk of physical and mental harm? Clearly, the answers to these questions are subjective and open to value judgments.

In attempting to resolve ethical dilemmas, always invoke the concept of shared responsibility and decision-making. Do not make the decision on your own; enlist others in the process. Get your supervisor's or administrator's advice and approval before you act on an ethical dilemma. Case Example 1.1 illustrates the difficult decisions involved in resolving ethical dilemmas.

CASE EXAMPLE 1.1: AN ETHICAL DILEMMA

Jill is a first-year MSW student who has been placed in an after-school program for emotionally disturbed children. The program is run by a comprehensive mental health agency that offers a wide range of services for children and adults. The agency is a subsidiary of a larger organization that owns and operates a number of inpatient and outpatient mental health facilities. The after-school program has two full-time social workers, a case aide, a half-time supervisor, and a quarter-time program administrator.

Approximately 20 children with emotional and behavioral problems are provided with on-site services 5 days a week and with in-home services once a week. Because of a technicality, the program lost its primary source of funding and was slated to close. Jill found out about the pending closing of the program from her supervisor. She was told not to tell the other staff or the children. The program administrator had decided that it was best for the children, their parents, and the staff not to know in advance about the closing.

Jill was concerned about the children's need to have enough time to deal with their feelings about leaving the program and about the parents' needs to have time to make other arrangements for the treatment and after-school care of their children. She also wondered how the lack of process about closing the program would affect the staff and their morale. Jill believed that the well-being of the children was being subjugated to the perceived needs of the agency. She suspected that the agency administrator felt that telling the children and their parents would upset them and that the children would act out more than usual during the time remaining in the program.

She also suspected that the agency administrator wanted to avoid having the parents put pressure on the agency to continue the program. It appeared to her that the closing policy was designed to protect the agency from disruption at the expense of the children and their parents.

Jill is faced with an ethical dilemma. She has been told by her supervisor to follow an agency policy that she believes is not in the best interests of her clients.

1. *What are Jill's options?*
2. *Is it advisable for her to apply guideline 4 and disregard agency policy?*
3. *What might be the consequences of such an action?*
4. *How should she attempt to resolve her dilemma?*

SAFETY

Understanding and following best practices regarding your personal safety is an important social work skill. Social workers interact with persons with severe mental health issues, abusive people, people with poor impulse control, substance abusers, and other potentially violent clients. Therefore, it is very important that you become knowledgeable about the safety procedures of your field placement agency and with safety best practices for your work with clients at your agency and in the community.

SAFETY GUIDELINES

An NASW (2013a) task force of leading social work professionals developed comprehensive safety guidelines for social workers (www.socialworkers.org/ LinkClick.aspx?fileticket=6OEdoMjcNC0%3D&portalid=0). The following discussion briefly summarizes the guidelines that pertain to your work with clients. Guidelines related to agency policies and procedures are not reviewed here. However, we encourage you to review them on your own and, if needed, to advocate for the development of agency policies and practices that enhance social worker safety.

NASW's (2013a) safety guidelines have four standards that focus on worker behavior: (a) use of mobile phones, (b) office safety, (c) risk assessment for field visits, and (d) transporting clients. The NASW guidelines show the recommended procedures for each of the four safety standards.

Field Reflection Question

How well do your field placement agency's safety policies and procedures correspond to those recommended by the NASW?

Become knowledgeable of the recommendations listed earlier and review them periodically throughout your field placement. Do not become complacent when it comes to safety. Following NASW safety guidelines should become a routine part of your social work practice.

The NASW guidelines, however, do not cover how to handle angry clients and de-escalate potentially threatening situations. The NASW (2013b) publication on managing angry clients has identified five strategies for de-escalating threatening interactions with clients (www.socialworkers .org/assets/secured/documents/practice/managingangerinclients .pdf).

The first strategy is to stay calm. Role-model a calm composure. Do not lean forward, make only minimal arm or hand movements, take deep calming breaths, and ask your client to remain calm. The second recommendation is to listen. Allow your client to vent and be heard. Third, remind your client that you are there to help. Emphasize why you are there and why you are working together. The fourth NASW recommendation is to empathize with your client and their feelings. Using empathy, communicate that you understand, and help the client feel heard. Finally, establish and maintain boundaries. Remind your client that you are respectful in your communication and that you expect the same in return. Indicate that you want to hear your client's concerns, but you need them to adhere to certain rules of communication, such as speaking in a calm voice and not using profanity (NASW, 2013b). If your field placement orientation did not cover de-escalation of hostile/angry clients, we strongly recommend that you and your field instructor discuss it in supervision.

CASE SUMMARY: "I AM PRAYING FOR MY SON"

PRACTICE SETTING DESCRIPTION

Topsham Rehabilitation and Healthcare Center in Virginia is a 134-bed long-term geriatric home and short-term rehabilitation unit. The building in which the facility is currently housed is much older than many of the long-term care facilities in the area, as it used to be part of a prison in the 1950s. The facility consists of five hallways: Three are long-term residential semiprivate and four-bed ward rooms, one hall is specifically for short-term residents filled with private and semiprivate rooms, and the final hall has a mixture of both short- and long-term private and semiprivate rooms. A large majority of the clientele in the facility come from lower- to middle-class socioeconomic homes. Because of the geographic location of the Topsham facility, the majority of residents come from factory or service industry jobs. The facility has an activities department, which facilitates various programs each day, as well as a complete kitchen and dietary staff, regulating and addressing the dietary needs of the individual patients. There is also a Physical, Occupational, and Speech Therapy department, which works 7 days a week for both restorative care for long-term residents and daily rehabilitation for short-term residents. On staff, there is a licensed social worker, an MSW student intern, and a social services assistant. There are three main courtyards in which the residents and patients may congregate, as well as large gathering spaces for activities and meals.

IDENTIFYING DATA

Ruth is a 75-year-old Caucasian female who is a very strict Catholic. Her religious views help define her beliefs and values. She moved into the facility about 2.5 years ago when her son decided that she should not be living alone. She ambulates in a wheelchair but is independent with all of her own activities of daily living. She also has mild dementia, which is the reason she was not eligible for an independent living facility.

Ruth was previously married and has one adult son. He lives in Florida and is homosexual. Her son is a pilot and is in a long-term relationship with a man he met while working at one of the airports. Ruth is in California, where she still owns a home. Her son decided that she should not live by herself, and placed her in Topsham Rehabilitation and Healthcare Center. Ruth is a college graduate and worked as an assistant at a law firm for many years. Although she was able to hold down a job in her later years, she had a very difficult time as a younger woman. Her husband was physically abusive to her and emotionally abusive to her son. She stayed with her husband until his death from a heart attack 20 years ago. Ruth was diagnosed with major depressive disorder and anxiety at a relatively young age. Her mental health issues and abusive relationship with her husband have contributed to her strained relationship with her son.

PRESENTING PROBLEM

Ruth expects that because of her status as her son's mother, he should take care of her and be involved in her life. He does not feel this way, although he does talk to her by phone on a regular basis. Ruth's relationship with her son is strained and a cause of concern for her. She feels that it is her place to give motherly advice to her son and expects him to behave and act in a certain way; when he does not, she attempts to make him feel guilty. Because of her strong Catholic beliefs, there have been many arguments regarding her son's homosexuality. Her frustration over her son and his "lifestyle" seems to be contributing to Ruth's increased depression and anxiety over the past 6 months.

ASSESSMENT

Ruth is a very bright woman who comes from a relatively affluent background. Her son speaks to Ruth on a regular basis, and they have a lot in common. The main strain in that relationship is his sexual orientation. Ruth uses humor as a coping mechanism, and because of her fun-loving nature, she is very well liked in the facility. This gives her a support system within the facility that she does not otherwise receive from her son. Although Ruth's spirituality can be a strength to get her through the day and to find a sense of purpose, her unwillingness to accept her son as a gay man and her rejection of his life partner create a huge barrier to having the kind of relationship she desires with her son. By refusing to accept her son's homosexuality and his relationship with his life partner, she is causing her son to distance himself from her. Instead, she refuses to bend and believes that if she preaches to him and prays for him enough, he will become heterosexual.

CASE PROCESS SUMMARY

In working with Ruth, I have focused on helping her improve her relationship with her son and her understanding of why her placement at Topsham is appropriate given her age and beginning stages of dementia. When we started working together, I asked Ruth what she would like to achieve in our work together. She stated that she wanted to understand why her son decided that Topsham was the best place for her and how to achieve a better relationship with her son. Recently, there has been a lot of hostility from Ruth regarding her son. When I attempt to challenge her or to get her to look at the situation from a different perspective, she shuts down or becomes very aggressive. Because of this, I realize how difficult it can be for a woman with her set of beliefs to grasp why her son is not married with children.

While working with Ruth, I have realized how difficult it can be to not be judgmental and impose my values and personal beliefs on how I approach our work. First, it is very difficult for me to accept that because of her strong religious beliefs, she cannot seem to accept that her son is homosexual. I grew up in a family that did not have strong spiritual ties but was very geared toward humanism and compassion for diversity, so I have a difficult time relating to those who use their beliefs to belittle or berate others.

Alex, MSW Student Intern

CASE DISCUSSION QUESTIONS

1. *In this case summary, identify a potential ethical issue facing Alex in her individual work with Ruth. Discuss why it is an ethical issue referencing the NASW's* Code of Ethics *and the CSWE's competency to demonstrate ethical and professional behavior. Describe at least three steps Alex needs to take to minimize the potential ethical issue.*

2. *In this case summary, identify at least one mezzo-level and one macro-level ethical issue. Discuss why each is an ethical issue by referencing the NASW's* Code of Ethics *and the CSWE's competency to demonstrate ethical and professional behavior. Describe how each ethical issue could potentially impact Alex's work with Ruth and what steps Alex could take to address the potential ethical issues.*

3. *In your field placement, describe an experience you have had that is similar to the ethical issues facing Alex. Discuss what you did to address the potential ethical issue. Discuss your effectiveness in dealing with the issue and what you would do differently when it comes up again.*

END-OF-CHAPTER RESOURCES

 A robust set of instructor resources designed to supplement this text is located at http://connect.springerpub.com/content/book/978-0-8261-3753-1. Qualifying instructors may request access by emailing textbook@springerpub.com.

CRITICAL THINKING QUESTIONS

1. Sara is a new field student at the county child protective services organization. During her second week of field placement, her supervisor begins assigning clients to her caseload. Sara reviews the list of clients with whom she is to make contact and notices she knows one of the names. A client whom her

supervisor had assigned to her is a next-door neighbor. What should Sara do? Why? What is the ethical concern?

2. Joanie is a field student at a hospital. While she is working in the ED, a patient who has been exhibiting suicidal and homicidal ideation is admitted and social work is called for a consult. Joanie has never worked with a client like this before and does not feel confident in her skills to assess for safety. What should Joanie do? Why? What is the ethical concern?

3. How do your personal values align with the core values of the profession? How are they similar? How are they different?

4. What should you do if your personal values conflict with the core social work values?

5. How do social workers' personal values impact their work with clients? What would you do if you have clients who behave in ways that go against your personal values and beliefs?

LEARNING ACTIVITIES

1. Consider your field placement and review the NASW safety guidelines. Based upon your review identify five to seven questions you can ask your field instructor about your agency's policies and procedures related to safety.

2. Reflect upon the core values of the social work profession that are presented in the NASW *Code of Ethics*. Consider how during your field placement you can aspire to upload each value. For each value identify 1 and 2 ways that you can live out that social work value.

ELECTRONIC RESOURCES

WEBSITE LINKS

 NASW Guidelines for Social Worker Safety: www.socialworkers .org/LinkClick.aspx?fileticket=6OEdoMjcNC0%3D&portalid=0

NASW *Code of Ethics*: www.socialworkers.org/About/Ethics/
Code-of-Ethics/Code-of-Ethics-English

NASW-MA Workplace Safety Resources: www.naswma.org/page/
SafetyPolicyRecs

VIDEO LINKS

The Placement Experience (3-minute clip of a student discussing
field work): www.youtube.com/watch?v=XYr1scwc2ZI

Professional Ethics and Values in Contemporary Social Work
Practice: www.youtube.com/watch?v=lImSqcEDOGs

Social Work Ethical Dilemmas: www.youtube.com/watch?v=xn
LvGuHv9zk

REFERENCES

Council on Social Work Education. (2022). *Educational policy and accreditation standards for baccalaureate and master's social work programs.* https://www.cswe.org/getmedia/94471c42-13b8-493b-9041-b30f48533d64/2022-EPAS.pdf

DuBois, B., & Miley, K. K. (2014). *Social work: An empowering profession* (8th ed.). Pearson.

Freund, A., Cohen, A., Blit-Cohen, E., & Dehan, N. (2017). Professional socialization and commitment to the profession in social work students: A longitudinal study exploring the effect of attitudes, perception of the profession, teaching, training, and supervision. *Journal of Social Work, 17*(6), 635–658. https://doi.org/10.1177/1468017316651991

Hepworth, D. H., Rooney, R. H., Rooney, G. D., & Strom-Gottfried, K. (2017). *Direct social work practice: Theory and skills* (10th ed.). Cengage.

National Association of Social Workers. (2013a). *Guidelines for social work safety in the workplace.* https://www.socialworkers.org/LinkClick.aspx?fileticket=6OEdoMjcNC0%3D&portalid=0

National Association of Social Workers. (2013b). *Managing clients who present with anger.* https://www.socialworkers.org/assets/secured/documents/practice/managingangerinclients.pdf

National Association of Social Workers. (2021). *Code of ethics.* https://www.socialworkers.org/About/Ethics/Code-of-Ethics/Code-of-Ethics-English

Reamer, F. G. (1990). *Ethical dilemmas in social service* (2nd ed.). Columbia University Press.

Understanding Your Agency and Community

CASE VIGNETTE

Lucy couldn't have been happier about her first field placement. She had found her "dream placement." The agency was close to her home, and the client population was exactly what she was looking for. And perhaps most importantly, the agency had an outstanding reputation in its field of practice.

But from the very first week at the agency, things seemed strained. Case files for her new caseload were incomplete or missing, and no one seemed to have any idea where they might be. Further, many of her coworkers, although quite kind and helpful to her, often appeared distracted or "edgy." And her field instructor seemed to have little time for her. She was distracted during their supervision and often cut it short saying she had emergencies that needed her attention.

Having a rewarding and successful field placement experience will be a challenge for Lucy. For that to happen Lucy will need to figure out how her agency functions in terms of communication patterns and leadership. It will also be important for her to understand the organizational culture and figure out ways to have her learning needs met within that culture.

LEARNING OBJECTIVES

By the end of this chapter, you will be able to:

- Identify your agency's vision, mission, and goals.
- Describe the agency's organizational auspices.
- Analyze the agency's organizational structure.
- Assess the organizational culture of your field placement agency.
- Define the community context of your field placement.
- Review secondary data sources on the geographic community.

LEARNING OBJECTIVES

- Research information of the target populations served by your field placement agency.
- Identify community resources and services.

UNDERSTANDING YOUR FIELD PLACEMENT AGENCY

A successful field placement experience does not happen automatically, but rather requires intentional effort and commitment on your part. One of your first tasks is to assess the lay of the land and find out everything you can about the agency and how it operates.

VISION, MISSION, AND GOALS

 A good starting place is the agency's vision, mission, and goal statements. Mission and vision statements capture the essence of the organization's beliefs and values. A vision statement explains the overall goal of the organization looking into the future, whereas the mission statement outlines the present plan to realize the vision (McQueary, 2014). Both the vision and mission statements can usually be found on an organization's website. See www.boardeffect.com/blog/what-difference-between-mission-vision-statements for a more detailed description of their differences.

Not all organizations will have a vision statement, but almost all will have a mission statement. Organizational goals are usually tied to the organization's mission statement. They are specific statements about what the organization hopes to achieve through its programs and services. Become familiar with your field placement's vision and mission statements as well as the organization's overall goals.

> **Field Reflection Questions**
>
> How does the mission of your field placement agency fit with your personal values and beliefs?
>
> How are they similar? Are there any differences? If there are differences, how will you manage the differences?

ORGANIZATIONAL AUSPICES

Another important aspect of your field placement agency related to its mission is its organizational auspices. The auspices of your field placement agency often determines the services provided as well as the target client population. Exhibit 2.1 is an example of an agency's vision, mission, goals, and objectives.

EXHIBIT 2.1

VISION, MISSION, GOALS, AND OBJECTIVES OF A COMMUNITY SUBSTANCE ABUSE TREATMENT AGENCY

VISION
The community we see is one in which all persons are free and empowered to make their own life choices, supported by caring families, neighbors, institutions, and government. All people can make these choices in part because they are free from the pain of addiction or unhealthy forms of dependence, but able to receive the care and treatment they need, without fear of punishment, stigma, or discrimination should life's pathways lead them in other directions.

MISSION
It is the mission of Seven Arrows to provide effective, compassionate, ethically sound, and stigma-free substance abuse treatment to all persons who suffer from the pain of addiction or unhealthy forms of dependence. We seek to provide our services to all persons in need, without regard to age, gender, race/ethnicity, sexual orientation, or past experiences. We also seek a variety of funding sources so that no person will be turned away from treatment because of inability to pay.

GOALS AND OBJECTIVES
Goal 1: Seven Arrows will provide a variety of effective, evidence-based substance abuse treatment services, both inpatient and outpatient, to all persons in need in the North Hills region.
Objective 1.1: Seven Arrows will provide inpatient, residential treatment services to a minimum of 250 clients per year.
Objective 1.2: Seven Arrows will provide methadone maintenance services for a maximum of 500 clients per year.
Goal 2: Seven Arrows will achieve the highest standards of quality through support of staff, nondiscriminatory practices, and community involvement.
Objective 2.1: Seven Arrows will provide a minimum of 100 hours of advanced training to each staff member each year.

One level of distinction is whether it is a governmental agency. Governmental agencies are operated and funded by municipal, county, state, or federal governmental bodies. Such agencies are mandated to provide specific types of services to specified client populations. These types of services are usually man- dated by public laws and/or governmental regulations. If your field placement is with a government agency or service, we recommend that you review the legislation that has mandated its services and that you research how its programs and services are funded. See https://blogs.loc.gov/law/2014/11/how-to-trace-federal-regulations-a-research-guide for a research guide on investigating federal rules and regulations.

If your field placement is not a governmental agency, then the distinction is whether it is a *not-for-profit* or *for-profit organization*. For-profit organizations are structured like any business and are in the business of providing social services

Field Reflection Questions

How does your field placement's funding source(s) affect service delivery to your clients? How does funding impact your work with clients?

to make money. In recent years, there has been a growth in for-profit organizations in the human services field (Schmid, 2008). They are often funded by government contracts, insurance reimbursement, and/or clients paying for the services received. If you are placed in a for-profit organization, find out how its programs and services are funded. Also, be very cognizant of how making a profit impacts the delivery of services and client-based decisions.

If your field placement agency is a nonprofit organization, then a common distinction is whether it is a *sectarian* or *nonsectarian organization*. Sectarian agencies have a religious affiliation, whereas nonsectarian organizations do not.

ORGANIZATIONAL STRUCTURE

One way to see how all the components of your field placement agency fit together is to review the agency's organizational structure. Often there is an organizational chart that lays this structure out visually. It will show you where the different programs are in the organizational structure and who reports to whom. Be clear on how your program or service fits into the organizational structure and how it fits into the administrative structure of the agency. Knowing the chain of command can help you successfully negotiate your field placement experience. See www.lucidchart.com/pages/tutorial/organizational-charts for descriptions of the various types of organizational charts.

Knowing the roles, functions, and purpose of your field agency's staff will help you successfully navigate your field placement experience. Human service organizations are typically composed of administrators, midlevel manager/supervisors, frontline workers, and a large variety of support staff (Kauffman, 2010). Social workers usually occupy administration, middle-management, and frontline positions. Frontline staff are those most concerned with delivering programs and services. Generally, administrators are concerned with the overall functioning of the organization. This often includes policy development, planning, personnel, resource development and acquisition, and compliance with external (and legal) requirements as well as leadership and setting the tone of the organization.

Supervisors (the middle line) serve as intermediaries between the administration and the frontline workers. Their task in the human services organization is to translate policies from the administration to their supervisees, communicate information both up and down the chain of command, oversee job functions, and provide guidance and support to frontline workers. The assumption is that the supervisor understands both the needs and the problems of the frontline workers, while also understanding the work requirements of the administration.

ORGANIZATIONAL CULTURE

Finally, we recommend that you keep your eyes and ears open to gain a sense of your field placement agency's *organizational climate* or *culture*. The adminis tration sets the informal climate of the organization. A climate where workers feel supported can go a long way toward overcoming the stress that is created by clients or the organizational environment. Conversely, a climate that feels oppressive and uncaring may make even pleasant work tasks feel stressful.

> **Field Reflection Questions**
>
> How would you describe the organizational culture of your field placement agency?
>
> What are the positive aspects of the organizational culture?
>
> What needs to change to improve the organizational culture for the staff?
>
> What could be changed to improve the culture for clients?
>
> How does the organizational culture impact your field placement experience?

Pay attention to how the administration communicates and interacts with the staff, how staff communicate and interact with each other, staff morale, and the general feel of working in the agency. Are the communication and interactions formal and hierarchical? Do the members interact in a friendly and supportive way? Do the staff have lunch together or do they eat alone? Are supervisors accessible and available for questions? Answers to these types of questions and understanding of the organizational culture will help you adapt your style to what is acceptable within your field placement agency. Your field instructor/supervisor will be the person to guide you in figuring out the norms of the agency. Observe, assess, and ask questions.

UNDERSTANDING THE COMMUNITY CONTEXT

DEFINING THE COMMUNITY

The community context of your field placement agency is variable. There are at least two major types of communities. These types are communities of place or geography, and communities of interest or affiliation (Hardcastle et al., 2011; Millington, 2010). Both types have borders or boundaries, membership, some commonality among participants, and some level of policies and rules to guide behavior. Although there is overlap in how these manifest in our country (Wilson, 2013), the major difference is that with a community of place you can physically point to the boundary. Communities of interest or affiliation have borders that are more generally conceptual. A quick example should serve to make this clear. The university community can be defined geographically based upon the property that it owns, or it can be defined conceptually by participation in university-sponsored activities. Community membership in both types can be established although the approach might differ. In the geographic definition, attending, residing, or working

Field Reflection Questions

Which definition of community best fits your field placement agency?

What role does community play in the functioning of your agency and its services?

How does the community context impact your work with clients?

at the university may be the demonstrable variable for identification. For the definition of community as interest group, this might expand to include people who give money to the university, people who attend sports events or cultural events, or even people who regularly read university newsletters.

As you begin your field placement, talk with the agency staff and your field instructor about how they view the community context of your agency and the services it provides. Do they view community as a defined geographic area? Or do they view the community in terms of a specific interest group or population? If community is viewed geographically, then figure out the geographic boundaries. If community is viewed by an interest group or affiliation, then identify the interest group. Once you have defined community your next task is to educate yourself about the community context of the field placement agency. How you go about this varies by type of community.

RESEARCHING THE COMMUNITY

 If a geographic definition of community best fits your field placement agency, then we suggest that you begin by gathering demographic information of the community. The types of secondary data available will vary depending upon how the geographic area is defined. The census data is a good place to start. The U.S. Census Bureau's website (https://data.census.gov/cedsci) allows you to search by ZIP code, city, county, and/or state to find a specific area's income levels, ethnicities, ages, and other social characteristics. Other types of information that might be available include health, housing, school, and crime statistics. These types of data may be available from local, county, and state websites. Your goal at this point is to try to get a comprehensive snapshot of the demographic characteristics of the geographic community served by your field placement agency. Understanding the composition of the community, its social characteristics and the social problems experienced by the community members will help you gain a better understanding of the life experiences of your clients and in turn increase your effectiveness.

If community is defined in terms of an interest group or affiliation, then your task is to research databases and the literature for information on population that defines your community. This also applies if you define community geographically. It is critical that you educate yourself about the cultural beliefs and values as well as the social problems experienced by the population groups served by your agency. We suggest you ask your supervisor and other frontline social workers about the clients they serve in the agency. What are the population or interest groups with whom you will be working? Ultimately your clients will educate you about their values, beliefs, and cultural traditions. At this point, your goal is to become as knowledgeable as possible about your client population. Developing expertise in information retrieval is an important skill that you will use throughout your field placement and social work career. Often an institution or agency will provide guidance in this area; for example, see https://blogs.helsinki.fi/students-digital -skills/3-information-seeking/3-2-information-retrieval for a comprehensive guide on information retrieval.

Currently, there are several searchable databases that contain summaries or abstracts of published journal articles in social work, psychology, education, social science, nursing, and other related disciplines. The major one in social work is *Social Work Abstracts,* and in psychology, *PsyLit.* Most libraries subscribe to several electronic databases. They can be searched using key words, authors, or titles. The search usually leads to article summaries or abstracts. The full text of articles of interest can then be reviewed in the library if available, or a copy can be requested through an interlibrary loan.

The internet has become an excellent source of information on a variety of social work topics. There are several search engines that are free and easy to use. One of the more powerful ones is Google. Searches are conducted the same way as with electronic databases, and usually lead to a list of "hits" with links to the identified websites. There are also several social work websites maintained by professional organizations and schools of social work that have links pages with addresses of websites of particular interest to social workers.

Caution, however, must be used with information obtained from the internet because there is no oversight or quality control. Anyone can post whatever they want. Care must be taken to verify the legitimacy of the website, qualifications of the author, and validity of the information. Nevertheless, there is a wealth of information relevant to social workers on the web, and the number of full text professional journals available online has increased dramatically during the past few years—a trend that will probably continue.

IDENTIFYING COMMUNITY RESOURCES

Identifying and obtaining needed resources and services are other important social work practice skills, especially for those working with disadvantaged and oppressed client populations. Resource mobilization and client advocacy are fundamental components of social work practice. As part of your field placement experience, we encourage you to actively develop relationships with other professionals in your field placement agency and in the community. Also, ask your field instructor about any resource directories or databases with information about community resources and services that are available in the community.

In addition to identifying and becoming familiar with community resources and services, we also recommend that you actively work on developing personal relationships with the various service provided in the community. Networking is a key to effective resource mobilization and client advocacy. Personal contact gets things accomplished. Formal requests for services and assistance are not as effective as presenting your case to someone you know and with whom you have a reciprocal relationship.

Developing a network begins by identifying relevant existing programs and services in the community and region. Most communities have published resource directories of human service organizations as well as blue page listings in the telephone directory. Identify key agencies and contact a social worker at each one to learn more about their programs and services and develop a relationship with a contact person at that organization.

Another networking strategy is to attend and join community coalitions and task forces related to your service area. Become an active member of community-wide efforts to address issues related to your professional work. Working with others builds relationships and expands your professional network. Strengthening your network increases your ability to effectively serve your clients (Poulin, 2010).

CASE SUMMARY: "MY DIFFICULT CLIENT"

PRACTICE SETTING DESCRIPTION

Circle for Change is a welfare-to-work program designed to address the barriers that participants may have to obtaining and maintaining employment. To do this, Circle for Change provides individual counseling; group counseling; computer, career, and life skills training; and General Education Development (GED) test preparation classes for participants without a GED or high school diploma. Clients are referred through the county Office of Employment and Training (OET). Women referred to the program are considered the "difficult clients" who have been on public assistance for many years and who have been unsuccessful in becoming gainfully employed after participating in numerous training programs.

The Circle for Change program uses an empowering collaborative approach to working with clients. It is a small program serving 10 to 15 clients during each 10-week session. The social work staff consists of a program coordinator, two MSW supervisors, and four MSW student interns. The program uses a team approach with all the social work staff working and interacting with the program participants. The program seeks to provide a welcoming and supportive environment for the participants.

The Circle for Change program is in an extremely disadvantaged community with many social programs. The community is predominantly composed of African American and Hispanic community residents. The poverty rate is very high, as are unemployment and teen pregnancy rates. The school district is ranked the lowest in the state and has been taken over by the state Department of Education. Drug use in the community is widespread and gang violence is a major issue with many residents feeling unsafe in their homes and neighborhood. By all measures the community is extremely disadvantaged with few resources or job opportunities.

IDENTIFYING DATA

Nadine is a 33-year-old African American woman who is currently unemployed and on public assistance. The county OET requires her to attend a job-training program for 12 hours a week and do community service at an approved site or conduct job searching for 18 hours a week.

Nadine dropped out of high school at age 16 to have her first child. She currently has five children ages 17, 14, 13, 10, and 7. All her children have different fathers, and none of these men are involved with their child's life either physically, emotionally, or financially. Nadine's oldest daughter is a junior in high school and expecting her first child before the end of the school year. Nadine has a very poor work history with many low-paying jobs of short duration. She has been on public assistance since the birth of her first child.

In addition to experiencing financial insecurity, she has also experienced periods of food insecurity and housing instability. She has a history of frequent moves to different rental units in her community with most of the moves precipitated by her inability to pay her rent.

PRESENTING PROBLEM

Nadine was referred to Circle for Change program from the OET. Participating in the program satisfies the requirement to attend a job training program. According to Nadine, her main problem is that she does not have a job, which stems from the fact that she does not have a high school diploma or a GED. After some time, Nadine indicates that she has "trust issues" and has a "fear of good things." She has coped with her financial situation by having a string of short-term positions and receiving assistance from welfare. Nadine also stated that she "does not get too close to nobody" because it takes her a long to time trust people.

Nadine and her caseworker at OET do not have a great relationship. The caseworker views Nadine as a "difficult client" and feels that Nadine's real issue is that she lacks motivation. The strained relationship is a problem because Nadine does not tell her caseworker anything personal about her life. Nadine has disclosed that she has witnessed her caseworker discussing other clients' personal business in front of other employees and clients. This has caused severe trust issues with Nadine and her caseworker. Nadine does not feel comfortable telling her caseworker when things come up in her life that impede her from fulfilling her requirements for her assistance, thus causing the caseworker to view her as lazy.

This was not Nadine's first welfare-to-work program. Nadine has been on public assistance off and on for many years. She has continually failed to retain employment. Nadine indicated that, while she enjoyed her last position of employment, she was forced to quit when she found out she was pregnant with her youngest child. Nadine has also stated that OET is part of the problem. They continually try to convince her to train to become a Certified Nurse's Assistant, although Nadine has no interest in doing such work. Nadine has said that she wants to find a job she really likes so she does not end up leaving it again.

Nadine has stated that her life is extremely stressful. Her oldest daughter is pregnant and planning to drop out of school when the baby is born. Her 14-year-old son has joined a gang and is working the corners selling drugs. He rarely attends school. Nadine has stated that one of her main goals is to have her daughter complete high school and to get her son off the streets and back into school.

Nadine, over time, indicated five distinct goals she wished to accomplish as part of her case management/individual counseling sessions at Coping Focus Counseling:

- *Work on trust issues.*

- *Obtain GED.*

- *Get an enjoyable job.*

- *Get two oldest children in school.*

- *Take time out for self-care.*

ASSESSMENT

Nadine has extraordinary economic difficulties. Currently her only income is that of public assistance through cash, food stamps, and medical assistance. She often has difficulty paying her utility bills because of her very low income. Nadine has stated that while her housing situation is comfortable, she does not like the area she lives in and wants to move when she is financially capable.

Nadine continually stated that she felt her biggest obstacle is her lack of education, which she is currently striving to change. Although Nadine is not highly educated, she is intelligent and eager to learn. Nadine picks skills up quickly and is also very good with computers. Nadine continually assisted other Circle for Change group members with their computer assignments and is also an excellent typist.

According to Nadine's caseworker, Nadine's main problem was that of motivation. However, Nadine consistently stated throughout her individual counseling sessions that she was motivated to change her life circumstances. Nevertheless, Nadine did not always take the necessary steps she needed to take to make that change happen. Through her work in her counseling sessions and her volunteer placement in a supportive environment, Nadine's motivation strengthened. As she was given opportunities to progress, she also made great advancements on some of her other goals, including one that was difficult for her to achieve: getting her children back into school. Although she has made great progress, Nadine does seem to have the tendency to put things off, especially things that cause her anxiety or are exceptionally difficult for her. She has indicated that she is confident in her ability to pass the GED exam, and time will tell if she is able to follow through on taking the test and beginning the full-time position that is waiting for her.

CASE PROCESS SUMMARY

Nadine was an active participant and successfully completed the Circle for Change program. She chose to continue individual counseling sessions after the program ended. She began working in an unpaid receptionist position as part of her 30-hour weekly requirement for assistance. Additionally, she successfully completed a GED preparation course. Nadine was offered a full-time receptionist position with benefits where she is currently volunteering, contingent on her successful completion of the GED test. She recently registered for the test and will be testing in less than a month.

Nadine made great strides in both of her more personal goals of taking time for herself and working on her trust issues. Nadine stated that her relationship with her counselor and other members of the Circle for Change program helped her to begin to trust people again. Nadine also began scheduling alone time for herself and has done an excellent job of setting aside at least 1 hour per week to focus on self-care.

Sara, MSW Student Intern

CASE DISCUSSION QUESTIONS

1. *Imagine that you have been placed with the Circle for Change program for your first MSW field assignment. Describe what you would do to better understand the program's community context. Be specific about how you would approach the task of educating yourself about the community and life experiences of the typical program participant.*

2. *Describe what you would do to understand your field placement agency. Be specific what and how you would approach the task of educating yourself about the program. What questions would you ask and what information would you ask to review?*

3. *Based upon the information provided in the case summary describe how Nadine's prior experiences and the community context might have impacted her financial, food, and housing insecurities. How have they impacted her parenting and trust issues?*

END-OF-CHAPTER RESOURCES

 SPRINGER PUBLISHING CONNECT™ | A robust set of instructor resources designed to supplement this text is located at http://connect.springerpub.com/content/book/978-0-8261-3753-1. Qualifying instructors may request access by emailing textbook@springerpub.com.

CRITICAL THINKING QUESTIONS

1. How does the organizational culture or climate impact client services? Identify as many positive and negative ways the organizational culture impacts the delivery of services to clients.

2. How do the funding streams of your field placement agency or program impact clients and service delivery? Identify positive and negative impacts.

3. How does the community context of your field placement agency affect your clients and their participation in the programs and services provided by your agency? Identify positive and negative ways the community context impacts the clients you serve.

LEARNING ACTIVITIES

1. Define the community served by your field placement agency. If you define community geographically, describe its demographic characteristics. If community is defined in terms of interest groups, prepare a summary sheet on the population or interest group based upon information you have derived from a search of the literature and from secondary data sources.

2. Identify the resources and community services that are available for your clients. Create a resource file that you can have for use with your clients. Make personal contact with your identified resources to learn more about the resource/service and to identify a contact person for future reference.

ELECTRONIC RESOURCES

WEBSITE LINKS

 Explore Census Data is the U.S. Census Bureau's portal for community-specific information. Search by ZIP code, city, county, and/or state to find a specific area's income levels, ethnicities, ages, and other social characteristics. https://data.census.gov/

 IssueLab is a service that lets you search thousands of social sector reports by subject. Many reports have helpful statistics such as demographic information. www.issuelab.org

 County Health Rankings & Roadmap provides data, evidence, guidance, and examples to build awareness of the multiple factors that influence health and support community leaders working to improve health and increase health equity. The Rankings are unique in their ability to measure the health of nearly every county in all 50 states. www.countyhealthrankings.org

CDC—WONDER manages nearly 20 collections of public-use data for U.S. births, deaths, cancer diagnoses, tuberculosis cases, vaccinations, environmental exposures, and population estimates, among many other topics. These data collections are available as online databases, which provide public access to ad-hoc queries, summary statistics, maps, charts, and data extracts. Most of the data are updated annually; some collections are updated monthly or weekly. https://wonder.cdc.gov

Community Commons is a collaborative initiative working to create healthy, equitable, and sustainable communities. The site has online databases on economy, education, environment, equity, food, health, housing, and transportation. www.communitycommons.org

VIDEO LINKS

Organizational Culture: www.youtube.com/watch?v=6AFn0vFtLC0

Types of Organizational Structures: www.youtube.com/watch?v=Vbcpr1TS9NM

Community Definitions: www.youtube.com/watch?v=ncfAz313Alc

Community Health: www.youtube.com/watch?v=BVv5Vw8kMSQ

REFERENCES

Hardcastle, D. A., Powers, P. R., & Wenocur, S. (2011). Chapter 4: The concept of community in social work practice. In D. A. Hardcastle, P. R. Powers, & S. Wenocur (Eds.), *Community practice: Theories and skills for social workers* (3rd ed., pp. 94–129). Oxford University Press.

Kauffman, S. (2010). Generalist practice with organizations. In J. Poulin (Ed.), *Strengths-based generalist practice: A collaborative approach* (3rd ed., pp. 254–321). Cengage Learning.

McQueary, A. (2014). 10 effective nonprofit mission and vision pages. *Wired Impact.* https://wiredimpact.com/blog/10-effective-nonprofit-mission-vision-pages

Millington, R. (2010, November 23). Different types of communities. *FeverBee Limited.* https://www.feverbee.com/different-types-of-communities

Poulin, J. (2010). *Strengths-based generalist practice: A collaborative approach* (3rd ed.). Cengage Learning.

Schmid, H. (2008). The role of nonprofit human service organizations in providing social services: A prefatory essay. *Administration in Social Work, 28*(3-4), 1–21. https://doi.org/10.1300/J147v28n03_01

Wilson, R. (2013, November 12). Another way to explain who we are: The 15 types of communities that make up America. *The Washington Post.* http://www.washingtonpost.com/blogs/govbeat/wp/2013/11/12/another-way-to-explain-who-we-are-the-15-types-of-communities-that-make-up-america

Maximizing Your Learning Opportunities and Documenting Your Competencies

CASE VIGNETTE

Ron, who is a first-year MSW student, has a field placement at an area agency on aging. He had worked at a social services agency as a case manager for 3 years before he began his graduate studies. In this field placement, he oversees the delivery and coordination of the various services being provided to elderly clients. As part of his field placement duties, Ron visits his clients in their homes and completes a comprehensive assessment, from which he develops a case management and evaluation plan. Although he has been a case manager in the past, he is excited about providing social work services to a different client population in a different service system with the opportunity to learn new skills.

Ron, however, is unsure how his performance as a social work intern will be evaluated. He has learned that he must develop a learning contract in collaboration with his field instructor and that the learning contract needs to focus on practice experiences related to professional competencies. He has also learned that at the end of the semester he will be evaluated on his proficiency on nine professional competencies. Ron realizes that a successful field placement is a requirement for staying in the MSW program and critical to his career goals. He wants to be sure that his learning contract and associated field placement experiences provide opportunities to address all the professional competencies and that his semester evaluation accurately reflects his learning and competency attainment.

How can Ron evaluate his professional practice regarding the nine competencies? How can Ron know whether he has successfully met the requirements for the competency?

LEARNING OBJECTIVES

By the end of this chapter, you will be able to:

- Identify the nine social work professional competencies and the role they play in social work education and accreditation.

LEARNING OBJECTIVES

- Describe the dimensions associated with the social work competencies.
- Conduct competency self-assessments and reflections on your client interactions or field placement experiences.
- Create a field placement learning contract with identified goals, objectives, activities, and data sources for evaluation.

ACCREDITATION AND PROFESSIONAL COMPETENCIES

The accrediting body for social work education programs in the United States is the Council on Social Work Education (CSWE) Commission on Accreditation (COA). The CSWE Commission on Educational Policy (COEP) creates educational policy for social work education and COA creates accreditation standards. The educational policy and accreditation standards together form the Educational Policy and Accreditation Standards (EPAS) that guide the accreditation of baccalaureate- and master's-level social work educational programs (Poulin & Matis, 2015).

SOCIAL WORK COMPETENCIES: EDUCATIONAL POLICY AND ACCREDITATION STANDARDS 2022

 Each of the nine professional competencies describes the knowledge, values, skills, and cognitive and affective processes that make up the competency at the generalist level of practice, followed by a set of behaviors that integrate these components. These behaviors represent examples of observable components of the competencies, whereas the preceding statements represent the underlying content and processes that inform the behaviors (CSWE, 2022). In the following, Competency 1 is shown as an example. The other competencies focus on diversity, justice, research, policy, engaging, assessing, intervening, and evaluating. An electronic copy of the 2022 EPAS can be found at www.cswe.org/getmedia/94471c42-13b8-493b-9041-b30f48533d64/2022-EPAS.pdf.

COMPETENCY 1: DEMONSTRATE ETHICAL AND PROFESSIONAL BEHAVIOR

Social workers understand the value base of the profession and its ethical standards, as well as relevant laws and regulations that may impact practice at the micro, mezzo, and macro levels. Social workers understand frameworks of ethical decision-making and how to apply principles of critical thinking to those frameworks in practice, research, and policy arenas. Social workers recognize personal values and the distinction between personal and professional values. They also understand how their personal experiences and affective reactions influence their professional judgment and behavior. Social workers understand the profession's history, its mission, and the roles and responsibilities of the profession. Social workers also understand the role of other professions when engaged in interprofessional teams. Social workers recognize the importance of lifelong learning and are committed to continually updating their skills to ensure they are relevant and effective. Social workers also understand emerging forms of technology and the ethical use of technology in social work practice. Social workers

- make ethical decisions by applying the standards of the National Association of Social Workers (NASW; 2021) *Code of Ethics*, relevant laws and regulations, models for ethical decision-making, ethical conduct of research, and additional codes of ethics as appropriate to context;

- use reflection and self-regulation to manage personal values and maintain professionalism in practice situations;

- demonstrate professional demeanor in behavior; appearance; and oral, written, and electronic communication;

- use technology ethically and appropriately to facilitate practice outcomes; and

- use supervision and consultation to guide professional judgment and behavior. (CSWE, 2022, p. 7)

COMPETENCY DIMENSIONS

McKnight (2013) proposes that competence is an "ongoing ability" to "integrate knowledge, skills, judgment, and professional attributes to practice safely and ethically" within one's professional scope (p. 460). The CSWE (2022) defines holistic competence as the demonstration of knowledge, values, skills, and cognitive and affective processes that include the social worker's critical thinking, affective reactions, and exercise of judgment regarding unique practice situations.

KNOWLEDGE

The knowledge dimension comprises your mastery of the substantive content of the competency. Social work curricula are constructed to provide students with coursework that includes readings, assignments, and discussions that educate students on the current knowledge related to each competency.

VALUES

The values dimension refers to the professional social work values (NASW, 2021). Although Competency 1 is about ethics and professional behavior, the other eight competencies have social work values dimensions as well. Understanding the values and ethics associated with the application of the different social work competencies is a fundamental aspect of ethical decision-making and professional social work competence.

SKILLS

The skills dimension refers to your ability to apply social work knowledge and values in your social work practice. Numerous skills are associated with each professional competency. Your field placement experience will provide you with an opportunity to apply, refine, and learn social work skills in practice situations.

COGNITIVE AND AFFECTIVE PROCESSES

This dimension has three associated subdimensions—critical thinking, affective reactions, and professional judgment. Critical thinking is the open-minded search for understanding. This process includes "providing evidence, examining the implications of the evidence, recognizing any potential contradictions and examining alternative explanations" (Heron, 2006, p. 221). Critical thinking is an intellectual, disciplined process of conceptualizing, analyzing, evaluating, and synthesizing multiple sources of information generated by observation, reaction, and reasoning. Affective reaction, by contrast, generally refers to the affective component of social work practice with clients (Rubaltelli & Slovic, 2008). It is the worker's emotional response to the client's presentation and situation and is tied to empathy and other affective processes. Affective reaction has relevance for social work competency, in that effective social work practice requires cognitive and affective understanding of the client as well as one's own feelings, emotions, and reactions (Poulin & Matis, 2015).

Professional judgment is about decision-making in social work practice. Thus, professional judgment is reasoned decision-making based on evidence, knowledge, analytical reasoning, and practice wisdom. It is a process of examining all facets of the case and making a reasoned decision supported by both objective and subjective evidence (Poulin & Matis, 2015).

The nine social work competencies and the associated dimensions are the interrelated components of professional social work practice. The competencies are interconnected; they do not stand alone.

Figure 3.1 shows a conceptualization of the various interrelationships among the nine professional social work competencies. The competencies in the outer ring of the circle are those that apply broadly to all practice situations. Ethical behavior, diversity, and justice competency are fundamental components of effective social work practice at all levels (Poulin & Matis, 2015). The competencies in middle ring

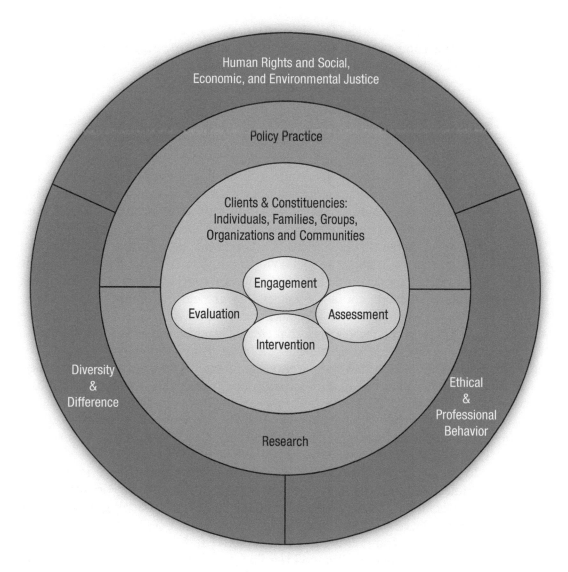

FIGURE 3.1 Social work competencies.

Source: Poulin, J., & Matis, S. (2015). Social work competencies and multidimensional assessment. *Journal of Baccalaureate Social Work, 20,* 117–135. https://doi.org/10.18084/1084-7219.20.1.117

of the figure, policy practice and research, are two areas of social work practice that are not client-based. These two competencies are informed by the competencies of diversity, justice, and ethical behavior and, in turn, inform social work practice with clients and constituencies. The compe-

Field Reflection Questions

How do you plan to incorporate cognitive and affective processes in your social work practice at your field placement?

How can you help structure your field placement supervision to ensure that you address your competencies in a multidimensional way?

tencies in the inner circle of the figure, engaging, assessing, intervening, and evaluating, are those related to social work practice with individuals, families, groups,

organizations, and communities. The diversity, justice, ethical behavior, policy practice, and research competencies all inform the social work practice competencies
with different clients and constituencies (Poulin & Matis, 2015).

THE LEARNING CONTRACT

The learning contract is an essential component of your field placement experience. Its purpose is to guide your learning and make it purposeful. Learning contracts usually specify activities or learning opportunities related to the social work
competencies. However, learning contract formats vary from program to program.
Therefore, this section will review the basic core components of a learning contract.

As a student in a generalist field placement, you must be proactive to ensure that
you have opportunities to master the social work competencies and develop the skills
needed for generalist practice, or to be ready for your specialization field placement.
Being proactive in your first couple of weeks at your field placement is not an easy
task. Nevertheless, it is important. Targeted and focused learning will not happen
automatically. There needs to be a plan that creates learning opportunities related to
the professional social work competencies and your individual learning needs. The
learning contract is the plan that shapes and directs your field placement experience.

Student field placements are a major component of social work education and
placements vary widely. There are a number of factors outside your control. One
area in which you do have control is your learning contract. It is where you and
your field instructor negotiate your field placement activities and learning opportunities that will contribute toward your professional development.

A key to having an excellent field placement learning experience is developing an individualized learning contract that identifies learning opportunities tied
directly to the social work competencies and your individual learning needs. To be
effective, the learning contract needs to be an ongoing component of your field placement experience. It is not something that is completed and then ignored or forgotten.
The learning contract must be reviewed regularly, and progress must be evaluated;
if learning opportunities related to all the social work competencies have not developed, then you must explore with your field instructor creative ways to make that
happen. It is your responsibility to monitor your learning contract and make sure
you have learning opportunities for each social work competency. Many of the competencies will be covered organically during your field placement activities. Others
might not. For those not covered, you will need to brainstorm with your field instructor ways to make that happen. Professional competence requires competence in all
nine areas and not just with some of the competencies.

DEVELOPING YOUR LEARNING CONTRACT

Most social work programs require a field placement learning contract. Your
school has a format and template that you must follow. Regardless of the template
for your school's learning contract there is a process you should follow. The first

step is to review the social work competencies and become very familiar with the core professional social work competencies. Your job as a social work student is to graduate as a competent social work professional. Your field placements are where you can engage in social work practice and associated activities related to the nine social work competencies. Before developing your learning contract, you need to have a clear understanding of what is expected of you as a professional social worker.

> **Field Reflection Questions**
>
> After completing a draft of your learning contract to what extent are your goals, objectives, and tasks ones that are truly yours and represent your learning needs?
>
> After completing your learning contract, what steps will you take to make it an active part of your field learning?

Having reviewed the professional competencies, your next step is to complete a self-assessment of your knowledge, skills, strengths, and challenges related to each competency. Ask yourself where you are in terms of your professional development and identify specific areas that need strengthening. Be honest with yourself. Your goal is not to show what you know but rather to identify areas that need further development. For each competency, develop two or three specific learning goals related to the competency. Your goals should be specific and based upon your self-assessment.

Having completed your competency self-assessment and identified potential learning goals, you are now ready to meet with your field instructor to identify field placement activities and learning opportunities related to each competency. The key is to identify activities that will provide learning opportunities related to the nine social work competencies and to the personal goals and challenges you have identified. Be comprehensive and identify as many activities as possible. This will help you and your field instructor design a field placement experience that proactively addresses your learning needs related to your professional growth and development. This is very different from just going to your field placement and letting whatever happens happen. Your field placement should be a structured learning experience. A comprehensive learning contract creates the structure and places the focus on your learning and professional development. Exhibit 3.1 shows a sample learning contract.

> **Field Reflection Questions**
>
> In your field placement how will you evaluate your knowledge related to each competency?
>
> Your skills?
>
> Your critical thinking and professional judgments?
>
> How can you help structure your field placement supervision to ensure that you address your competencies multidimensionally?

EVALUATION OF YOUR FIELD PERFORMANCE PROCESS

The evaluation of your field performance is done by your field instructor. Typically, your field instructor conducts your end of the semester evaluation and your grade for the semester is submitted by your faculty field liaison. Your

EXHIBIT 3.1

SAMPLE LEARNING CONTRACT

Brief Description of Agency Setting:
The community agency is a safe space for women and children escaping violence. The program provides temporary emergency assistance with other difficulties such as budgeting, credit complications, legal questions and obstacles, mediation, and so forth. The agency has 32 beds within 10 different rooms. The residents have access to laundry facilities, computers with internet access, a full kitchen, dining room, television room, and public transportation. There is a children's program that offers homework assistance and summer camp as well as other activities. The crisis hotline is also operated from within the agency and is staffed 24 hours a day. Crisis hotline advocates provide support, safety planning, and referrals.

Competency 1: Demonstrate Ethical and Professional Behavior

Social workers understand the value base of the profession and its ethical standards, as well as relevant laws and regulations that may impact practice at the micro, mezzo, and macro levels. Social workers understand frameworks of the ethical decision-making and how to apply principles of critical thinking to those frameworks in practice, research, and policy arenas. Social workers recognize personal values and the distinction between personal and professional values. They also understand how their personal experiences and affective reactions influence their professional judgment and behavior. Social workers understand the profession's history, mission, and roles and responsibilities. Social workers also understand the role of other professions when engaged in interprofessional teams. Social workers recognize the importance of lifelong learning and are committed to continually updating their skills to ensure they are relevant and effective. Social workers also understand emerging forms of technology and the ethical use of technology in social work practice. Social workers

- make ethical decisions by applying the standards of the NASW *Code of Ethics*, relevant laws and regulations, models for ethical decision-making, ethical conduct of research, and additional codes of ethics as appropriate to context;
- use reflection and self-regulation to manage personal values and maintain professionalism in practice situations;
- demonstrate professional demeanor in behavior; appearance; and oral, written, and electronic communication;
- use technology ethically and appropriately to facilitate practice outcomes; and
- use supervision and consultation to guide professional judgment and behavior.

Goal 1: To be become proficient in my ability to apply the NASW *Code of Ethics* in my social work practice with my clients.
Objective 1 (Knowledge): I will strengthen my knowledge of the NASW ethical standards.
Objective 1 Activities and Due Dates:

- I will read agency guidelines on professional behavior; appearance; and oral, written, and electronic communication (no later than the second week of field placement).
- I will attend agency Health Insurance Portability and Accountability Act (HIPAA) training (no later than the third week of field placement).
- I will study the NASW *Code of Ethics* (no later than the fourth week of field placement).
- I will review and discuss guidelines for resolving ethical dilemmas with my supervisor (no later than the fourth week for field placement).

Objective 1 Data Source: Competency Reflection Log (CRL) summaries and reflection notes on documenting completion of the activities and subsequent discussions in supervision.

EXHIBIT 3.1

SAMPLE LEARNING CONTRACT (*continued*)

Objective 2 (Behavior): I will apply ethical standards and principles, in consultation with my field instructor, in responding to ethical dilemmas I encounter with clients and/or colleagues.

Objective 2 Activities and Due Dates:

- I will review ethical standards and ethical dilemmas in supervision with my field instructor (begin no later than the third week of field placement and ongoing as the need arises).
- I will bring all possible ethical dilemmas to my supervisor for consultation and guidance (ongoing as the need arises).

Objective 2 Data Source: CRL summaries and reflection notes on my field instructor's observations and feedback on my ability to apply ethical guidelines in resolving an ethical dilemma with clients and/or colleagues.

Objective 3 (Cognitive/Affective): I will engage in self-reflection to help me effectively manage my personal values and value conflicts with my clients.

Objective 3 Activities and Due Dates:

- I will discuss my personal values and value conflicts with my supervisor to help guide my professional judgment and behaviors (begin no later than the third week of field placement and ongoing as the need arises).

Objective 3 Data Source: CRL summaries and reflection notes on supervisory sessions where we discussed my use of self-reflection related to managing personal values and value conflicts.

Note: An electronic template of a learning contract is available by accessing Springer Publishing Connect™ via the instructions on the opening page of this book, and clicking on the drop down Show Supplementary, Student Materials, Learning Contract Template.

field instructor will evaluate you using an instrument provided by your school. Field evaluation instruments vary from school to school. What they all have in common is evaluating your performance on the nine social work competencies. Regardless of the instrument used by your school, the bottom line is that your field instructor, in collaboration with you, will complete your performance evaluation, which will determine if your pass field or not. Therefore, it is incumbent upon you to make sure your field instructor has data necessary to make an informed evaluation of your performance. We also believe that you must be proactive to make sure this happens. Assuming that your field instructor remembers what you did and how well you did your various tasks and activities related to each competency is risky.

Agency practice is very demanding these days. Being a field instructor is an added demanding responsibility to an already busy schedule. Your field instructor is there to provide guidance and constructive feedback. Your field instructor will tend to view your performance in terms of your assigned tasks and agency needs. Viewing your performance in terms of the social work competencies requires a different lens and perspective. We believe that to facilitate your learning and to ensure an accurate competency-based evaluation, you, the student intern, need to organize and provide data on your performance to your field instructor. There are several ways this can be accomplished.

In developing your learning contract be sure to build into the evaluation component sources of data for your field instructor's evaluation. Some potential sources of data for your field instructor are (1) observation of your interactions with clients and/or colleagues, (2) your reflection notes, (3) review of your written work, and (4) insights gained through your participation in supervision sessions. Regardless of the data source one common thread is that the data need to be reviewed, discussed, and processed with your field instructor during supervision. To help make sure competency conversations take place in supervision be sure to include them on your weekly supervision agendas. Remember, it is your responsibility to help structure your supervision to include processing your field experiences and client interactions related to the social work competencies.

ASSESSING YOUR PROFESSIONAL COMPETENCE

Competency is a complex concept that focuses on your ability to do, not just what you know (Bogo et al., 2014). It involves "the demonstration of competence informed by knowledge, values, skills and cognitive and affective processes that include the social worker's critical thinking, affective reactions, and exercise of judgment that inform performance" (CSWE, 2022, p. 7). Your social work program will evaluate your performance in your field placement and your competency attainment most likely using some type of field placement measure.

We believe that engaging in a process of ongoing and continuous self-assessment is a critical part of your field placement evaluation. Social work professionals must continually engage in a process of reflection and self-assessment as part of their ethical practice in providing the best possible services to their clients. Social work students in field placement must also engage in a process of reflection and self-assessment. Reflection and self-assessment are critical components of learning and your professional development.

The sample Competency Skills Self-Assessment (CSSA) form shown in Exhibit 3.2 and the sample Competency Reflection Log (CRL) shown in Exhibit 3.3

EXHIBIT 3.2

SAMPLE COMPETENCY SKILLS SELF-ASSESSMENT FORM

Student:_____Mary Sones_____
Date: ___9/21/22_____ Semester: _____ Fall _____
Agency: _____Do Good Works_____

Instructions: Rate your level of mastery of the practice behaviors associated with each social work competency. Base your ratings on your self-assessment of your social work practice skills. Select the rating score that best reflects your current ability to perform the behavior in practice situations. If you have not had an opportunity to perform a practice behavior, give that practice behavior a score of zero.

EXHIBIT 3.3

SAMPLE COMPETENCY REFLECTION LOG

Instructions: The CRL is designed to help you keep track of your client interactions and field experiences that are related to the nine professional competencies (CSWE, 2022). The key to developing your professional competencies is to be aware of how your client interactions and field experiences are related to the different competencies and to reflect upon those experiences using this log. Another key to competency development is to discuss your experiences in an ongoing basis with your field supervisor. Doing so will help you gain a deeper understanding of the competencies and how they are interrelated.

Each professional competency, as defined by CSWE, is described in the CRL. The narrative descriptions of the competencies define them. The competencies are complex with multiple components and practice behaviors. CSWE identified five competency dimensions—knowledge, values, skills, affective reactions, and cognitive processes. The CRL covers all of the dimensions except knowledge. The practice behaviors listed below the competency descriptions represent the skill dimension.

For each interaction or field experience that you record in your CRL, select the appropriate competency, briefly describe the interaction and its context, identify the social work values and ethical principles that are most directly related to the interaction, identify the practice behaviors related to the competency that you used and reflect upon the effectiveness of your actions, describe your affective reactions that you experienced and how they affected your practice decisions, and describe your cognitive processes and how they affected your practice decisions. Insert additional rows as needed for each recorded interaction. Toward the end of each semester, complete an overall summary on your progress on the four dimensions of each competency. Assess your mastery of each competency, describing your strengths and challenges relative to the values, skills, affective reactions, and cognitive processes.

Competency 1: Demonstrate Ethical and Professional Behavior
Social workers understand the value base of the profession and its ethical standards, as well as relevant policies, laws, and regulations that may affect practice with individuals, families, groups, organizations, and communities. Social workers understand that ethics are informed by principles of human rights and apply them toward realizing social, racial, economic, and environmental justice in their practice. Social workers understand frameworks of ethical decision-making and apply principles of critical thinking to those frameworks in practice, research, and policy arenas. Social workers recognize and manage personal values and the distinction between personal and professional values. Social workers understand how their evolving worldview, personal experiences, and affective reactions influence their professional judgment and behavior. Social workers take measures to care for themselves professionally and personally, understanding that self-care is paramount for competent and ethical social work practice. Social workers use rights-based, anti-racist, and anti-oppressive lenses to understand and critique the profession's history, mission, roles, and responsibilities and recognize historical and current contexts of oppression in shaping institutions and social work. Social workers understand the role of other professionals when engaged in interprofessional practice. Social workers recognize the importance of lifelong learning and are committed to continually updating their skills to ensure relevant and effective practice. Social workers understand digital technology and the ethical use of technology in social work practice.

Competency 1 Practice Behaviors. Social workers working with clients and constituencies in micro, mezzo, and macro practice situations

(continued)

EXHIBIT 3.3

SAMPLE COMPETENCY REFLECTION LOG (*continued*)

- make ethical decisions by applying the standards of the NASW *Code of Ethics*, relevant laws and regulations, models for ethical decision-making, ethical conduct of research, and additional codes of ethics within the profession as appropriate to the context;
- demonstrate professional behavior; appearance; and oral, written, and electronic communication;
- use technology ethically and appropriately to facilitate practice outcomes; and
- use supervision and consultation to guide professional judgment and behavior.

Describe the client interaction or field experience, and the context of the interaction or field experience.	Reflect upon your substantive competency knowledge related to the client interaction or field experience.	Identify the practice behavior(s) you used and reflect upon your effectiveness. How well did it/ they work and why?	Identify the social work values and ethics relevant to the client interaction and reflect upon how the identified values/ethics influenced your practice decisions.	Describe your affective reactions and their use in making your practice decisions.	Describe your cognitive processes and how your critical thinking influenced your practice decisions.
Date: 9/21/2022 Context: A new participant who joined my substance abuse treatment group is someone I know personally from my neighborhood. Learning Contract: NASW *Code of Ethics* Learning Objectives: Apply ethical standards and principles, in consultation with my field instructor. Engage in self-reflection to help me effectively manage my personal values and value conflicts with my clients.	I am knowledgeable about the NASW *Code of Ethics* generally but not fully knowledgeable about all the ethical standards. I understand the standard on privacy and confidentiality, but I am not as clear about the standard on conflicts of interest.	I used two practice behaviors: (a) make an ethical decision by following the ethical standard on privacy and confidentiality; and (b) use supervision to guide professional judgments. I think I was effective with the first practice behavior because I did not acknowledge knowing the new member. By doing so, I maintained her privacy. I felt (affective reaction) that violating her privacy would be inappropriate and that she would acknowledge me if that was what she wanted (self-determination).	Several social work values and ethics are relevant to this situation. The social work value of respecting the dignity and worth of the person applies. My presence in the group could cause embarrassment for my former neighbor. Three ethical standards also apply to this situation. Ethical Standard 1.06a—Conflict of Interest could possibly apply. Having a personal relationship with a group member could interfere with my professional discretion and impartial judgment.	Seeing someone in the group who I knew from my neighborhood growing up made me feel uncomfortable. I felt uncomfortable for the client and for myself. Initially, I was unsure how to handle the situation.	When I realized I knew the new participant, I immediately knew that I had to decide about acknowledging our relationship. I reviewed in my mind the NASW *Code of Ethics* and was confident that I had to respect her privacy, because acknowledging her could be embarrassing and I did not know her preferences. Based on that, I made the decision to not acknowledge that we knew each other. I feel this was the correct decision because she did not acknowledge me, and my supervisor supported my decision.

EXHIBIT 3.3

SAMPLE COMPETENCY REFLECTION LOG (*continued*)

		Discussing the situation with my supervisor was also effective. I got additional clarification on how to handle similar situations in the future and clarification of the conflicts of interest standard related to dual relationships. We developed a strategy for future group meetings with the new participant.	Ethical Standard 1.06c—Dual Relationships applies. Social workers should try to avoid all forms of dual relationships. Ethical Standard 1.07—Privacy and Confidentiality could also apply to this situation. I would need to guard against sharing information about the group member's past from our former relationship. Recognizing these ethical concerns as potential ethical violations helped me recognize potential ethical violations and guard against them.		

Note: An electronic template of the CRL is available by accessing Springer Publishing Connect™ via the instructions on the opening page of this book, and clicking on the drop down Show Supplementary, Student Materials, Competency Reflection Log.

CRL, Competency Reflection Log; CSWE, Council on Social Work Education; NASW, National Association of Social Workers.

are designed to help you with the task of self-reflection and assessment of your development for each of the nine professional competencies (for copies of both forms covering all the social work competencies, access Springer Publishing Connect™ via the instructions on the opening page of this book, and click on the drop down Show Supplementary, Student Materials, Competency Reflection Log, or Competency Self-Assessment: Skills Dimension).

We suggest that you complete the CSSA at the beginning of your field placement as a baseline and then near the end of your first and second semesters in placement. This will serve as a pre- and posttest rating of your practice skills.

We also suggest that you keep throughout your field placement an ongoing CRL for each competency. When you have a client interaction or field placement experience related to a professional competency, you record it in the appropriate CRL and briefly reflect upon that experience. You can then use your reflection in supervision with your field instructor to enhance your learning related to the competency. This ongoing qualitative assessment of your progress on each competency with help keep the focus of your learning on the professional competencies. It will also give you a record and information that you can bring to your field placement evaluation meeting with your field instructor.

COMPETENCY 1: DEMONSTRATE ETHICAL AND PROFESSIONAL BEHAVIOR

Professional values, ethics, ethical dilemmas, personal and professional values, professional judgment, interprofessional relationships, use of technology, use of supervision, at the micro, mezzo, and macro levels of practice:

How would you rate your ability to perform the following practice behaviors? Would you say you:

0	1	2	3	4
Have not had any opportunity to use the practice behavior.	Have very limited ability to incorporate the practice behavior in most practice situations.	Have a beginning ability to incorporate the practice behavior in some practice situations.	Have the ability to incorporate the practice behavior in most practice situations.	Have the ability to incorporate the practice behavior in all practice situations.

• Adhere to the core social work values and NASW ethical principles	3
• Make ethical decisions by applying the ethical standards of the NASW *Code of Ethics* and relevant laws and regulations	2
• Use ethical decision-making models to resolve ethical dilemmas	0
• Follow ethical standards in conducting research studies	0
• Use refection and self-regulation to manage personal values and maintain professionalism	2
• Use reflection to understand how affective reactions influence practice decisions and professional judgment	3
• Demonstrate professional behavior and appearance in oral communication	4
• Demonstrate professional behavior in written and electronic communication	4
• Demonstrate understanding of the roles and responsibilities of all disciplines when engaged in interprofessional teams	1
• Use technology ethically and appropriately to facilitate practice outcomes	2
• Participate in professional development and trainings	0
• Use supervision and consultation to guide professional judgment and behavior	3

Note: The practice behaviors associated with each competency in the CSSA have been expanded from those shown in the CSWE EPAS to better capture the complexity of the competencies. The EPAS's practice behaviors are intended to be examples of how the competency is put into actual practice. They are not intended to represent all the possible ways the competencies could be applied in practice situations. An electronic template of the CSSA form is available by accessing Springer Publishing Connect™ via the instructions on the opening page of this book, and clicking on the drop down Show Supplementary, Student Materials, Competency Self-Assessment: Skills Dimension.

CASE SUMMARY: "AGAINST MY VALUES"

PRACTICE SETTING DESCRIPTION

Transitions is a group home run by a nonprofit social services agency that contracts with the county's public children and family services agency to provide housing and social work services to female teenagers who are aging out of foster care. A wide range of counseling, life skills, case management, and educational services are offered to prepare the participants for independent living. Transitions serves eight teenagers ages 15 to 19 at any one time, and the average stay for those who complete the program is about 2 years. All the teenagers have been in long-term foster care, and most have lived in several foster homes while growing up.

The group home has a BSW-level social worker who serves as the house parent and oversees running the house. There are three case aides—one during the day and two during the evening hours. Social workers based at the parent agency are assigned to provide counseling services and run life skills groups and educational programming for the participants. As a first-year MSW student, I am completing my generalist field placement at Transitions. My primary roles as an intern are to provide case management and mentoring services to three of the teenagers residing in the group home. My field instructor is the social worker assigned to provide counseling services to the Transitions residents.

IDENTIFYING DATA

Mary is a 17-year-old African American female who has been in foster care since the age of 5. She was placed in care because of parental neglect. Her mother was addicted to heroin and would leave Mary and her younger sister unsupervised for hours at time. There was also suspicion of abuse by one of her mother's numerous paramours. During Mary's 12 years in foster care, her mother's parental rights were terminated but Mary was never adopted. She lived in six different foster homes before she was placed in the Transitions group home when she was 15 years old. Mary struggled in school and had frequent suspensions for behavior issues and truancy. Although she was at grade level for her age, academically she was performing well below her grade level. Mary dropped out of high school when she turned 16 years of age.

Mary has not had contact with her mother since her termination of parental rights when Mary was 8 years old. She had occasional visits with her younger sister but has not had any contact with her for the past 5 years. Mary's relationships with five of her former foster parents are strained or nonexistent. She maintains phone contact and occasionally visits her first foster mother. Mary has few friends and has trouble getting along with her peers. She is not close to any of the other group home residents.

The Transitions house parent, the case aides, and some of the social workers view Mary as hostile and manipulative. They give her a wide berth and tend to not confront her if she is angry or acts out. They make no real effort to engage with her, develop relationships, or encourage her participation in the life skills or educational groups. The social worker, my field instructor, who is assigned to Mary, meets with her occasionally, but he reports that she is essentially unwilling to engage in a counseling relationship. Mary is one of my three assigned internship clients. My field instructor has asked me to try to develop a relationship with Mary and help her engage in the services offered by the program. He warned me that this will be a challenge, but he is hopeful that she can be reached.

PRESENTING PROBLEM

Mary has been in the group home for 2 years and is scheduled to transition to independent living in 1 year. She is a high school dropout with poor academic skills. She has shown little to no progress in strengthening her basic life skills and has not made any progress in terms of obtaining the educational resources she needs to improve the skills she would need for most types of minimum wage jobs.

In the group home, Mary is basically allowed to reside there but not to participate in the services offered. She does not have a positive relationship with any of the staff or group home residents. Most of the time, Mary displays indifferent or negative attitudes and responds angrily or is dismissive to any efforts to engage with her. At the most fundamental level, the presenting problem is that Mary is not prepared for independent living and she is not participating in the life skills, educational services, or counseling services that are designed to strengthen her ability to successfully make the transition out of foster care. In addition, Mary's poor interpersonal and relationship skills will hinder her transition to independent living.

ASSESSMENT

It appears that the staff are willing to tolerate Mary's hostile behavior and isolation rather than engage in any type of confrontation with her. I believe that Mary is tolerated and allowed to stay in the group home because there are no other options for her. Her social worker and my field instructor, however, has not given up on Mary: He has hope that she can be reached and engaged in a helping relationship.

Mary had a difficult early childhood with a neglectful parent. Mary most likely did not form a secure attachment with her mother. Attachment issues were further compromised by having lived with six different foster parents during her childhood and adolescent years. It appears that Mary formed a trusting relationship with her first foster parent, but that trust was broken when she was removed from the home and placed in a second foster home. With each subsequent move, her willingness or capacity to form secure attachments, in all probability, diminished. It is hard for Mary to trust. She perceives relationships in terms of disappointment and abandonment. This has resulted in her being very guarded in the group home and unwilling to form relationships with the Transitions staff and her peers.

Mary has been in the foster care system since she was 5 years old. During this time, she has had only one positive parental figure—her first foster mother. Other than during that relationship, Mary most likely received very little parental guidance throughout her journey in foster care. She has been provided with shelter, but not the parental guidance and role modeling that would prepare her for adulthood. As she nears her transition out of foster care and into so-called independent living, she is probably feeling very scared and anxious. Her hostile behavior is her defense from her fears. It is scary to imagine being on one's own at the age of 18 without any family or support system. Mary adopts her hostile and indifferent "I don't care about anything" attitude as a way of protecting herself from her internal fears. Mary's trust issues make it hard for her to share her feelings and be vulnerable with the staff or her peers. She instead lashes out to others and turns inward— isolated, alone, and, more likely than not, very anxious about being on her own and making her way in life as an independent young adult.

CASE PROCESS SUMMARY

Prior to my first meeting with Mary, I discussed her background, her behavior in the group home and program, as well as my field instructor's assessment of what might be influencing Mary's behavior and nonparticipation. Cognitively, I felt that I had a pretty good handle on what to expect in my first meeting with Mary. The case aides also advised me to give her plenty of space and not to force a conversation. They agreed that doing so would just cause a hostile and angry reaction from Mary. During my first week of placement, I had observed Mary being very disrespectful to the staff, argumentative with her peers, and not held accountable for her actions. I did not have any direct interactions with Mary. When Mary was assigned to me in week 2, I was tasked with introducing myself and discussing my role and how we will work together. I was a bit nervous and apprehensive about my ability to engage with my assigned client.

*My plan was to initiate a casual conversation with Mary in which I would introduce myself, discuss my role, and offer my help in any way possible. I wanted to keep it casual and informal and hopefully set up a time to meet. I approached Mary in the living room where she was listening to music with her headphones. No one else was in the room. Once I got her attention, I asked whether I could talk with her for a few minutes. She replied with an angry "Who the f*** are you?" I introduced myself and said I was a social work intern. Mary replied, "I am in a bad mood, and I hate social workers. Get the f*** out of my face and leave me alone."*

Emotionally, I was not prepared for the way Mary treated me. I tried to behave professionally and not respond negatively, but inside I was offended, angry, and judgmental. I tried not to show it, but I am confident my nonverbals revealed how I felt and the effect her behavior had on me. I grew up in a religious home where my parents emphasized respecting others and appropriate behavior when interacting with adults. As a parent myself, I, along with my husband, have tried to instill these values in our children. I found Mary's behavior extremely offensive. I also felt that it was wrong that Mary was allowed to behave this way in the group home with no consequences or accountability. I was also very discouraged that the initial meeting had been a complete failure.

I processed the interaction and my self-reflections in supervision with my field instructor. We discussed how my personal values were influencing my feelings about Mary and our working together. We discussed human behavior and the social environment, person-in-environment, and attachment theory to better understand Mary's behavior. We also discussed ways I might manage my personal feelings and how to become more empathic about Mary's challenges and the reasons behind her hostile and defensive behavior. We used qualitative assessment of the interaction to identify ways to improve my practice effectiveness with Mary.

Janet, MSW Student Intern

CASE DISCUSSION QUESTIONS

1. *Based on the preceding case summary, describe how you would manage the conflict between Janet's personal values and Mary's behavior. Discuss how you would cognitively, behaviorally, and emotionally manage your feelings of being disrespected and of being personally offended by Mary's behavior.*

2. *Describe a client interaction you have had that is like what Janet experienced in her first meeting with Mary. Describe the interaction, your internal processing, and what you did to engage your client and improve your practice effectiveness.*

3. *In the case summary, identify two mezzo-level organizational issues that Janet could possibly address during her field placement. Describe at least one organizational intervention that she could pursue to improve service effectiveness and staff morale. Briefly describe how you would conduct a qualitative evaluation of the effectiveness of your proposed intervention.*

4. *In the case summary, identify two macro-level issues that have impacted Mary's life and her current situation as an unprepared teenager aging out of foster care. Identify three change goals and describe how Janet might go about developing a macro-level intervention to address the identified goals.*

END-OF-CHAPTER RESOURCES

A robust set of instructor resources designed to supplement this text is located at http://connect.springerpub.com/content/book/978-0-8261-3753-1. Qualifying instructors may request access by emailing textbook@springerpub.com.

CRITICAL THINKING QUESTIONS

1. What social justice issues are associated with the client population served by your field placement agency? How do the social justice issues impact the clients served by your field placement agency?

2. How does the social work competency on human rights and social, economic, and environmental justice impact your social work practice in your internship?

3. How do the macro competencies in the outer ring of Figure 3.1 interact with the practice competencies in the inner ring of Figure 3.1? How would you describe the relationships among the various social work competencies?

4. How does the use of self-reflection in assessing your professional competence differ from qualitative program evaluations? How are they similar?

LEARNING ACTIVITIES

1. Review the CSWE (2022) EPAS and professional competencies. Complete a self-assessment of your competency for each of the nine social work competencies using the SCSA and CRL. Rate and briefly describe your self-assessment of the knowledge, values, skills, and cognitive/affective dimensions for each competency. For each competency prepare a summary that highlights your strengths and areas that need improvement. Identify activities and strategies that you will use to strengthen your competency proficiency.

2. Review your self-assessment and action plan with your field placement supervisor. Incorporate your self-assessment, action plan, and supervisory feedback into developing your learning contract. If you have already completed your learning contract, make any necessary changes based upon this learning activity.

ELECTRONIC RESOURCES

WEBSITE LINKS

Council on Social Work Education—2022 Educational Policy and Accreditation Standards (EPAS 2022): www.cswe.org/getmedia/ 94471c42-13b8-493b-9041-b30f48533d64/2022-EPAS.pdf.

VIDEO LINKS

Developing Learning Contracts: www.youtube.com/watch?v =XbHQ8JpyOak

Developing Goals and Objectives: www.youtube.com/watch?v=MAhs-m6cNzY

 Evaluating Your Social Work Practice: www.youtube.com/watch?v=ZYt4SWD_-uM

 Critical Thinking: www.youtube.com/watch?v=HnJ1bqXUnIM

 Reflective Practice: www.youtube.com/watch?v=1W8pqWU35BQ

REFERENCES

Bogo, M., Rawlings, M., Katz, E., & Logie, C. (2014). *Using simulation in assessment and teaching: OSCE adapted for social work*. Council on Social Work Education.

Council on Social Work Education. (2022). *Educational policy and accreditation standards for baccalaureate and master's social work programs*. https://www.cswe.org/getmedia/94471c42-13b8-493b-9041-b30f48533d64/2022-EPAS.pdf

Heron, G. (2006). Critical thinking in social care and social work: Searching student assignments for the evidence. *Journal of Social Work Education, 25*, 209–224. https://doi.org/10.1080/02615470600564965

McKnight, S. E. (2013). Mental health learning needs assessment: Competency-based instrument for best practice. *Issues in Mental Health Nursing, 34*, 459–471. https://doi.org/10.3109/01612840.2012.758205

National Association of Social Workers. (2021). *Code of ethics*. https://www.socialworkers.org/About/Ethics/Code-of-Ethics/Code-of-Ethics-English

Poulin, J., & Matis, S. (2015). Social work competencies and multidimensional assessment. *Journal of Baccalaureate Social Work, 20*, 117–135. https://doi.org/10.18084/1084-7219.20.1.117

Rubaltelli, E., & Slovic, P. (2008). Affective reactions and context-dependent processing of negations. *Judgment and Decision Making, 3*, 607–618. http://journal.sjdm.org/71204/jdm71204.pdf

Using Supervision to Guide Professional Development and Behavior

Elaine is a BSW student placed at a community crisis center. The agency provides 24-hour mobile crisis response to the community, a walk-in clinic for individuals experiencing a crisis, and a referral case management support team to link individuals to resources available in their community. Elaine is very excited to be at this placement because she has also been interested in mental health and thinks she is going to learn a lot during her time at this agency. She feels like she is learning so much every single day at her placement.

Every Thursday afternoon, Elaine meets with her field supervisor, Erin, who is an MSW at the agency. Elaine and Erin spend their time in supervision discussing the events of the week thus far. They talk about how many clients Elaine was able to help at the walk-in clinic or how many calls she went out on with the mobile crisis team. Elaine and Erin also talk about how Elaine helped the clients she encountered that week. Erin will often ask Elaine to share her rationale for why she did what she did with the client. Sometimes, Elaine is not sure of the answer, so she tells Erin that she "doesn't know." Erin understands that as a social work student, Elaine is not going to have all of the answers and part of her role as the field supervisor is to assist Elaine in making connections between what she has learned from her social work courses and what she is currently doing in her field placement.

Elaine values her time in supervision because she knows that Erin has been a social worker for many years and has a lot of experience helping clients. Elaine feels that she is learning how to be a better social worker by talking with Erin about how to approach a client situation. Often, Erin will share how she would address a situation. By discussing her thought process, Elaine finds a new way to think about a situation with her own clients. Through supervision, Elaine can enhance her professional identity and confidence in her ability to be a self-regulating, independent social work professional.

- *Why do you think that Elaine appreciates supervision so much?*

- *How might Elaine's perspective on her field experience change if Erin did not make time for Elaine to process her experiences?*

- *How do you think the role of your field supervisor influences your field placement experience?*

LEARNING OBJECTIVES

By the end of this chapter, you will be able to:

• Describe the supportive dimensions of social work supervision.

• Describe the administrative dimensions of social work supervision.

• Describe the educational dimensions of social work supervision.

• Identify and describe your preferred learning style.

• Identify ways that you can increase trust in the supervision relationship.

• Evaluate your current supervisory relationship.

• Distinguish between mentoring supervision and employment supervision.

SOCIAL WORK SUPERVISION

We have discussed how field is the signature pedagogy of the social work profession. At the heart of field placement is supervision, which is portrayed in the opening case vignette. Social work supervision can be traced back to the early days of the profession in the early 20th century, when it was used with early charity workers in New York (Kadushin & Harkness, 2014). Supervision within social work has long been a means to pass along practice wisdom from the trained professional social worker to the learner. It is through social work supervision that you, the student, can practice and improve your social work skills in a real-world setting. Social work supervision is a collaborative process in which both you and your supervisor work together to enhance your practice skills and develop your professional self (National Association of Social Workers [NASW] & Association of Social Work Boards [ASWB], 2013). Through social work supervision, your professional social work identity can mature (Field et al., 2016). Social work supervision serves to ensure that you are developing the appropriate skills necessary to be an ethical and competent social work practice professional (Caras, 2013). Through your field placement, you will have the opportunity to critically engage in practice settings to enhance your social work skills; your social work supervision is a central component to this critical engagement (Zuchowski, 2016).

To supervise is to direct, watch over, or keep an eye on the work of another. Thus, in supervision, the supervisor oversees and monitors the actions of the supervisee. Social work supervision goes beyond this basic definition, however, to include a dynamic engagement between the supervisor and the supervisee. Good-quality supervision provides a foundation for the developing social worker. As a field student, you are encouraged to make the most of your weekly supervisions to lay a strong foundation for your future as a professional social worker.

The role of your weekly supervision is to enhance your learning and develop your professional self as the upcoming social worker. Supervision is a space to explore what you are doing well and areas for ongoing growth and development. It is important that you are open to feedback in the supervision process. Social work supervision in field can serve many purposes:

- assessing your growth related to the nine social work competencies established by the Council on Social Work Education (CSWE)

- developing your professional self and increasing your sense of professional autonomy

- encouraging personal development by helping you explore how your personal values and beliefs align and merge with those of the profession

- promoting professional values within all elements of practice

- enabling you to reflect upon ethical and legal considerations related to social work practice

It is very important that you and your supervisor are on the same page regarding expectations for supervision. Your school will have requirements for supervision that must be followed. Beyond that, it is often helpful if you and your supervisor early in your time together discuss the plan for supervision. Developing a supervision agreement can be helpful during your field placement (Field et al., 2016). A supervision agreement serves to ensure that both parties are clear on what to expect from each other throughout the supervision relationship. Caras and Sandu (2014) suggest that "supervision requires a learning alliance, which empowers the person to acquire relevant skills and knowledge for his profession. This alliance aims to develop interpersonal skills in supervision relationship" (p. 76). Social work supervision is multidimensional and can have multiple functions or purposes, so it is important that both partners are clear on what they expect from supervision. Often, field supervisors have had students earlier and are familiar with the social work supervision requirements in field. If they are new to supervising social work students, your field faculty liaison can assist them in better understanding the role of supervision in field education.

It is very important that you are participating in regular supervision every week with your field supervisor. If, for whatever reason, you are not participating in supervision at your field placement, you should let your faculty liaison know right away.

As the student you must be actively engaged in the supervision process. You must do more than show up to supervision. Good supervision will require you to prepare. One way that you can prepare for your weekly supervision is to keep a document wherein you write down any questions that come up for you during the week, such as your Competency Reflection Log (CRL). It is easy to forget something if it is not written down, so having the list of questions prepared before supervision will be useful. Also, your learning contract is an excellent tool to prepare for supervision. Each week, before supervision, take a minute to review your learning contract. Identify any goals that you may have accomplished in the past week and be prepared to discuss these with your supervisor. Not only will this make sure that you are accomplishing the tasks outlined in the contract, but it will also assist your supervisor in evaluating your progress during the internship as well. Using the Supervision Form in Exhibit 4.1 could also assist you in preparing for your weekly supervision and be an excellent way to keep track of your learning.

DOMAINS OF SUPERVISION

Social work supervision can be thought of in terms of three primary domains: support, administration, and education (Kadushin & Harkness, 2014; NASW & ASWB, 2013). Exhibit 4.2 provides an overview of each domain of social work supervision.

EXHIBIT 4.1

SUPERVISION FORM

Date of supervision:

What work did you complete this week at field placement?
What learning contract activities have you addressed this week?
Reflect on feelings and reactions from this week at the field placement. What were some feelings and reactions you have had?
Connect your coursework to your experiences at your field placement this week. What was at least one connection?
What social work skills and theories did you use this week?
How did you apply or integrate the NASW *Code of Ethics* into your field placement this week?
Which competencies did you use this week?
What plans do you have for upcoming weeks at your field placement based on this week?
What questions do you have for your supervisor?

Note: An electronic template of the Supervision Form is available by accessing Springer Publishing Connect™ via the instructions on the opening page of this book, and clicking on the drop down Show Supplementary, Student Materials, Supervision Form.
NASW, National Association of Social Workers.

EXHIBIT 4.2

DOMAINS OF SOCIAL WORK SUPERVISION

Support	Administration	Education
• Address stress and other hazards of helping (burnout, vicarious trauma, and compassion fatigue)	• Agency policies and procedures • Job tasks • Job functioning	• Incorporation of theory, models, and frameworks • Professional development and training

The three dimensions of support, administration, and education are all necessary during your social work supervision during your field placement.

Social work supervision serves to provide support to you, the learning social worker. As a social work student, receiving support in supervision is vital for your success in the field experience. In fact, support is very important within the entire profession of social work. At times, practicing social work can be quite demanding and stressful. It is important to learn ways to diminish and manage stress whenever possible. Through supportive supervision, you, as the developing social worker, can address situations, experiences, or processes that are difficult for you. Together with the support of your field supervisor, you can brainstorm and problem-solve potential solutions to ameliorate such conditions. There may be simple changes that you are able to make that your supervisor can help you see. In the event that it is something beyond your control, your field supervisor may be able to provide suggestions on ways to cope with or better manage the stressor.

Social work supervision also covers administrative processes. Through supervision, you can review agency policies and procedures. You can review macro-level policies that relate to your practice as well. Likewise, reviewing professional ethical values and standards is part of administrative supervision. Administrative supervision is often a central component of employment supervision, which we discuss later in this chapter. Within administrative supervision, work tasks and assignments are often explored to ensure that the agency's mission, goals, and objectives are being met and clients are being served appropriately, both effectively and efficiently.

Finally, social work supervision can serve as an educational process. Educational supervision seeks to increase your knowledge, skills, and training and help push you toward mastery of the social work competencies. Educational supervision is a pivot aspect of field supervision, as you are a student, and still learning how to be a professional social worker. As a developing social worker in field, you can take all of the theoretical concepts that you learned in your social work courses and implement them while engaging in the helping process. It is necessary to understand not only *what* to do in a situation with a client, but also *why* you are doing it. The *why* is often connected to theories, perspectives, models, or evidence-based practices that have been found to be well suited for the situation you are experiencing as a social worker. Good social work practice is grounded in research and derived from the wealth of practice knowledge available to us.

> **Field Reflection Questions**
>
> Consider your field supervision sessions. To what extent do you cover each of the three domains of supervision?
>
> Is there a domain that could be strengthened?

> **Field Reflection Questions**
>
> Reflect on your supervision sessions with your supervisor; which of the domains of supervision did you cover?
>
> Is there a domain that you do not address in supervision?
>
> How can you be sure to incorporate all three domains in supervision?

EXHIBIT 4.3

LEARNING STYLES

Learning Style	Definition	Preferences
Visual	These learners prefer to use images to help them with organization information.	Charts, graphs, maps, logic models, visual organizers, pictures, videos
Auditory	These learners prefer to receive new information by listening and speaking.	Verbal commands, presentation lectures, discussions
Kinesthetic	These learners prefer to use hands-on learning activities to understand information.	Tactile experiences, hands-on learning, learning by doing and then reflecting
Solitary	These learners prefer taking in new information on their own at first.	Self-study
Social	These learners prefer working interactively to gain new information.	Group projects

LEARNING STYLES AND LEARNING STYLE ASSESSMENT

Field Reflection Questions

How do you learn best? Which type of learning style represents your preferred style?

Are there any struggles or barriers that you will need to address related to your preferred learning style and the setup of your field placement?

As social workers, we appreciate that every person is a unique individual and, as a result, we respect differences. Differences can present in a variety of ways. For example, students learn in a variety of ways. Maybe you have noticed that you do better in a class when the instructor shows videos, or maybe you need to read something for it to sink in, or maybe you need to actually try it out on your own to really understand what is being taught. Those differences refer to individual learning styles. Exhibit 4.3 outlines some common learning styles.

It is important to understand which learning style (or styles) seems to fit you most. Understanding how you learn best requires some self-reflection. Note that your preferred learning style may vary depending on the content that you are learning. For example, in a subject that you really enjoy, you may have a good fit within one learning style; in contrast, in a subject that is more difficult or challenging for you, a different learning style may be more beneficial. Knowing how you learn best can help you during your field placement. You should communicate with your field instructor what your preferred learning style is so that you can discuss ways to help you get the most out of your field placement. Also, because there may be times you will need to take in information in a nonpreferred way, your field instructor can help you to problem-solve ideas to get the most out of those experiences as well. Remember that your field placement is part of your social work *education*. You are still a student. You are still learning. Embrace that reality during your field placement and recognize that you are not always going to have all of the answers and will be learning every day how to become a better, more competent social worker. While you are still learning, it is important to make the most of your time as a student and learn as much as you can during this process.

TYPES OF SUPERVISION

The various models of supervision can range from a collaborative engagement to a more authoritarian process. Different styles of supervision provide different opportunities. Collaborative supervision encourages both the supervisor and the supervisee to engage in a dyadic process together, co-creating the supervision relations on an ongoing basis. In this type of supervision, the supervisee is often asked to prepare materials to share and discuss in the supervision session. In contrast, in the authoritarian supervision process, the supervision is more hierarchical. Going beyond styles of supervision, there are other distinctions regarding types of supervision that we discuss.

MENTORING SUPERVISION

The supervision we have been discussing thus far in this chapter relates to mentoring supervision. Mentoring supervision is supervision using a process to enhance the skills of the supervisee. This type of supervision is required weekly during your field education. Mentoring supervision is also the type of supervision required if you plan to pursue professional clinical licensure later in your career.

EMPLOYMENT SUPERVISION

Employment supervision, though similar, differs from mentoring supervision. It varies from organization to organization. The primary purpose of this type of supervision is to review agency-specific policies, procedures, and other organizational matters. There is often an element of case consultation or sharing of issues, concerns, or progress for clients among team members. Often, this type of supervision lacks an emphasis on professional growth and enhancement.

As a profession, social work values ongoing supervision. Throughout your future career, you can seek out supervision from a licensed social work professional to assist you in deepening your professional skillset. The NASW maintains an active list of members who provide supervision services to social workers on its website.

GROUP SUPERVISION

Most often, social work supervision is provided in an individual context, with just the supervisor and the supervisee being present. Sometimes, however, supervision occurs in a group format. The goals of supervision remain the same whether supervision is provided on a one-on-one basis or in a group. The distinction comes from the number of supervisees participating. Benefits of group supervision include having multiple learners who can share experiences and provide support to one another. A potential drawback of group supervision is that a learner may feel reluctant to be completely open and share some experiences in a group setting. If you are involved in group supervision, it is important that you feel comfortable with your group so that you can get the most benefits from your time in supervision. Often, supervisors who facilitate group supervision will create ground rules for group supervision that help everyone feel safer when sharing experiences, thoughts, and feelings in this setting. Sometimes, these ground rules include such things as respecting one another, treating what is said in super-vision as confidential, promoting open communication with the use of "I-statements," and emphasizing the principle that there are no stupid questions.

Field Reflection Questions

Compare and contrast group and individual supervision. What do you think would be the benefits of each for you at your current field placement?

What, if any, would be the drawbacks to each for you?

STAGES OF SUPERVISION

There are various stages in the supervision process. As the supervisee it can be helpful to understand this because it can normalize the process. There are various models to understand supervision including the developmental stages of supervision and attachment-informed supervision (Vassos et al., 2018). The Integrative Developmental Model of Supervision developed by Stoltenberg and McNeill (2010) provides a developmental approach to understanding the stages a learner goes through during the supervision process (see Exhibit 4.4).

Field Reflection Questions

Considering the stages of supervision in Exhibit 4.4, which level best depicts where you are currently?

How can supervision help you to get to the next level?

STUDENT/SUPERVISOR MATCH

Your relationship with your field supervisor is a very important aspect of your time in field. It is with your field supervisor that you will meet weekly to conduct your

STAGES OF SUPERVISION

Level 1	Level 2	Level 3
• Limited experience • Confusion • Anxiety • Concerns about being incompetent • Little to no self-efficacy • Little to no autonomy • Motivated to learn and grow	• Less focus on self-preoccupation, more focused on clients • Increased confidence • Better able to read emotional cues from clients • Questioning fit in the profession • Still growing • Increased autonomy	• Stable • Autonomous • Reflective • Deliberate practice • Solid sense of professional self

Source: Based on Stoltenberg, C. D., & McNeill, B. W. (2010). *IDM supervision: An integrative developmental model for supervising counselors and therapists* (3rd ed.). Routledge. https://doi.org/10.4324/9780203893388

social work supervision. The quality of the relationship between you and your field instructor is based on many factors. One factor is how well you and your supervisor are matched. As with any type of relationship, certain qualities and characteristics can enhance a relationship. Regarding your professional supervisory relationship, there can be similarities that bring you and your field instructor closer. Sometimes there may be no obvious similarities other than the fact that both of you love social work, but that is often enough to make a terrific match. A great deal of research has demonstrated that the quality of the relationship between the field student and the field supervisor is associated with student learning and satisfaction from the field placement (Cleak et al., 2016; Cleak & Smith, 2012; Tangen & Borders, 2016).

As social workers, we appreciate that relationships are very significant. The NASW *Code of Ethics* (2021) states that we "understand that relationships between and among people are an important vehicle for change" (Ethical Principles, para. 5). The relationship with your field supervisor is no different. Having a secure, stable relationship with your field supervisor is critically important and related to your overall success in field (Bennet et al., 2012; Bogo, 2015). As with any relationship, there are ways that you can strengthen your relationship with your field supervisor. Qualities at the heart of the social work supervision relationship are trust, sharing, and vulnerability.

Although we certainly encourage you to have a strong, open relationship with your field supervisor, it is also important to maintain a professional attitude. Your relationship with your field supervisor should remain strictly professional throughout your field experience. Just as we as social workers should avoid dual relationships with clients, while completing your field experience, you should avoid dual relationships with your field instructor. The NASW *Code of Ethics* (2021) sets forth ethical standards regarding supervision and consultation that outline the nature of the professional supervisory relationship (see Exhibit 4.5).

EXHIBIT 4.5

NASW ETHICAL STANDARD 3.01: SUPERVISION AND CONSULTATION

a. Social workers who provide supervision or consultation (whether in-person or remotely) should have the necessary knowledge and skill to supervise or consult appropriately and should do so only within their areas of knowledge and competence.

b. Social workers who provide supervision or consultation are responsible for setting clear, appropriate, and culturally sensitive boundaries.

c. Social workers should not engage in any dual or multiple relationships with supervisees in which there is a risk of exploitation of or potential harm to the supervisee, including dual relationships that may arise while using social networking sites or other electronic media.

d. Social workers who provide supervision should evaluate supervisees' performance in a manner that is fair and respectful.

Source: National Association of Social Workers. (2021). *Code of ethics.* https://www.socialworkers.org/About/Ethics/Code-of-Ethics/Code-of-Ethics-English

NASW, National Association of Social Workers.

TRUST, SHARING, AND VULNERABILITY

Field Reflection Questions

What is the level of trust in your supervision relationship?

How can you increase the level of trust?

For social work supervision to be most beneficial, it is important that there is trust between the supervisor and the supervisee. Trust involves many factors but is tied especially closely to the social work value of integrity. Related to the value of integrity, we can increase trust by being honest and truthful. We can follow through with what we say we are going to do and be dependable and reliable.

Open, honest sharing is important in social work supervision. It is important to use your time in supervision not as a time to try to impress your supervisor by saying what you think the "right thing" is, but rather as a time to sort through your thoughts and feelings in an effort to become a competent social work professional. At times, you may need to explore your own personal thoughts, feelings, and beliefs in supervision regarding how they are impacting your practice as a social worker. You may also need to discuss situations or experiences with clients or systems that you work with during your placement that are personal triggers for you. Although social work supervision often involves discussing personal issues, it is not to be confused with personal therapy. Unguru and Sandu (2017) suggest that though counseling and supervision are similar, a distinction is that the supervisor is more engaged in sharing their perspectives and experiences with the supervisee than what would typically be shared in a counseling session.

Social work supervision requires self-reflection not only on elements of social work practice, but also on the practitioner's thoughts, feelings, and behaviors. Effective social work professionals must engage in continuous self-reflection. We must be mindful of how our thoughts, feelings, and behaviors influence our practice. We discuss self-reflection in more depth in Chapter 5.

Brown (2017) has suggested the mnemonic "BRAVING" to better understand trust. In this acronym, the "B" stands for maintaining boundaries. As social workers, we know that

> **Field Reflection Question**
>
> How can you distinguish between supervision and personal therapy?

boundaries are very important. We talk about having healthy boundaries with our clients quite often. Regarding social work supervision, it is also important to have boundaries. One way to have clear boundaries in your field supervision is to maintain a professional relationship and be clear on each other's roles and responsibilities during the field process. The "R" in the mnemonic stands for reliability. As you may recall from a research course you have taken, being reliable refers to consistency; thus, we can develop trust by being consistent. As we have discussed, one way we can do this is to demonstrate the social work value of integrity: We can do what we say we are going to do. By following through on our words with actions, we demonstrate integrity, and show that we are reliable. The "A" in the mnemonic stands for accountability. Being accountable requires that you are responsible for what you have done (or maybe did not do). The "V" represents the concept of a vault. By definition, a vault is a storage compartment. In Brown's analogy, the vault refers to holding information as secret or in confidence. To have a relationship of trust, we should not share things that are meant to be kept confidential. The "I" represents integrity. As social workers, through the NASW (2021) *Code of Ethics*, we understand integrity to mean being "continually aware of the profession's mission, values, ethical principles, and ethical standards and practice in a manner consistent with them" while being honest and responsible (Ethical Principles, para. 6). The "N" stands for nonjudgment. Trust requires that we integrate a nonjudgmental stance and attitude into our professional persona. Finally, the "G" stands for generosity. Brown suggests that generosity means we give the benefit of the doubt to the person we are in relationship with. By being generous, we assume goodwill toward the person and try not to take offense or become defensive.

Once you have a foundation of trust in your supervisory relationship, you can proceed with sharing and vulnerability. Sharing is a necessary aspect of supervision. Sometimes, it can be difficult to determine what to share. Sometimes, we may not want to share certain things because they make us feel vulnerable. Vulnerability refers to a state of being open or exposed to possible attack. It can be scary. Despite that, vulnerability is necessary for many things in life, including true connection and feeling emotions such as joy. Brown (2012) defines vulnerability as "uncertainty, risk, and emotional exposure" (p. 34). Vulnerability is connected to having the courage to speak our truth (Brown, 2012). As a field student, you may at times feel vulnerable during your field placement. For example, if you are presented with a task to complete at the agency and you do not know how to do it, you may feel vulnerable about saying you do not know and asking for help. We encourage you to remember that during your field placement (and throughout your social work career), it is okay to be vulnerable. It is okay not to have all of the answers. It is okay to ask for help. In fact, the NASW *Code of Ethics* lists competence as one of our values—it is our duty to ask for help when it is needed to ensure we are meeting the expectation of competence in our work.

SUPERVISORY RELATIONSHIP INVENTORY

There are many measures available that you can use to assess your supervisory relationship with your field supervisor (Tangen & Borders, 2016). We have provided an inventory that you can take to rate your current supervisory relationship with your field supervisor (see Exhibit 4.6).

Field Reflection Questions

Has there been a time in your field placement thus far when you had to share something that made you feel vulnerable?

What was that experience like for you?

What did you learn from that experience?

If you score 20 or higher in all three categories in Exhibit 4.6, then it is safe to assume that field supervision is working well. If you score less than 20 in any category, you should evaluate the scores and decide whether the low score is problematic. For example, getting a low score on the administrative component might not indicate a problem given the amount of time in the placement. Maybe you do not need a lot of supervision related to agency policies and procedures. If your assessment identifies areas that you would like to strengthen, we strongly recommend you share the results with your field instructor so you can discuss ways to address the concern. The purpose of the inventory is to increase your awareness of the three components of field supervision and, if needed, begin a conversation with your field instructor on ways to strengthen any area that is not being addressed to meet your learning needs.

PROBLEM-SOLVING

Field Reflection Questions

After completing the Supervisory Relationship Inventory, what did you learn about your current supervisory relationship?

Where can your relationship be improved?

How can you facilitate these improvements?

Social work supervision can be an amazing opportunity to engage in problem-solving with your field supervisor. Furthermore, through good supervision, you can increase your social work problem-solving skills. In fact, the International Federation of Social Workers has defined social work as a profession that seeks social change, problem-solving, and empowerment (International Federation of Social Workers, 2012).

In supervision, it is important to share situations with your supervisor before they become full-blown problems whenever possible. By addressing a situation before it becomes a problem, you can brainstorm potential solutions. Open communication before difficult situations arise is the most preferable way to problem-solve (Edmondson, 2014). Often, your field supervisor can share their practice wisdom and previous experiences with you to indicate what they have learned on

EXHIBIT 4.6

SUPERVISORY RELATIONSHIP INVENTORY

The following questions are about what you and your supervisor do in your sessions together. Answer each question by circling the response that best describes your interactions with your field instructor using the following rating scale.

1 Not at all	2 A little	3 Some	4 A lot	5 A great deal

Administration: To what extent:

A1. Have you and your supervisor discussed their expectations for your field placement?

1	2	3	4	5

A2. Do your supervisory sessions focus on documentation and required paperwork?

1	2	3	4	5

A3. Do your supervisory sessions focus on administrative issues and agency policies?

1	2	3	4	5

A4. Do your supervisory sessions focus on tasks you need to accomplish?

1	2	3	4	5

A5. Have you and your supervisor discussed how your progress is going to be assessed?

1	2	3	4	5

Education: To what extent:

E1. Have you and your supervisor reviewed your progress on the learning goal(s) identified in your learning contract?

1	2	3	4	5

E2. Do your supervisory sessions focus on clinical/case issues?

1	2	3	4	5

E3. Have you and your supervisor discussed your work and progress on the nine social work competencies?

1	2	3	4	5

E4. Does your supervisor help you reflect upon your feelings, reactions, and use of self in working with your clients?

1	2	3	4	5

E5. Does your supervisor help you think more clearly about your clients/cases?

1	2	3	4	5

Support: To what extent:

S1. Do you feel your supervisor cares about you?

1	2	3	4	5

(continued)

EXHIBIT 4.6

SUPERVISORY RELATIONSHIP INVENTORY (*continued*)

S2. Does talking with your supervisor have a calming, soothing effect on you?

1	2	3	4	5

S3. Do you feel that your supervisor provides you with emotional support?

1	2	3	4	5

S4. Does talking with your supervisor give you confidence in your abilities?

1	2	3	4	5

S5. Are you willing to take risks and talk about your mistakes and struggles with your supervisor?

1	2	3	4	5

Scoring	Score
Administration: sum of items A1–A5	
Education: sum of items E1–E5	
Support: sum of items S1–S5	
Total: sum of A, E, and S items	

Note: An electronic template of the Supervisory Relationship Inventory is available by accessing Springer Publishing Connect™ via the instructions on the opening page of this book, and clicking on the drop down Show Supplementary, Student Materials, Supervisory Relationship Inventory.

the job. By engaging in supervision and discussing such issues with your supervisor, you can benefit from their experiences and insights.

We understand, though, that on occasion, things may happen and, as a result, you will be facing a problem. If you find yourself in a predicament during your field placement, it is important that you reach out to your field supervisor as soon as possible to problem-solve together. Even if the problem arose from something that you did (or failed to do), trust us: It is best to address the situation with integrity and directly address it with your field supervisor quickly.

In addition to problems that arise with clients, during your social work supervision, you and your field supervisor can problem-solve to identify and address other possible problems that may arise while you are a field student. Being a field student is a time of excitement and anticipation; you are one step closer to becoming a professional social worker. However, we fully understand that students today face many challenges and are often balancing a variety of commitments, trying to make it through the semester. It is common for field students to often be juggling or attempting to balance multiple demands between field, coursework, family, employment, and so forth (Hemy et al., 2016). Remember, your social work supervision can provide support as you face these challenges. Coupling support and problem-solving, together with input from your supervisor, you may be able to find ways to better balance the demands you are facing and incorporate ways to take care of yourself while undergoing this process.

PERFORMANCE IMPROVEMENT PLAN IMPLEMENTATION

Now and again during a field placement there is a need to implement a performance improvement plan. This is a strategy to support you, the learner, in meeting your educational goals. Sometimes the initial reaction of a learner to a performance improvement plan is negative. We strongly encourage you to reframe that perspective and instead view this plan as a way to help you get the most out of your placement and to help address areas for growth. In Exhibit 4.7 you can see a performance improvement plan template. This is often a document that is completed by your site supervisor and reviewed with you and shared with your faculty liaison as well. Should you

EXHIBIT 4.7

PERFORMANCE IMPROVEMENT PLAN TEMPLATE

Performance Concern *Detail specific dates and examples of where the standards have not been met.*	Expected Standard of Performance *Detail what is expected of the student in terms of their performance—what does "good" look like?*	Improvement Actions *Detail what actions need to be taken to meet expected standard of performance.*	Support *Detail what has been agreed on in terms of support required to achieve the expected standard of performance.*	Review Date *Specify date(s) that performance will be reviewed.*
Student is not maintaining professionalism related to attendance at field placement. On 9/17, 9/20, 9/24, and 9/28 the student arrived 2 hours late at the site and had not informed anyone they would be late.	Student is expected to arrive on time for their shifts at the field placement. In the event the student needs to adjust their schedule, they must reach out in advance to the site supervisor and follow the procedure to request a schedule change.	Student will arrive on time. Student will reach out in advance if they need to change their schedule. Student will follow agency procedures for a schedule change.	Student will review their schedule and make sure they are able to prioritize their schedule at their field site. Student will problem-solve any barriers to this and make the necessary changes to address any barriers.	This plan will be reviewed again on 10/30.

Student: _____   Date: _____

Field Instructor: _____   Date: _____

Faculty Field Liaison: _____   Date: _____

Note: An electronic version of the Performance Improvement Plan template is available by accessing Springer Publishing Connect™ via the instructions on the opening page of this book, and clicking on the drop down Show Supplementary, Student Materials, Performance Improvement Plan Template.

encounter the need for a performance improvement plan, it is important to reach out to your faculty liaison to review your school's procedure regarding this Exhibit 4.7.

CASE SUMMARY: "IT IS OKAY TO NOT KNOW"

PRACTICE SETTING DESCRIPTION

Hope is a BSW student who is completing her field placement at Redstone Hospital. Redstone Hospital is a 300-bed community hospital in a rural area of Ohio. This hospital is the only hospital in a three-county radius. The hospital has a social work staff of five full-time and three part-time social workers. Hope's field supervisor, Christa, is a full-time social worker with over a decade of experience working at Redstone Hospital. Christa's primary responsibility is covering the ED.

IDENTIFYING DATA

While covering the ED, the social worker must be prepared to deal with a variety of situations. The medical staff will often call upon the social worker for a consult if there is a suspicion of abuse or neglect. The social worker will also be called if there is a concern that the patient is experiencing a mental health crisis or has a substance abuse problem. Sometimes, the social worker is called to a patient's room to assist with locating resources for the patient or arranging transportation for the patient to return home if they are not being admitted to the hospital. As you can see, the social workers who cover the ED could be called in for a consult on a variety of issues at any time. When Hope's placement first started, she and Christa went on all consults together. As Hope and Christa became more comfortable, Hope would start going on consults on her own and then report back to Christa regarding the patient.

PRESENTING PROBLEM

One evening Hope was working with Christa covering the ED. The night had been a very busy one so far. It seemed as if the social workers were being requested for everyone in the ED. While Christa was in the social work office looking to find a bed in a rehab facility for a patient who came in high and was willing to get treatment, a request for another consult came in from the medical staff, requesting a social worker right away for a patient who needed transportation home. Christa asked Hope whether she wanted to work on finding a bed at a rehab or whether she felt comfortable going to see the resource consult. Hope had never had to find and secure a bed at a rehab facility before. She thought it would be easier to go and talk to the patient who needed transportation because she had done that before.

When Hope arrived at the patient's room for the consult, she was startled by the patient, who was standing on her bed. The patient was talking so fast that it was hard for Hope to understand what she was saying. The patient kept talking with an urgency that alarmed Hope. When she had said she would take this consult, she thought that she was going to find out where the patient lived and get some bus tickets to take care of the problem. Hope was not sure what was going on with this patient, but she knew that she needed more than just bus tickets. Hope hesitated for a moment because she did not know what she was going to do. She thought for a second and then paged Christa to come and meet her in the patient's room.

Christa arrived right away. As soon as Christa got to the room, Hope apologized for not knowing what to do and calling her to come down. Christa patted Hope on the shoulder and said, "You knew exactly what to do. You knew your limits and you asked for help when you needed it. I am proud of you."

ASSESSMENT

The next day, during their regular group supervision, Christa brought up the incident from the night before. At first, Hope thought that maybe Christa changed her mind and was upset with her for not knowing what to do. Christa asked Hope to talk about how she came to the decision to call for her to come and help on that case. Hope thought for a second and then realized that, even though she felt like she should have known what to do and did not want to admit she did not know what to do to help this patient, Christa had never made Hope feel bad for asking for help or not knowing what to do. Hope explained that she felt safe asking Christa for help because she knew that Christa would be supportive and nonjudgmental.

CASE PROCESS SUMMARY

After supervision, Hope thought about the past 2 days and how much she had been learning at Redstone Hospital with Christa. She realized that she was learning so much because she was asking for help when she was not sure what to do. Christa would always help her in the moment and then spend time talking about the situation during their next supervision session. Hope knew that it was safe to share and be vulnerable with Christa because she had a strong foundation of trust with Christa. Hope felt lucky to have Christa as her field supervisor because she knew she was learning a lot.

Hope, BSW Student Intern

CASE DISCUSSION QUESTIONS

1. *Hope felt comfortable asking Christa for help because they had a strong supervisory relationship. How do you think this scenario would have been different if Hope felt her supervisory relationship with Christa was poor?*

2. *Sometimes, it can be difficult to ask for help. Has there been a time in your field placement when, like Hope, you were in over your head and were not sure what to do? How did you respond?*

3. *The day after Hope asked Christa for help, they discussed the situation again in supervision. Why do you think it is important to process specific client situations in supervision? Is there a benefit to talking about such situations soon after they happen? If so, what are those benefits?*

END-OF-CHAPTER RESOURCES

 A robust set of instructor resources designed to supplement this text is located at http://connect.springerpub.com/content/book/978-0-8261-3753-1. Qualifying instructors may request access by emailing textbook@springerpub.com.

CRITICAL THINKING QUESTIONS

1. Describe the supervision you participate in at your field placement. How does your supervision help your growth as a social worker?

2. How would you rate your supervisory relationship with your field supervisor? How does your relationship with your field supervisor influence your field placement experience?

3. In what ways can you improve your professional supervisory relationship by using trust, sharing, and vulnerability?

4. How do you balance appropriate self-disclosure and being open during your social work field supervisions?

5. How can you use what you now know about your preferred learning style to assist you in getting the most out of your field supervision? What is one way that you can incorporate your preferred learning style into each dimension of supervision?

6. If you were having problems with your supervisory relationship during your field placement, what would you do? How would you try to address the situation? With whom would you talk about this issue?

LEARNING ACTIVITIES

1. Consider your field placement and the expectations for professionalism in that setting. Identify those expectations in a list. Rate yourself on each expectation on a scale from 1 to 10 on how well you are meeting that expectation (with 1 being not at all and 10 being exceeding). Consider your ratings and identify ways that you can improve your professionalism. Discuss this with your supervisor in your next supervision and see if your self-ratings match their ratings of you.

2. Reflect on your supervisory relationship with your field instructor. Complete the Supervisory Relationship Inventory. Identify the strengths in your relationship and consider areas for growth. Develop two goals to improve your supervisory relationship and share those with your supervisor in your next supervision.

ELECTRONIC RESOURCES

WEBSITE LINKS

NASW & ASWB—Best Practice Standards in Social Work Supervision (2013): www.socialworkers.org/LinkClick.aspx ?fileticket=GBrLbl4BuwI%3D&portalid=

Social Work Podcast Titled "Supervision for Social Workers" (2008): https://socialworkpodcast.blogspot.com/2008/01/super vision-for-social-workers

Article: "Supervisor, Beware: Ethical Dangers in Supervision" by Claudia J. Dewane (2007): www.socialworktoday.com/archive/ julyaug2007p34.shtml

VIDEO LINKS

NASW Presentation on Supervision (2010): www.youtube.com/watch ?v=HQmRpV0xXgc

Brené Brown, social work researcher, discusses "The Power of Vulnerability": www.ted.com/talks/brene_brown_on_vulnerability

Tips on Preparing for Clinical Supervision: www.youtube.com/ watch?v=UJa2CDiQYT8

REFERENCES

Bennet, S., Mohr, J., Deal, K. H., & Hwang, J. (2012). Supervisor attachment, supervisory working alliance, and affect in social work field instruction. *Research on Social Work Practice, 23*(2), 199–209. https://doi.org/10.1177/1049731512468492

Bogo, M. (2015). Field education for clinical social work practice: Best practices and contemporary challenges. *Clinical Social Work Journal, 43*(3), 317–324. https://doi.org/10.1007/s10615-015-0526-5

Brown, B. (2012). *Daring greatly.* Gotham Books.

Brown, B. (2017). *Braving the wilderness: The quest for true belonging and the courage to stand alone.* Random House.

Caras, A. (2013). Ethics and supervision process: Fundaments of social work practice. *Procedia—Social and Behavioral Sciences, 92*(10), 133–141. https://doi.org/10.1016/j.sbspro.2013.08.649

Caras, A., & Sandu, A. (2014). The role of supervision in professional development of social work specialists. *Journal of Social Work Practice, 28*(1), 75–94. https://doi.org/10.1080/02650533.2012.763024

Cleak, H., & Smith, D. (2012). Student satisfaction with models of field placement supervision. *Australian Social Work, 65*(2), 243–258. https://doi.org/10.1080/0312407X.2011.572981

Cleak, H., Roulston, A., & Vreugdenhil, A. (2016). The inside story: A survey of social work students' supervision and learning opportunities on placement. *British Journal of Social Work, 46*(7), 2033–2050. https://doi.org/10.1093/bjsw/bcv117

Edmondson, D. (2014). *Social work practice learning.* Sage.

Field, P., Jasper, C., & Littler, L. (2016). *Practice education in social work: Achieving professional standards* (2nd ed.). Critical Publishing.

Hemy, M., Boddy, J., Chee, P., & Sauvage, D. (2016). Social work students "juggling" field placement. *Social Work Education, 35*(2), 215–228. https://doi.org/10.1080/02615479.2015.1125878

International Federation of Social Workers. (2018). *Global social work statement of ethical principles.* https://www.ifsw.org/global-social-work-statement-of-ethical-principles

Kadushin, A., & Harkness, D. (2014). *Supervision in social work.* Columbia University Press.

National Association of Social Workers. (2021). *Code of ethics.* https://www.socialworkers.org/About/Ethics/Code-of-Ethics/Code-of-Ethics-English

National Association of Social Workers & Association of Social Work Boards. (2013). *Best practice standards in social work supervision.* https://www.socialworkers.org/LinkClick.aspx?fileticket=GBrLbl4BuwI%3D&portalid=0

Stoltenberg, C. D., & McNeill, B. W. (2010). *IDM supervision: An integrative developmental model for supervising counselors and therapists* (3rd ed.). Routledge. https://doi.org/10.4324/9780203893388

Tangen, J. L., & Borders, D. (2016). The supervisory relationship: A conceptual and psychometric review of measures. *Counselor Education and Supervision, 55*(3), 159–181. https://doi.org/10.1002/ceas.12043

Unguru, E., & Sandu, A. (2017). Supervision: From administrative control to continuous education and training of specialists in social work. *Romanian Journal for Multidimensional Education, 9*(1), 17–35. https://doi.org/10.18662/rrem/2017.0901.02

Vassos, S., Harms, L., & Rose, D. (2018). Supervision and social work students: Relationships in a team-based rotation placement model. *Social Work Education, 37*(3), 328–341. https://doi.org/10.1080/02615479.2017.1406466

Zuchowski, I. (2016). Getting to know the context: The complexities of providing off-site supervision in social work practice learning. *British Journal of Social Work, 46*(2), 409–426. https://doi.org/10.1093/bjsw/bcu133

Using Reflection and Self-Regulation to Promote Well-Being Through Self-Care

CASE VIGNETTE

Mary has been at her social work placement field site, a local crime victims center, for about a month. She was initially really excited about her placement because in addition to social work, she was always intrigued by the criminal justice system. Mary thought that working at the crime victims center would be a great way to merge her two interests. She would be supporting clients who have been victims of crimes.

Mary has a small, but growing, caseload and sits in on the rape survivor support group that meets twice a week. During the support group, the survivors process their experiences and share sometimes graphic details of what they have experienced.

Mary is starting to get headaches more often than ever before and she feels very tired. Her sister recently told her that she seems so "on edge" lately. Mary chalks all of this up to being a busy student who has a lot on her plate. She has needed to ask for time off from her part-time job and field placement because she has been so exhausted and not feeling like herself.

Mary has been staying in a lot more than usual. She used to be quite social and enjoy going out on the weekends with her friends. One night, after some coaxing from her friends, Mary went out with a couple of her girlfriends. While out, someone came over and started talking to one of her friends; Mary yelled at this person and told the person to get away right now. Her friends do not understand what is wrong with Mary and why she overreacted in such a way. Mary is not sure why she responded that way, either.

- *What do you think is going on with Mary?*

- *How do you think her field placement is influencing these changes in her?*

- *What should Mary do?*

LEARNING OBJECTIVES

By the end of this chapter, you will be able to:

- Describe reflection, self-regulation, and self-awareness as it relates to being a professional social worker.

- Describe various potential hazards (vicarious trauma, burnout, and compassion fatigue) as they relate to social work practice.

- Describe self-care.

- Identify self-care strategies that you can implement.

- Identify personal supports.

- Develop a personal self-care plan.

PROMOTING PERSONAL WELL-BEING

As social workers, we often encourage our clients to advocate for themselves. We encourage our clients to be empowered to speak up regarding what they need. We understand the importance of self-care for our clients. However, at times, we lose sight of the importance of self-care for ourselves.

The importance of self-care for social work professionals cannot be understated. It is as vital as ongoing training. To truly be competent professionals, we need to engage in regular self-care. Despite the understanding that self-care is important and necessary, many helping professionals, including social workers, continue to be depleted in this area.

KNOW THYSELF

To be an effective professional social worker, you will need to engage in reflection and self-regulation. When we are thinking deeply or carefully about something, we are engaging in reflection. Self-regulation refers to our ability to maintain or control ourselves regarding our thoughts, feelings, and behaviors. Successful reflection and self-regulation require self-awareness. It is impossible to engage in reflection and self-regulation if you are unaware of your thoughts, feelings, and behaviors.

SELF-AWARENESS

Self-awareness is a term used to describe the recognition of personal thoughts, feelings, and behaviors. Some people naturally seem to do a better job at self-awareness than others, but do not worry: Self-awareness is something that you can practice and improve. Being present in the moment and practicing mindfulness (which we talk about later in this chapter) are ways that you can improve your self-awareness.

Field Reflection Questions

Practice some self-awareness right now. What are you thinking about?

What emotions are you experiencing?

What feelings or sensations do you notice in your body?

How do we get to know our *self* better? Ideally, your education, especially your social work courses, will have served as a catalyst for self-exploration and critical thinking. Throughout your social work education, you have learned about the use of self in your practice classes. In addition to what you learn in the classroom, you may have gained insights into yourself from a variety of other sources. Maybe you have received feedback from people you are close to or maybe you have sought your own avenues to get to know yourself better through books, groups, or activities designed with such a purpose. Self-awareness, or personal knowledge about the social worker's self and needs, can be achieved in a variety of ways (Bogo, 2010). Throughout your field experience, you can explore your self-awareness and use of self in the following ways: field supervision, process recordings, feedback from others (including field supervisors, faculty members, colleagues, peers, and clients), and personal reflection.

Everyone has a bad day every now and then; however, as social workers, we are mandated by the National Association of Social Workers (NASW) *Code of Ethics* (2021) to hold our commitment to the clients we serve in the highest priority. It is inappropriate, and unethical, to allow your personal issues to interfere with your client's treatment. So, what are social workers to do? Self-awareness is a strategy that can be one potential solution (see Case Example 5.1). By being self-aware, you can identify concerns before they become an issue in treatment. Through self-awareness, you can be alert to and care for your own needs to ward off the hazards of helping in the form of burnout, compassion fatigue, and vicarious trauma. One way you can care for your own needs is by engaging in consistent self-care.

CASE EXAMPLE 5.1: SELF-AWARENESS

When Sara was a young girl, her father was diagnosed with cancer. He battled cancer for much of her adolescence. Based on her experiences in the hospital setting, Sara knew that when she grew up, she wanted to work in a hospital to help others who were going through the same thing. While in college working on her BSW degree, Sara was assigned a field placement at a local hospital to support patients and families in the oncology unit. One day, while completing rounds, Sara walked into the room of a new patient who looked very much like her father. Immediately Sara was flooded with a wave of emotions and felt her stomach getting tight. Sara took a deep breath and did a quick scan of herself. She recognized that this man looked very much like her father, and that her mind and body had just transported her back to her adolescence when she watched her dad battle the same disease.

What Should Sara Do?

This situation, much like many other situations in social work, does not have a clear black-and-white solution. There are a lot of other variables that impact what Sara should do next in this situation. Sara was aware of her response, and she obviously has good insight because she was able to recognize what triggered this reaction. If Sara can contain her personal feelings and not let them interfere with her work with the client, she can proceed. If she does not feel that she can support the client, for whatever reason, then she should reach out to another social worker for support. Either way, using supervision to process this experience is strongly recommended. Supervision is an amazing tool in the toolkit for social workers (refer to Chapter 4 for more on supervision).

HAZARDS OF HELPING

Hazards are dangers or risks that can be potentially harmful. Sometimes we encounter hazards through our work environments or working conditions. Nearly all professions have some potential hazards. The potential hazards of helping professions (see Exhibit 5.1), such as social work, that we must safeguard against are burnout, vicarious trauma, and compassion fatigue. These phenomena are found within helping professions and are at times referred to as "the cost of caring." In addition to our training, the gear that we can put on to protect us from these hazards is self-care. Self-care serves to buffer us against these hazards and serves as a defense. Self-care cannot prevent these hazards, much like an umbrella cannot prevent the rain, but it can help negate the impact of these hazards.

It is important to note that these factors are potentially hazardous—not all helping professionals will be impacted by these phenomena during their careers. A multitude of factors will influence whether an individual will be negatively impacted by any one of these hazards (we talk about some of these factors later in this chapter). It must be stated that not all stress is bad. Some stress is a good thing; it can keep us motivated and performing optimally. Optimal levels of stress can encourage us and help us in many aspects. Where we must be careful is when stress goes beyond the optimal range and becomes detrimental and counterproductive. Excessive stress can lead to decreased motivation, feelings of hopelessness, lack of productivity, and fatigue.

BURNOUT

Burnout is often described as a state of exhaustion affecting the person mentally, physically, and spiritually because of ongoing exposure or involvement in the helping profession (Newell & Nelson-Gardell, 2014). Burnout can impact our mind by challenging our worldview or imposing a hopelessness. It can also impact our body and physical functioning. Burnout is a gradual process that intensifies over time. Burnout impacts all aspects of a person's well-being. The symptoms of burnout are outlined in Exhibit 5.1.

EXHIBIT 5.1

HAZARDS OF HELPING

	Burnout	Vicarious Trauma	Compassion Fatigue
Onset	Gradual	Rapid	Rapid
Symptoms	• Exhaustion, tired, lack of energy • Unable to cope, overwhelmed • Easily frustrated, cynical related to job (coworkers, clients) • Difficulty concentrating, lack of creativity	• Intrusive memories, flashbacks • Distressing dreams • Hypervigilance, exaggerated startle response • Avoidance • Memory distortions, difficulty concentrating • Negative worldview (thoughts that the world is unsafe)	• Mental fatigue • Decreased empathy • Depleted levels of compassion for clients • Can lead to mental health concerns if untreated

CASE EXAMPLE 5.2: BURNOUT

Kevin is completing his foundation MSW social work field placement in a community mental health center. The center is in an area with high levels of poverty and crime. Most clients who seek treatment at the center have experienced multiple traumas. Kevin has his own caseload and sees about five or six clients a day for individual therapy. At the end of the day, Kevin feels exhausted, mentally and physically, but he often has unfinished paperwork that he brings home with him. When he goes home, he does not want to talk to his partner. Rather, he wants to just "zone out" on the couch, eat his dinner, and stream TV reruns before he must start on the paperwork from the day. One night, when Kevin is utterly overwhelmed by his work, he decides he cannot keep this up. He does not enjoy his placement or seeing his clients anymore. Some days he feels so exhausted that he does not know how he will make it through the day, much less his field placement.

What Should Kevin Do?

In this scenario, we see the way that burnout can impact a social worker. Using supervision to discuss and process what is going on with Kevin might be helpful. Kevin and his supervisor can explore some of the factors that are probably adding to his level of burnout, such as the size of his caseload and his need to take paperwork home. The supervisor may be able to provide Kevin with strategies to address his paperwork issue so that he can get his work done at the office; then he can have a break from work at home in the evenings. One thing is for sure, Kevin needs support to be able to support his clients.

VICARIOUS TRAUMA

Vicarious trauma, sometimes called secondary traumatic stress (STS), describes when the worker is traumatized because of being exposed to the traumatic experiences of clients. The manifestation of vicarious trauma in the worker can mirror the symptoms of posttraumatic stress disorder (PTSD) within the victimized client. If the worker has been vicariously traumatized, they may experience symptoms of PTSD including reexperiencing the trauma in the form of nightmares and intrusive thoughts, avoiding reminders of the trauma, problems sleeping, hypervigilance and increased arousal or startle responses, altered cognitive functioning, or regression.

Vicarious trauma is not a diagnosis in the *Diagnostic and Statistical Manual of Mental Diseases* (5th ed.; *DSM-5*). However, under the diagnosis of PTSD in the *DSM-5* (American Psychiatric Association, 2013), exposure to the traumatic event can take several forms, including direct exposure, witnessing the traumatic event in person, learning of the traumatic event from someone with whom you are close, or firsthand repeated exposure to details of a traumatic event. Vicarious trauma overlaps with the firsthand repeated exposure to details of a traumatic event.

Symptoms of vicarious trauma can be categorized into the following areas: cognitive behavioral, affective, somatic, and spiritual. Cognitive behavioral symptoms include such things as feeling irritable or preoccupied, withdrawing from others, poor concentration and memory, and experiencing changes in sleep or appetite. Affective symptoms encompass a variety of emotional reactions that can range from being numb and shutdown to feeling angry and hostile. Somatic symptoms refer to experiences of the body. There are a myriad of somatic symptoms that can occur as a result of vicarious trauma. Some include headaches, muscle aches, and stomach distress. Spiritual symptoms related to vicarious trauma may include the individual questioning their worldview and feeling hopeless or lost.

It has been suggested that vicarious trauma can alter a worker's worldview (Cox & Steiner, 2013). For example, a social worker who works primarily with victims of violent crimes may begin to have beliefs that the world is unsafe—Case Example 5.3 illustrates such a scenario. As a social work placement field student, it is imperative that if you notice any of the symptoms noted in this chapter or start to feel traumatized by the work that you are doing, you immediately speak with your supervisor and your faculty liaison about your experiences. You will not be judged for your experience; rather, you can be supported and given the tools and supports that you need to address it head-on.

CASE EXAMPLE 5.3: VICARIOUS TRAUMA

Jessica is a social work intern completing her foundation MSW field placement at a sexual assault support center. Her daily responsibilities include conducting intake assessments with all new clients who come to the center. Each day, Jessica usually meets with three to four victims of sexual assault who share their experiences with her. Jessica begins to have nightmares and intrusive thoughts that resemble the stories that the clients have told her. She also notices that she feels more on edge when she goes out in the community. Jessica is afraid to tell her supervisor about these feelings because she is worried that they reflect poorly on her performance and potential to become an effective professional social worker.

If you were Jessica's coworker and she shared her feelings with you, how would you handle this situation?

What would you encourage Jessica to do?

COMPASSION FATIGUE

The final occupational hazard we discuss in this chapter is compassion fatigue. In comparison to burnout and vicarious trauma, compassion fatigue is a broader term used to describe the overall experience of mental fatigue within the worker because of ongoing treatment and the chronic display of empathy with individuals who are, in some way, suffering (Newell & Nelson-Gardell, 2014). To understand this better, it may be helpful to explore compassion on a deeper level.

Compassion can be defined as an awareness or understanding of what another person is going through that is accompanied by a strong desire to help that person in order to reduce or eliminate their suffering. At the core, compassion means to suffer with or be concerned regarding the suffering of another person. Individuals demonstrating compassion often have a desire to help. It is no secret that there is suffering in the world. Frankly, many of you have chosen the field of social work to ameliorate such suffering. Many within the profession of social work feel "called" to make a difference (Newell & Nelson-Gardell, 2014). Although it is a noble pursuit to make a difference, we must realize that the negative effects of chronic exposure to traumatic, violent, and stressful experiences or stories can take a toll on the worker. When this chronic exposure begins to overwhelm the individual, compassion fatigue can develop.

Unlike burnout that occurs gradually, compassion fatigue can have a much more rapid onset (Melvin, 2012). Compassion fatigue, when left untreated, can evolve into other more serious conditions. Various research suggests that other serious mental health concerns and illnesses could occur because of compassion fatigue. Compassion fatigue not only impacts the individual but can impact the organization as well. It is no secret that some portions of the helping profession experience higher rates of turnover in employees. This can be due to compassion fatigue. It can also impact other aspects of organizational performance and productivity.

RISK AND PROTECTIVE FACTORS

The hazards that we have just discussed—burnout, vicarious trauma, and compassion fatigue—are real conditions that exist within all helping professions, including social work. Although these are real occupational hazards, as we have said, not all workers will experience them. There are a variety of factors to consider when exploring why some workers are affected by these hazards and others can avoid them. In doing so, it is important to consider personal risk and protective factors.

A risk factor is some sort of characteristic or attribute that makes an individual more susceptible, or vulnerable, to developing or being influenced by something. Risk factors that indicate individuals may be at a higher likelihood of developing these hazardous conditions include the following:

- *The nature of the work*: The population with which you work can be considered a risk factor. If you are working in a setting where you are exposed to high volume of difficult or traumatic cases, you may be more vulnerable. This also includes working within a setting where you are exposed to high-risk experiences and meet with resistance from the client systems. An example would be working within an agency when, at times, families are not cooperative and view the helper's role in a negative light.

- *Organizational factors*: Characteristics of the organization where you work may increase the likelihood of developing an occupational hazard. Having high caseloads and a lack of supervision can result in feeling chronically overwhelmed and may even trigger feelings of helplessness. Poor morale within an agency can foster isolation and lack of unity and support. Insufficient training and support can be extremely detrimental to the workers as they are unprepared to appropriately handle what may come their way through the course of their employment.

- *Unrealistic expectations*: It is a noble pursuit to wish to change the world, but we must be realistic in our endeavors. It is unreasonable to think that within 1 week on the job, you will be able to eradicate all of the world's social problems. It is important to maintain perspective, be realistic in your goals, and celebrate small victories. Just as you work to establish achievable goals with your clients, you should also strive to set such goals for yourself and your work.

- *Poor boundaries*: A boundary is an invisible line that marks limits. Within social work, we are called upon by our code of ethics to always maintain appropriate professional boundaries with clients. It is the responsibility of the worker at all times to be alert to and, when possible, avoid dual relationships. Understanding boundaries is a cornerstone of the social work profession. Regarding burnout, vicarious trauma, and compassion fatigue, boundaries are important both with clients and with the job itself. With clients, the social worker must establish and maintain healthy boundaries for their mutual benefit. With the job itself, the social worker must be mindful to not take the work home and establish a separation between their personal and professional lives.

- *Personal issues*: Unresolved emotional issues can derail your social work practice. It is important to be aware of your personal experiences and seek out support to address concerns so that they do not interfere with your professional work. Unaddressed personal issues can lead to barriers in treatment that will halt work with those whom you should be serving. Furthermore, it is necessary that you are aware of any countertransference responses that arise while you are working as a social worker. Countertransference refers to a situation in which your personal feelings are projected onto the client or become entangled in the work you are doing with your clients.

Protective factors can serve as a buffer warding against the development of occupational hazards. These factors, which can mediate against potential hazards, include such things as routine self-care practices, thoughtful self-awareness (reflection and self-regulation), appropriate training, and healthy, clear boundaries.

> **Field Reflection Questions**
>
> Which risk factors are present for you at this time in your placement?
>
> Is there anything you can do to lessen these?
>
> Which protective factors are present for you?
>
> Are there any protective factors you can add?

Support is a protective factor that is quite important. As a field student, you may draw upon support from others in many ways. Personal support may come from your family and friends. Sometimes it is difficult trying to manage your time with friends and family while completing your schoolwork and field hours, but we encourage you to stay connected with your personal supports, as they represent a protective factor that will help you to be a better social worker. Peer support is another form of support available to you as a field student. In your field class, you have a group of other social work students who are going through the same process as you are right now. It can be very helpful to have a peer who is having the same experience to provide support and encouragement. The shared experience is something that can quickly bond you and allow you to be there to help each other throughout your time in field. As we discussed at length in the previous chapter, supervision is another source of support while you are in your field placement. Using your field supervisor and any other organizational supports available to you is an excellent way to increase your personal protective factors.

Personal resilience is a protective factor that can support you throughout your social work career. Resilience is a general term used to describe your ability to bounce back or overcome adversity. It is something that can be fostered and nurtured within an individual. Resilient individuals are resourceful and adaptive, maintain a sense of hopefulness and a positive outlook despite circumstances, can draw upon appropriate coping strategies, and use supports.

SELF-CARE

We have talked about the necessity of being self-aware, but it is equally necessary to take care of yourself so that you can be effective in taking care of others. As social workers, we must take care of ourselves to be effective in our professional practice. Once you are aware of what is going on within you, the compassionate next step is to care for yourself. Returning to an earlier example of self-awareness, when you recognize that you are hungry, the simplest way to take care of that need is to eat something. It is not uncommon for social workers to get busy at work helping others and to skip lunch, dismissing their own feelings and needs. Self-awareness allows us to acknowledge our needs, and self-care requires us to take care of these acknowledged needs.

DEFINING SELF-CARE

Self-care is a term used to describe the habits, routines, and activities that an individual engages in to promote well-being, support health, and maintain balance in their personal and professional lives (Lee & Miller, 2013). It refers to a continuum of activities that seek to reduce stress and promote optimal well-being. Self-care is intentional. It is "an empowering tool that allows practitioners to take ownership of their health and wellbeing holistically and with consideration to both their personal and professional lives" (Lee & Miller, 2013, p. 96). Self-care is especially important for helping professionals such as social workers.

Self-care strategies can serve as a buffer against hazards of burnout, vicarious trauma, and compassion fatigue, which we discussed earlier in this chapter. Adopting this perspective serves to empower social workers to enhance their own well-being and address their own needs. It is important that we as social workers honor our well-being and take steps to ensure that we are functioning as best as we can so that we can fully support the clients we serve.

SELF-CARE ACTIVITIES

Self-care is best viewed as a holistic, multidimensional construct encompassing the following areas: physical, psychological, emotional, social, spiritual, and leisure (Lee & Miller, 2013). Self-care practices, which are sometimes called "rituals," can take on many forms. Most often, self-care focuses on three dimensions of individual well-being: the mind, body, and spirit. When we use the term self-care, we are referring to the integration of all these dimensions. Holistic well-being is an umbrella term that is used to capture our functioning about this. It is necessary that all parts (or dimensions) of us are being cared for to be in a state of wellness.

Self-care rituals (Figure 5.1) are quite subjective and individualistic, reflecting personal preferences and interests (Brown, 2020). For example, one person may find running to be extremely enjoyable, whereas another person may despise running but find a similar joy in drawing. With that in mind, the following are some examples of self-care strategies for the mind (emotional or psychological self-care),

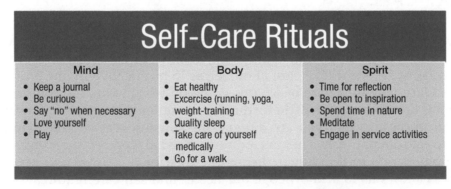

FIGURE 5.1 **Examples of self-care rituals.**

body (physical self-care), and spirit (spiritual self-care) that you may wish to consider for yourself. A great place to start when considering which self-care rituals are appropriate for you would be to take a self-care inventory. There are a variety of inventories available that you can use to rate yourself and determine which areas of self-care are current strengths and which areas of self-care you could improve. Exhibit 5.2 is a simple self-care inventory for you to use to explore your current levels of self-care. It is important to be honest with yourself when completing the self-care inventory, as this gives you a baseline to start assessing your current self-care behaviors.

EXHIBIT 5.2

SELF-CARE INVENTORY

Use this inventory to determine your current levels of self-care for each dimension. Please note that this is not an exhaustive list of self-care activities, but rather a sample of potential self-care activities. At the end of each section, you will see lines marked "other." If you have a self-care strategy that you engage in that is not on the list, please add it in the spaces provided. For each activity, please use the following scale:

3: I do this really well (frequently).
2: I occasionally do this.
1: I rarely do this.
0: I never thought to do this (never).

Physical Self-Care	0	1	2	3
Eat three meals a day				
Chose nutritious foods				
Drink water				
Rest				
Get enough sleep				
Go to the doctor when sick				
Go to the doctor for routine preventive/wellness visits				
Exercise				
Walk				
Stretch				
Other: _____				
Other: _____				
Emotional/Psychological Self-Care	0	1	2	3
Express thoughts and feelings				
Ask for help				
Maintain healthy boundaries				

(continued)

EXHIBIT 5.2 (*continued*)

Take personal responsibility				
Obtain personal therapy or coaching				
Engage in self-awareness				
Emotional/Psychological Self-Care	0	1	2	3
Journal				
Color, draw, create				
Read				
Practice self-compassion				
Other: _____				
Other: _____				
Spiritual Self-Care	0	1	2	3
Pray				
Spend time in nature				
Participate in a community				
Reflect				
Engage in service				
Set intentions				
Practice mindfulness				
Meditate				
Other: _____				
Other: _____				

Note: An electronic template of the Self-Care Inventory is available by accessing Springer Publishing Connect™ via the instructions on the opening page of this book, and clicking on the drop down Show Supplementary, Student Materials, Self-Care Inventory.

SELF-CARE FOR THE MIND

Rituals that promote psychological and emotional well-being are part of this category of self-care. Lee and Miller (2013) assert that the target of this dimension of self-care is to "maintain a positive and compassionate view of the self and negotiate the demands that arise from the intersection of the individual and environment" (p. 99). As social workers, the core of our work involves providing compassion for others. Despite this compassion we can hold for others, often it is more difficult to display the same compassion toward ourselves. We are often our own toughest critics. One simple self-care strategy for the mind would be to demonstrate more compassion toward yourself.

To be able to help others fully, we ourselves must be willing to ask for help (Brown, 2020). As a field student, you will need to ask for help during your placement;

you do not need to know all the answers all the time. Use this time in field to practice getting comfortable asking for help and assistance when you need it.

Other self-care strategies for the mind include things such as recognizing personal strengths, problem-solving, journaling thoughts and feelings, and seeking individual treatment to address personal issues when appropriate. These strategies closely tie back into the concepts of reflection and self-regulation that we discussed earlier in this chapter. By promoting self-care of the mind, it can serve to promote self-awareness, which we know is critically important for effective professional social work practice.

Self-Care for the Body

Our bodies are fascinating and complex machines. Let us consider another machine—a car. You routinely put gas in your car and from time to time take your car to the garage to get a tune-up so it can continue to take you where you want to go. Our bodies also require fuel and regular tune-ups and routine maintenance to keep us functioning at our best.

Goals for physical self-care target optimizing physical function and personal safety (Lee & Miller, 2013). Examples include such things as eating well-balanced meals throughout the day, getting enough quality sleep at night, exercising your body, and addressing medical illnesses and injuries by seeking medical attention when appropriate.

Self-Care for the Spirit

Caring for the spirit encompasses all activities that ignite an inner passion or resonate deep within yourself. For some, spiritual self-care practices are tied to their religious practices. However, it is noteworthy that in this context, the concept of spirit does not have to be viewed within the context of religious beliefs.

Mindfulness is one strategy of spiritual self-care that has grown in popularity in recent years. For social workers, some posit that mindfulness training can allow the worker to attend to clients and encourages a sense of acceptance and openness that enhances the helping relationship (Gockel et al., 2012) more closely.

So, what is mindfulness? For some, the first picture in their mind may have been of a monk sitting cross-legged on the floor engaging in chanting and breath work. Yes, this is one type of mediation, but it is just that—one type. There are a variety of mindfulness exercises that involve all the senses for individuals across the life span. There has been much attention focused on mindfulness practices that can be used in everyday life for the average individual. All mindfulness activities revolve around the focus of being present in the current moment. Mindfulness encourages us to experience the world through all our senses—what we are seeing, tasting, hearing, smelling, and feeling. Mindfulness is about self-acceptance as well. It is recommended that mindfulness is practiced regularly to fully reap its many benefits. Some links to resources on mindfulness are given at the end of this chapter for you to try out. Remember, just like self-care rituals, mindfulness is not a "one size fits all" proposition. Try a few different types of mindfulness strategies to see what works best for you.

SUPPORTIVE RELATIONSHIPS

The value of support should not be understated. After all, we are *social* workers, not *solitary* workers; the word "social" is in our title for a reason. We as a profession understand the value and importance of human relationships. The NASW *Code of Ethics* (2021) cites the importance of human relationships as one of the professions' guiding principles.

Throughout your field placement, you have several relationships that can support you throughout this process. The first and foremost is your relationship with your field supervisor. The role of the field supervisor is one defined by support. Field supervisors are not only tasked with providing you with an orientation to the organization and overseeing your daily tasks. They are also charged with creating a meaningful learning environment in which you can engage your social work skills while being supported by trained practitioners. In addition, your weekly supervision with your field supervisor is designed to be the time when you can not only review routine questions related to the job, but also seek support as you grow throughout the field process.

Another supportive relationship you have while you are in field is with your faculty liaison. This staff member has been assigned to assist you during your field journey. The role of the faculty liaison includes being available to support both you, as the student, and the field supervisor. Your faculty liaison is a great resource of support if you have something you want to discuss related to the field.

Field can, at times, be difficult. Who better to understand what you are going through than those who are going through it with you right now? Your social work peers are a great source of support during the field process. The shared experience of field can serve as a bond for your connection.

Field Reflection Questions

Which supportive networks do you have in your life that you can rely on for support?

Be sure to include both personal and professional support systems.

Make a list of your supports. How are these people helping you?

How could they be more supportive of you?

DEVELOPING A SELF-CARE PLAN

As you have read, self-care is necessary to serve as a buffer against the helping profession hazards. We started this chapter by asking you to approach self-care with curiosity; now we ask you to approach self-care with creativity as we discuss developing a self-care plan.

What is a self-care plan? Well, it is simply a written plan of which self-care rituals you are going to incorporate into your life. You can reflect on the self-care inventory that you completed earlier in this chapter to give you a good place to

---

EXHIBIT 5.3

SELF-CARE PLAN

Tara's Self-Care Plan

In the space below each dimension of self-care, list two to three rituals that would promote care of yourself.

Mind	Body	Spirit
• Color a mandala once a week. • Keep a gratitude journal every night.	• Eat three meals a day. • Go for a walk at least three times a week. • Drink eight glasses of water each day.	• Read an inspirational story or passage every morning. • Meditate twice a week.

Note: An electronic template of a Self-Care Plan form is available by accessing Springer Publishing Connect™ via the instructions on the opening page of this book, and clicking on the drop down Show Supplementary, Student Materials, Self-Care Plan.

---

start in developing your self-care plan. There are a variety of formats available for self-care plans, which range from quite simple to more reflective and engaging. A quick online search for "self-care plans" will result in a myriad of options. No matter the template, a basic self-care plan should address the dimensions of self-care (mind, body, spirit) and allow you space to identify which rituals you plan to complete. Exhibit 5.3 provides an example of a simple self-care plan.

After completing your plan, it is important to set yourself up for success. Consider which barriers are present that may hinder your ability to stick with your plan. Once you have identified these barriers, develop strategies to address them so that you can stick with your plan. For example, you may identify time as a barrier to engaging in self-care because you are a busy student who is trying to manage the demands of coursework and field work with other demands from your personal life. One possible strategy to address this time barrier is to schedule time in your day to take some time to engage in self-care. You may schedule just 5 minutes a day to sit and meditate or 30 minutes early in the morning to go for a jog. Self-care is effective only when it is being practiced: It does no good to have an amazing self-care plan if you cannot implement it.

One strategy that may be helpful is to find a self-care partner. Having someone to support you in your self-care endeavors and to help hold you accountable for taking care of yourself can be a great motivator. Just as you are probably more likely to go to the gym or exercise class if you have a workout partner, you will be more likely to engage in self-care if you have a self-care partner. Identify your self-care partner and have a conversation with them about where you are and where you would like to be with your self-care. Ideally, if your self-care partner is engaging in their own self-care, you can be mutually supportive of each other. Talk with each other about what type of support motivates and encourages you most and decide how you will check in with each other to hold each other accountable. Something as simple as a text message to touch base can serve this purpose.

Think of your self-care plan as a compassionate contract with yourself. It has been said that you cannot give what you do not have, so for us, as social workers, to give compassion to our clients, it is important for us to show compassion to ourselves. Consider your self-care plan an ever-evolving document that demonstrates your commitment to try and take care of your *self*. Because it is something that will change over time, it is important to revisit this plan periodically to see what you need to adjust. Take another self-care inventory and then revisit your plan every couple of months.

CONNECTING SELF-CARE TO YOUR PLACEMENT

We have defined and discussed the importance of self-care in the social work profession. It is important that you begin practicing self-care during your field placement. Just as you are developing and refining your practice skills, this is a time to consider and work on your self-care as this is a necessary dimension to your long-term practice as a social work professional. Being a student can be a stressful experience. You may be juggling coursework, hours at your placement, and other responsibilities such as relationships and work. However, practicing self-care has been shown to reduce stress in students (O'Neill et al., 2019).

CASE SUMMARY: "I CAN'T CRY NOW . . . SOMEONE ELSE IS DYING"

PRACTICE SETTING DESCRIPTION

Prairie Homecare and Hospice Services is a small organization that operates in a rural community in Pennsylvania. The staff consists of several nurses and medical staff, but there are only two full-time social workers to support all of the clients, who currently include more than 150 patients. This is the first time that Prairie Homecare and Hospice is hosting a social work field student. As the field student, I am going to work with both the social workers and eventually have my own small caseload of clients.

IDENTIFYING DATA

Early on in my field placement, my days were spent totally with the two social workers. I would ride with them to and from client visits, and we would cofacilitate sessions with the patients and their families. I did feel comfortable from the beginning, especially with the elderly female patients. I guess I felt this way because they reminded me of my own grandmother, who had lived with my family for the past 12 years until about 6 months ago, when she passed away after a long bout with cancer. My grandmother and I were always really close. When my parents worked, she would be at home to take care of me and my sisters. Due to my comfort around these older women, my supervisors thought I was ready to have my own caseload. I started off with 10 clients of my very own. Of the 10, nine were older women, eight were on hospice.

Now that I had a caseload of my own, I did not spend as much time with my supervisors. Because our work involved so much traveling, I would really see them only at the start of each day for a few minutes and then on Friday afternoon for our weekly supervision. They kept telling me how great I was doing and that they were hearing great things about the work I was doing with the clients. Because I was doing such a good job, they quickly increased my caseload—in fact, they doubled it. Now I have 20 clients whom I am responsible for seeing and documenting. I think I should be grateful to have so much responsibility because it must mean I am doing a good job. The only problem is some days I feel like I am running around in circles driving from one home to the next without any breaks.

PRESENTING PROBLEM

About 2 weeks after being assigned 20 cases, one of the first cases that had been assigned to me, Mrs. Charlotte, started taking a turn for the worse as her health declined. Mrs. Charlotte was one of my favorite patients to visit, probably because she looked so much like my grandmother, and she said I was like the granddaughter she never had. Previously, my visits with Mrs. Charlotte were filled with laughter and chatting, but recently she has mostly been sleeping. The lead nurse says, "It won't be long now."

For a couple of weeks, I continue to see all my clients, but it seems like everyone is getting sicker. I am starting to get angry that my patients are not recovering. I wonder what they are doing wrong or why they will not go back to the hospital to try and get better. I am frustrated that I cannot make them better. I do not know what I am doing wrong!

This week has been the worst. First, on Monday morning I learned about another patient passing away over the weekend. While I was sitting in the staff meeting, my work cell phone rang that I was needed by the family at Mrs. Charlotte's house. I got there as fast as I could, but I was too late. She was gone. Mrs. Charlotte passed away and I was not there for her. As I stood on her porch, talking to the nurse from my office, I could feel tears welling up inside of me. My stomach hurt. I remembered that I was here as a social work intern, and I told myself internally that I should not cry. To remain professional, I quickly took a deep breath, said goodbye to the nurse, and got in my car. I thought I would be able to cry in my car once I pulled away. As soon as I got in the car, my phone rang, it was a different office nurse telling me that another one of my clients was close to passing and the family was requesting a social worker. When I hung up the phone with her, I plugged the address into my GPS and started driving to where I was needed. I thought to myself, "I can't cry now; someone else is dying."

That week, three clients on my caseload passed away. I guess I should have expected it because I am working for a hospice after all.

ASSESSMENT

For the past week, I have been feeling irritable and I am just so tired. It does not seem to matter how much sleep I get; I just want to stay in bed and sleep some more. I also noticed that I have been thinking about my grandmother a lot recently. During supervision this week, both the social workers at the agency who I work with met me. They shared that they bet the past week was hard for me experiencing several losses of patients. I did not want to seem bothered by it, so I quickly downplayed my reaction to it and said, "Oh, it's fine, just part of the job." One social worker nodded and said, "Sometimes our patients do pass away, but a loss is still hard, even if we expect it to happen." There was something about how she said and how she looked at me in such a comforting way that I lost it right there in her office. I started to cry. When she asked me about my tears, I said this past week has reminded me a lot about my grandmother. She handed me a box of tissues and we started unpacking some of my reaction.

CASE PROCESS SUMMARY

Through my supervision, I was able to process with my supervisor that in part my reaction was due to some of my own unresolved feelings surrounding my grandmother's death that I had not yet dealt with. I realized that I should have asked for help earlier, when my caseload started feeling overwhelming. I also saw that maybe I was having some counter-transference reactions with Mrs. Charlotte and that is why I felt so attached to her. I also learned through supervision that it is okay to have feelings as a social worker. Feelings are normal and natural, but it is important to be aware of these feelings and to process them in a place like supervision so that they do not interfere in my practice with my clients. I plan to start journaling about my feelings and taking breaks throughout the day to do things I enjoy, such as going for a walk at lunch or listening to my favorite music while driving in my car.

Alice, MSW Student Intern

CASE DISCUSSION QUESTIONS

1. *In what ways could Alice have promoted personal well-being better in the scenario?*

2. *Based on the scenario, how do you think Alice did in managing her personal experiences and professional behaviors? If you were Alice, what would you have done differently?*

3. *If Alice wanted to talk to her supervisor about what she was feeling (before the supervisor brought it up), how could she have initiated that conversation? What should that conversation look like?*

END-OF-CHAPTER RESOURCES

 A robust set of instructor resources designed to supplement this text is located at http://connect.springerpub.com/content/book/978-0-8261-3753-1. Qualifying instructors may request access by emailing textbook@springerpub.com.

CRITICAL THINKING QUESTIONS

1. In your field placement, how can you use reflection and self-regulation to maintain professional social work behavior? On days that are exceptionally difficult, which strategies can you use to promote well-being in a professional environment?

2. What would you do if you began to recognize signs of vicarious trauma in a fellow student at your field placement? Which steps would you take and why?

3. How can you use reflection and self-regulation to promote well-being through self-care for yourself? How would you describe self-care to someone who is unfamiliar with it? How could you encourage it for others? How do your personal experiences influence your professional judgment and behavior as a social work field student?

4. How do you use reflection and self-regulation to manage personal values and maintain professionalism in the field?

5. How can you improve your self-awareness as a professional social worker?

6. How can you ensure that you will engage in self-care not only as a field student but also as a practicing social work professional after graduation?

LEARNING ACTIVITIES

1. Consider your field placement site and the work that you are doing and the organizational expectations. How could a social worker protect themselves from the hazards of helping in your practice setting? What might be some organization risk and protective factors related to these hazards?

2. Evaluate your own self-care practices by completing the exercises shared in this chapter. Consider how you can improve or continue to engage in self-care regularly to promote holistic well-being. Develop a self-care plan and share it with one other person for accountability.

ELECTRONIC RESOURCES

WEBSITE LINKS

Self-Care Starter Kit, from University at Buffalo's School of Social Work: http://socialwork.buffalo.edu/resources/self-care-starter-kit.html

The American Institute of Stress Home Page: www.stress.org

The *Mindful* website provides various media exploring mindfulness. www.mindful.org

The Compassion Fatigue Awareness Project provides links to self-assessments (PROQOL, compassion fatigue self-test, life stress self-test) that can be done online or on PDF versions. https://compassionfatigue.org/self-tests.html

VIDEO LINKS

Ted Talk Featuring Megan McCormick Discussing Her Own Self-Care Journey: www.youtube.com/watch?v=sUKKJapwUXc

Social Work Tech Video 5—Self-Care Plan: www.youtube.com/watch?v=GWwwPb6akqA

Health Equity Institute's "Release: Self-Care for Trauma Workers" features trauma workers discussing burnout, vicarious trauma, and self-care. www.youtube.com/watch?v=CoLupPSmmoU&index=3&list=PLoqWbfSB28TspN27SF9DVdufULmyvj39E

"What is Compassion Fatigue?" Dr. Frank Ochberg discusses both compassion fatigue and burnout. www.youtube.com/watch?v=VubmnvCl9sk

"Social Work and Compassion Fatigue Webinar" by Maretter Monson: www.youtube.com/watch?v=7kBHNpUMo0g

REFERENCES

American Psychiatric Association. (2013). *Diagnostic and statistical manual of mental disorders* (5th ed.). https://doi.org/10.1176/appi.books.9780890425596

Bogo, M. (2010). *Achieving competence in social work through field education*. University of Toronto Press.

Brown, M. E. (2020). Hazards of our helping profession: A practical self-care model for community practice. *Social Work*, *65*(1), 38–44. https://doi.org/10.1093/sw/swz047

Cox, K., & Steiner, S. (2013). Preserving commitment to social work service through the prevention of vicarious trauma. *Journal of Social Work Values & Ethics*, *10*(1), 52–60. https://jswve.org/download/2013-1/articles(2)/52-60-Preserving%20Commitment%20to%20Social%20Work%20Service.pdf

Gockel, A., Burton, D., James, S., & Bryer, E. (2012). Introducing mindfulness as a self-care and clinical training strategy for beginning social work students. *Mindfulness*, *4*(4), 343–353. https://doi.org/10.1007/s12671-012-0134-1

Lee, J. J., & Miller, S. E. (2013). A self-care framework for social workers: Building a strong foundation for practice. *Families in Society: The Journal of Contemporary Social Services*, *94*(2), 96–103. https://doi.org/10.1606/1044-3894.4289

Melvin, C. S. (2012). Professional compassion fatigue: What is the true cost of nurses caring for the dying? *Journal of Palliative Nursing*, *18*(12), 606–611. https://doi.org/10.12968/ijpn.2012.18.12.606

National Association of Social Workers. (2021). *Code of ethics*. https://www.socialworkers.org/About/Ethics/Code-of-Ethics/Code-of-Ethics-English

Newell, J. M., & Nelson-Gardell, D. (2014). A competency-based approach to teaching professional self-care: An ethical consideration for social work educators. *Journal of Social Work Education*, *50*(3), 427–439. https://doi.org/10.1080/10437797.2014.917928

O'Neill, M., Yoder Slater, G., & Batt, D. (2019). Social work student self-care and academic stress. *Journal of Social Work Education*, *55*(1), 141–152. https://doi.org/10.1080/10437797.2018.1491359

Developing Your Professional Competencies

Demonstrating Ethical and Professional Behavior

CASE VIGNETTE

Jocelyn is completing her BSW field experience as a case manager with a large human services organization. She meets with clients to establish goals and then works with the clients to achieve these goals. Often, she is helping her clients with housing, healthcare, and social and vocational goals. Much of Jocelyn's time is spent communicating with other professionals over the phone, in person, or electronically. She often collaborates with other professionals and participates in interdisciplinary team meetings for many of her clients. Jocelyn needs to follow up with other professionals who are also working with her clients to monitor progress toward goals. She often has to request information and documentation from other providers to include in her records.

People have always told Jocelyn that she is a very social and outgoing person. Jocelyn is excited about all the communication she will have with other service providers because she loves to talk to people. She thinks that this is going to be easy because she is so social. As Jocelyn meets new service providers with whom she needs to collaborate, she adds them to her Facebook account so that they can chat with each other over Messenger. Within a couple of weeks, Jocelyn has added more than 20 service providers on her personal Facebook page. Despite now using her personal Facebook account to connect with other professionals, Jocelyn continues to post about her personal social life, including nights out with friends, stories about how stressed she is with school, and how she feels about her coworkers at her field site.

- *Is Jocelyn communicating like a professional?*

- *What, if any, ethical concerns arise from Jocelyn's current communications?*

COMPETENCY 1: DEMONSTRATE ETHICAL AND PROFESSIONAL BEHAVIOR

Social workers understand the value base of the profession and its ethical standards, as well as relevant laws and regulations that may impact practice at the micro, mezzo, and macro levels. Social workers understand frameworks of ethical decision-making and how to apply principles of critical thinking to those frameworks in practice, research, and policy arenas. Social workers recognize personal values and the distinction between personal and professional values. They also understand how their personal experiences and affective reactions influence their professional judgment and behavior. Social workers understand the profession's history, its mission, and the roles and responsibilities of the profession. Social workers also understand the role of other professions when engaged in interprofessional teams. Social workers recognize the importance of lifelong learning and are committed to continually updating their skills to ensure they are relevant and effective. Social workers also understand emerging forms of technology and the ethical use of technology in social work practice.

Social workers

- make ethical decisions by applying the standards of the National Association of Social Workers (NASW) *Code of Ethics*, relevant laws and regulations, models for ethical decision-making, ethical conduct of research, and additional codes of ethics as appropriate to context;

- use reflection and self-regulation to manage personal values and maintain professionalism in practice situations;

- demonstrate professional demeanor in behavior; appearance; and oral, written, and electronic communication;

- use technology ethically and appropriately to facilitate practice outcomes; and

- use supervision and consultation to guide professional judgment and behavior. (Council on Social Work Education [CSWE], 2022, p. 7)

LEARNING OBJECTIVES

By the end of this chapter, you will be able to:

- Describe professional oral, written, and electronic communications.
- Distinguish between professional and casual (informal) communications.
- Describe elements of an effective case note.
- Complete a process recording.
- Compose professional email correspondence.
- Describe the ethical use of technology regarding social work practice.
- Develop a personal social media policy.
- Identify the NASW ethical standards related to technology.

ORAL COMMUNICATION

Most of us have heard the phrase "it is not what you said, but how you said it" at some point in our lives. Words are powerful, and how they are used is something we must be considerate of in all contexts. As social workers, we must constantly behave professionally. As professionals, our communication—whether it be oral, written, or electronic—should demonstrate our professionalism. Professionalism is possessing competence or expertise expected in one's field. For social workers, the CSWE outlines the competencies that you must possess to be a professional social worker and that are discussed throughout this text.

PROFESSIONAL SPEAKING

To be an effective professional social worker, you must be aware of the spoken language you are using. In this role, it is important to distinguish between casual and formal speech. Casual speech has its place, but as professional social workers, we should use formal speech in most circumstances to present our best professional selves. Formal speech for professional social workers is usually the adoption of the speech of the dominant culture. In the dominant U.S. culture, this means use of proper elocution (clear speech, proper pronunciation), appropriate speed and tone (inflection), and proper syntax. When engaging in formal speech, you should avoid words that are informal (e.g., *hey, yeah, kinda, nah, gonna,* and *ain't*). Slang terms should be avoided, as they may be misunderstood. When speaking professionally, you should remember your manners as well. Use terms such as *please, thank you,* and *you are welcome.* If you are not accustomed to speaking formally, you should practice. As with anything, practice can improve your performance and help you in getting more comfortable with professional speaking.

JARGON AND ACRONYMS

CBT, BHRS, RTF, ADHD, OCD, LTSR, EBP, IOP, DBT—sometimes social work can feel like a bowl of alphabet soup! All these letters mean something, but they lose their meaning if you do not know what they stand for (see Case Example 6.1). First and foremost, if during your field placement you come across an acronym that you do not understand, *ask.* It may also be helpful to keep a list of commonly used acronyms for your placement, especially while you are settling in and getting familiar with the jargon that professionals are using. These acronyms and other forms of professional jargon all have their place, but we need to be cautious when using this type of language in our communication. We need to be sure not to just throw out a list of jargon and acronyms to our clients or others who are not familiar with our professional terminology.

ORAL AND POSTER PRESENTATIONS

Field Reflection Question

What are some common acronyms or jargon used at your field placement?

As we will discuss in depth in the research chapters of this text, it is important for social workers to be engaged in research-informed practice and practice-informed research. A critical piece of this relationship with research is sharing findings with other professionals. One way to share these findings with others is through presentations. Presentations most frequently occur at conferences and can be categorized as oral or poster. Oral presentations involve a lecture. Poster presentations involve having a visual aid displaying the major points of the research and a more casual conversation with the audience. Students are often invited and encouraged to present their findings at conferences to gain valuable experience presenting their research. This is something we would encourage each of you to consider doing during your MSW education. Whether making an oral or poster presentation, there are several things to consider in order to demonstrate professionalism. When presenting, you must be aware of your professional self as it is expressed in a variety of ways (through what you say, your presentation materials, and your appearance). We have discussed the importance of professional speech previously; it is also important to make sure that your speech is inclusive and to avoid any terms or slang that can be exclusionary or offensive (we will explore this idea further in a later section on bias-free writing). Your presentation materials should demonstrate professionalism. They should follow standards related to the format you are presenting whether it be through an electronic format with a slideshow shared from your computer or a poster. Review your presentation for errors and correct any that you notice. It is often helpful to have someone else review the presentation for you as well to check for any mistakes you may have missed. Also, you will want to be sure to follow American Psychological Association (APA) guidelines and cite your sources appropriately. Lastly, when considering your professional appearance, consider how to dress in such a way that demonstrates your commitment to professionalism and does not distract from the content of your presentation.

CASE EXAMPLE 6.1: OVERWHELMED BY ACRONYMS AND JARGON

Jim has an MSW field placement as a mobile family therapist. His MSW supervisor handed him a stack of charts for the clients he will be shadowing this week. As Jim started to look at the first chart, he read, "The IP has been dx with OCD by Dr. Rudd. F/U in 2 weeks for med mgmt." He stopped and read that sentence again (and again), but it did not make sense to him. He was afraid to ask his supervisor about it because he felt self-conscious thinking it was something that he should have already known. By the time Jim made it through the fourth chart, he was pretty discouraged because he did not feel as if he was able to understand what was going on with any of the clients he was supposed to be seeing this week.

What Should Jim Do?

As we have said earlier (and will say again), your field placement is a time for learning and growing as a social worker. You are not expected to have all the answers. It is okay to ask for help, support, or, in this case, clarification when you are presented with something you do not understand. Your field supervisor is there to help you with issues just like this.

(And in case you were wondering, the sentence given earlier can be translated to "The identified patient [client] was diagnosed with obsessive-compulsive disorder by Dr. Rudd. Follow-up in 2 weeks for medication management.")

WRITTEN COMMUNICATION

Written communication is all around us; we read articles, books, and emails all the time. As a college student, you most certainly have had your share of written assignments, many of which assessed your ability to effectively communicate

Field Reflection Questions

How would you assess your current communication skills? Are you stronger at oral or written communication? Why?

How can you improve your communication skills?

your thoughts and ideas through written words. For social workers, good writing skills are crucial to demonstrate professionalism. Rai and Lillis (2013) assert that "writing plays a central role in social work practice" (p. 1), and we could not agree more. In this section, we discuss several ways in which social workers will need to express themselves through written communication, including case notes, process recordings, and biopsychosocial assessments. Later we talk about electronic communication that involves written communication as well.

BIAS-FREE WRITING

As social workers we are called upon by our *Code of Ethics* to demonstrate cultural awareness. This cultural awareness applies to all aspects of ourselves including our written communication. One way that we can demonstrate cultural awareness is to engage in bias-free writing. Bias-free writing seeks to be inclusive in written language and promotes principles of diversity, equity, and inclusion. When using bias-free writing we are being conscious to not exclude members of our audience related to any area of diversity or difference. One example of this would be the use of pronouns when writing. As social workers we recognize that there are a variety of different expressions of gender identity. If our writing makes assumptions about an individual (or group of individuals) by using pronouns such as "he" or "she," we are excluding a group of individuals who do not identify as either of those options. The APA provides several great resources on their website related to the use of bias-free language in professional communication (see https://apastyle.apa.org/style-grammar-guidelines/bias-free-language).

AMERICAN PSYCHOLOGICAL ASSOCIATION STYLE GUIDELINES

As a social work student, you are most likely quite familiar with the APA and APA guidelines. APA formatting is a means by which written style and grammar maintain professionalism across various disciplines. APA Style is not stagnant, as it revises and changes over time. At the time of this publication, we are presently in the seventh edition of APA formatting. This formatting outlines all aspects of the writing process from page numbers, titles, and headings to use of language and, of course, citations and references. It is beyond the scope of this text to dive into all APA style guidelines; however we do encourage you to review them thoroughly as they are critical for success in professional communication. In addition to the *Publication Manual of the American Psychological Association* (APA, 2020), there are many other resources including your institution's writing center, and online APA resources.

CASE NOTES

In social work, it is often said, "If it is not documented, it did not happen." Clear, accurate, and timely documentation is necessary for effective social work practice. Documentation not only is critical to ensure continuity of care and measure change over time, but is often necessary for reimbursement from third-party payers such as insurance companies and other funding sources.

As social workers, our written words are quite powerful, so we must recognize the latent power and be considerate of this when documenting information. McDonald et al. (2015) suggest that social workers must constantly be mindful that "*how* and *why* we write as well as *what* we write reflects our commitment to the values and ethics of professional practice" (p. 360). Your documentation of client interactions becomes a lasting record that can follow clients long after your helping relationship with them has been terminated. Social workers must be sure that we are using our best written communication skills to document in a way that is ethical and professional.

Each social services agency will have its own documentation requirements for case notes, and it is important that you familiarize yourself with these forms and requirements early on during your field placement. If you are unsure what the requirements are at your field placement, ask your field supervisor right away. Although specifics for case note requirements will vary from agency to agency, there are several things that we, as professional social workers, should always consider.

Professional social workers provide clear documentation. Clarity in our writing refers to it being easy to understand or interpret. Our documentation is direct.

We should avoid ambiguous writing that could lead to misinterpretations. Also, clear documentation is complete, without any missing gaps or interactions that are unaccounted for within the chart. For example, if a social worker documents that during the visit she witnessed a "touching event between siblings," this could have multiple meanings. Did the social worker witness an event that was heartfelt and kind, or did the social worker witness a sexual or physical interaction between siblings that involved inappropriate personal contact? This example, which McDonald et al. (2015) cite in their work, illustrates the necessity for clarity in written communication. Had the social worker been referring to a heartfelt interaction and another worker read the documentation and mistook it for inappropriate physical touching, that misunderstanding could lead to significant difficulties for the family involved. We should try to avoid language such as this that can have different meanings and can easily be misinterpreted.

Professional social workers provide accurate documentation. At the heart of ethical written communication is the truth. Lying, misleading, or fabricating information is forbidden. Our documentation should reflect the whole truth, even when it may not be pleasant. Sometimes, social work students fear that if they document that a client is having negative experiences or not progressing in treatment, it will negatively reflect upon them, so they do not accurately document what the client is experiencing. First, client progress, or lack thereof, does not necessarily reflect your ability to be an effective social worker. A variety of factors influence client progress throughout treatment. By not accurately documenting the client and their situation, you are breaking the core social work value of integrity and doing a disservice to your client (and yourself as the helper). Professional social workers must always practice with integrity, which includes being honest in our written communication.

To meet the previous two standards of documentation—clear and accurate—our documentation must also be timely. Timely documentation serves multiple purposes. First, the sooner we can document our interactions with clients, the more likely our documentation is to be clear, accurate, and complete. It is natural to lose details of interactions as time passes. As professional social workers, we must make every effort possible to capture the details that are important for our clients' records so that we can effectively document those details in our case notes. Whenever possible, you should complete your documentation immediately following a client interaction. Should you not have the time or ability to document immediately, we recommend that you jot down some notes of the details you feel should be included in the case note so that you can reflect on your notes later when you sit to write them. If you are finding it difficult to complete your field documentation in a timely manner, this is an important conversation to have with your field supervisor. Together you can review your schedule and documentation requirements and then brainstorm solutions.

In addition to being sure that your documentation is clear, accurate, and timely, one common record-keeping practice is writing a SOAP note. In a SOAP note, S is for subjective observations, O is for objective data, A is for assessment, and P is for plan (Hepworth et al., 2017). Subjective observations refer to how the client views their situation or experience. You can document this by writing, "client reports that

. . ." or "parents voiced concerns about . . ." within your case notes. In contrast, objective data refer to facts and descriptions—the things you see, hear, smell, count, or measure in some other way. The assessment section of the case note should include your clinical judgments, impressions, and diagnosis information. The last section of the case note should include your plan or intended next steps in working with this client, including any expectations for the worker or the client. Exhibit 6.1 shows a sample SOAP note.

EXHIBIT 6.1

SAMPLE SOAP NOTE

Client Name: Carolyn D.   Date/Time: 3-1-2018 11:15 a.m. to 12:00 p.m.

Met with client to continue cognitive behavioral therapy (CBT) intervention to address symptoms of depression. Client arrived on time and reported feeling "a little bit down" today. Client appeared to be unkempt and dressed much more casually than had ever previously presented. Eye contact was minimal and at times, client appeared tearful during session. Client stated she has "no energy" to take care of herself regarding showering and washing her hair. Social worker readministered a depression inventory previously taken by the client. On this date, the client's score indicates a rise in depressive symptoms from 2 weeks ago. Social worker plans to collaborate with client's psychiatrist regarding the recent medication adjustment made and share client's current presentation to ensure continuity of care. Social worker and client will continue to use CBT interventions to address depressive thoughts but will meet more frequently (weekly instead of every other week).

PROCESS RECORDING

A process recording is a tool used in social work education and supervision to assist the learning social worker in exploring client–worker dynamics and examining the use of self in the helping process. Process recordings are often very detailed written works but can at times include audio or visual recordings as well. They have long been used in social work education to examine what was said and done in the helping process while exploring the motives, thoughts, and behaviors associated with the interaction. Formats for process recordings can vary, but most include the following elements:

- background information
  - description of the setting (place, date, time) in which the interaction took place
  - first names of parties involved
- purpose
- content
  - description of the interaction (verbal and nonverbal; see Exhibit 6.1 for a sample of how to display the content of a process recording)
- impressions and assessment
  - social worker's comments and feelings about what happened and why
- plans
  - future plans with this client
- issues, questions, and problems
  - any questions the social worker has regarding the interaction or content

Tips for Success

For process recordings to be most beneficial, we recommend that you complete them as soon as possible after the interaction, while your recollections and reactions are as fresh as possible. As we discussed earlier, timely documentation is highly desirable because of its ability to capture the most accurate details of the interaction. We also recommend that you take full advantage of the educational benefits of process recordings by being as honest as possible when reconstructing the interaction and your reactions. Do not try to include what you think is the "right thing" to write down. Rather, use the process recording for its intended purpose, as a tool to help you reflect on your practice skills and become a more effective and efficient social work professional. Most social work programs that require students to complete process recordings also require that the process recording be reviewed by the field instructor and discussed in supervision. Process recordings are helpful learning tools only if you are honest and open to feedback. Exhibit 6.2 shows a sample of the beginning of a process recording.

ELECTRONIC COMMUNICATION

We are living in a technologically advanced era. Many of us always have technology with us. Our ability to be electronically connected is greater than ever before. As with most things in life, technology comes with both advantages and potential disadvantages. As professional social workers, we must be able to successfully navigate the use of technology in electronic communication in its various forms.

EXHIBIT 6.2

SAMPLE PROCESS RECORDING

Jenna, an MSW field student who is placed at a local hospital, prepared the following process recording. In the example, the social work student, Jenna, and her field supervisor, Janet, received a page from the ED requesting a consult. After reviewing the patient's information in the electronic medical record, the social workers determined the purpose of this session. The social workers planned to meet with Nick (a 10-year-old Caucasian male) and his biological mother in the ED to discuss an incident of assault between siblings to assess the situation and gather pertinent information.

Interview Content (May Also Include Client Behavior— That Is, Nonverbal Communication)	Client's Feelings/ Affect	Student's Gut-Level Feelings	Analysis of Your Intervention and Identification of Any Themes or Issues in This Section
Jenna: We were called in by the doctors to talk with you a little bit. Can you tell us what brought you to the hospital tonight?	Mother is upset.	Nick does not seem to be in much pain; mother is very emotional.	Gather information to be able to best assist the family.
Mom: My children were fighting; Nick got kneed in the head.	Mother is tearful.	Mother seems very upset for such a minor injury. There are probably more family dynamics the team needs to uncover.	
Janet: So, Nick, can you tell us a little about your siblings? Brothers? Sisters?	Nick is looking down, avoiding eye contact with social workers.	Nick appears to be shy.	Nick had been in a fight with his younger sister. Get details from Nick.

Our professional code of ethics addresses the use of technology in social work practice. Technology can be used in a myriad of services, including, but not limited to, counseling, therapy, advocacy, education, supervision, research, and evaluation, as well as program administration. All principles and standards set forth by the NASW *Code of Ethics* should be followed whether the interactions, relationships, or communications occur in person or electronically (NASW, 2021).

SOCIAL MEDIA

Twitter, Facebook, Instagram, Snapchat, LinkedIn, and other similar apps and sites are great ways to stay connected with family and friends. They are commonplace today for most people; however, we, as social workers, need to be aware of our social media presence. Social media serve as more than just a means to connect with others; Westwood (2014) suggests that social media have an "awareness angle which brings important social issues and the impact of social inequalities" to light (p. 3). It is estimated that social workers use social media at high rates to share professional information in the form of blogs, podcasts, and articles (Hitchcock & Battista, 2013).

Before your next tweet, post, link, or snap, consider your digital footprint, including whether it is demonstrating the professionalism of a social worker. In this age of technology, we must be mindful of our digital footprint. The term *digital footprint* refers to the online record trail we leave on the World Wide Web. We suggest that you take a moment to Google yourself and see what comes up; you may be surprised. Knowing what is online is the first step in being able to manage your online identity.

Privacy settings are something else that are important to consider. With technology being so easily accessible, it is easy for others to search for you online. Regardless of privacy settings, we urge you to post with caution. Bottom line: If you would not want the picture or post to be put on a billboard on the side of the highway, we strongly suggest that you reconsider posting it online. Once it is out there, it is very difficult, if not impossible, to totally erase.

EMAIL

With email so readily accessible on mobile devices, it is sometimes easy to forget that this form of communication also requires professionalism from social workers. When composing or responding to an email, although it may be convenient to respond quickly, we urge you to take a moment and consider your message.

How can you increase professionalism in an email? First, thoughtfully consider your subject line; do not leave it blank. The subject line does not have to be (and should not be) a novel, but it should identify the purpose of the email. Then, start your email off with a salutation or greeting. Something as simple as "Good morning" or "Dear (name)" is a great way to start off your email. This starts your message off right.

When typing your email, be sure to use appropriate grammar and punctuation. Capitalize the appropriate words and use professional language (avoid the pitfalls we have been discussing in this chapter so far). At the end of your email, include a closing such as "Sincerely" or "Thank you" and do not forget to include your name. With email, it is often taken for granted that the person knows who the email is coming from; the recipient probably does, but that does not negate your responsibility to send a professional message.

Remember, how you email in your personal life is one thing; how you email as a professional social worker is a completely different matter. Always proofread your emails before sending them to catch typos or autocorrect errors that may be hiding in your message. Exhibit 6.3 illustrates a simple professional email message for your review.

EXHIBIT 6.3

PROFESSIONAL EMAIL EXAMPLE

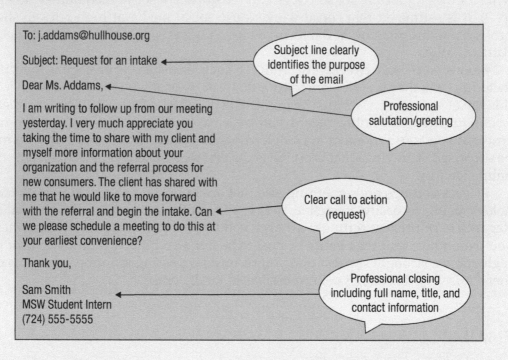

As a student in field, you most likely have access to your campus-issued email that you can use for correspondence. It is important to consider what email address you will be using when you begin applying for social work jobs and networking. Be mindful that your email address should be professional. Shy away from using email addresses such as 2cute4u@mymail.com or superherogamer2003@yourmail.com. Although these might be fine for your personal correspondence, something more professional might be a better choice for your career. A professional email choice may be as simple as your first and last name or first initial and last name.

When communicating electronically, it is important to be mindful that at times our message can be lost in translation (Park et al., 2014). When communicating electronically, we do not have access to tone of voice, inflection, or other nonverbal cues to help us interpret the messages we receive. To be sure that our electronic communication is professional, we should try to follow general "netiquette" rules (Khani & Darabi, 2014). Netiquette refers to appropriate and clear electronic communication. Write emails that avoid sarcasm or harsh rhetoric, use appropriate formality, and avoid all caps, excessive punctuation, or emojis (Park et al., 2014).

VIRTUAL PRACTICE

Though virtual practice, sometimes referred to as telehealth, has been around much longer than the recent pandemic, the impact of COVID-19 increased its use exponentially. Social workers relied on virtual practice options to stay connected with clients during stay-at-home orders and to prevent the spread of disease. Virtual practice looks different depending on your social work role. Regardless of your role, there are several importance considerations to keep in mind when working with clients remotely through a virtual platform. It is very important that the social worker still maintain a professional presentation despite practicing virtually. The social worker should dress professionally. The social worker should also consider their surroundings and make sure that they are viewed in a professional setting. Making sure that the background is tidy and does not distract the client is important. The social worker must also be mindful to avoid unintended self-disclosures through things such as photographs in the background. Considering privacy and confidentiality is paramount when conducting virtual sessions. The social worker should be in a private space that ensures client privacy. The social worker can wear headphones to promote this as well. It is important to fully discuss the benefits and limitations of virtual practice with clients when starting this type of work so that the client can make an informed decision regarding their choice to participate.

PROFESSIONAL AND ETHICAL USE OF TECHNOLOGY

It is important that as professional social workers, we are caring and genuine with our clients. In demonstrating that connection, we may be friendly toward our clients, but we must be clear that although we are friendly, we are not our clients' friends. Throughout this text, and your social work education, you have learned about establishing and maintaining appropriate boundaries. The responsibility for the development and maintenance of boundaries falls totally upon the social worker. So as the social worker, you need to establish and be clear about these professional boundaries with your clients. It is inappropriate to be friends with clients on social media. Social work professionals should not accept requests and invitations from clients on social media platforms because the social worker is responsible for maintaining appropriate boundaries with clients and avoiding potentially hazardous dual relationships (NASW, 2021). Furthermore, social workers should not engage in personal communication with clients through any electronic forum.

According to Loue (2016), "social workers are increasingly relying on the internet to provide information to clients/patients, to seek advice about patients, to provide mental health treatment, and as part of an ongoing supervisory or consultant relationship" (p. 1). With a growing focus on telehealth services and a rise in app-based video conferencing to connect with helping professionals, social workers must be aware of the benefits and potential limitations of such advances (see Exhibit 6.4).

EXHIBIT 6.4

PROFESSIONAL USE OF TECHNOLOGY

Benefits	Limitations
• Offers services to those who may be unable to access in-person services (because of transportation issues, for example)	• Potential breaches in confidentiality because of hacking and lack of encryption
• Can be more convenient (related to client scheduling)	• Lack of connectivity or access to technology in some areas (particularly rural regions) as well as the possibility for technology failures
• Services are often less expensive for clients	
• Increased access to professionals (no longer limited to those in the geographic area)	• Lack of in-person interaction/connection
• Real-time monitoring	• Cost of technology (devices, internet access)
• The ability to respond rapidly	
• Ease of communication	

 Furthermore, several social work professional organizations came together recently to release technology standards for social workers. The NASW, Association of Social Work Boards, CSWE, and Clinical Social Work Association set standards for technology use in social work practice (see www.socialworkers.org/includes/newIncludes/homepage/PRA-BRO-33617.TechStandards_FINAL_POSTING.pdf).

PROFESSIONAL ONLINE IDENTITY

Developing a professional online identity is another important step to consider. For some social workers, developing this professional online identity is necessary (especially if they deliver services electronically). Curington and Hitchcock (2017) suggest that professional social workers who use social media for professional purposes should create a professional online identity, post for professional reasons, and create a social media policy. Your professional online identity is different from your personal online identity, which we discussed earlier in this chapter. Your professional online identity may use social media platforms, blogs, business websites, or other online forums. Through these forums, you are clearly identifying yourself as a professional social worker. Because this is a professional presentation, your postings should be aligned with social work values and principles while following guidelines set forth by professional organizations. As this is a professional presentation, you should develop a social media policy regarding how you use technology and your response to various situations (see Exhibit 6.5 for tips on developing a professional social media policy).

EXHIBIT 6.5

TIPS FOR DEVELOPING A PROFESSIONAL SOCIAL MEDIA POLICY

Your social media policy serves to "to inform clients, constituents, colleagues and others about when, how and why you use social media in a professional capacity" (Curington & Hitchcock, 2017, p. 10). Your social media policy is a personal policy in which you will include standards that are applicable to your professional situation; however, it is recommended that you include risks and benefits of the use of technology in professional practice (refer back to Exhibit 6.4). Your social media policy should include (at least) the following:

- the goals of your technology presence
- your policies related to friending, following, and contacting clients
- identification of the professional standards from which your policy is derived
- ethical concerns created using technology
- how you hope to use technology in your professional practice

CONFIDENTIALITY AND PRIVACY

As professionals, we must always consider the intended and unintended consequences of behaviors. When using electronic communication and the assistance of technology, we must be aware of our limitations to safeguard information. Currently, it is common to hear about hackings and data breaches, but we must never get too accustomed to these terms to forget what that means for us as social workers and for the clients we serve. When serving vulnerable populations and dealing with sensitive and confidential information, we must take all steps possible to protect the information of our clients. We should follow all state and federal guidelines related to privacy and compliance. There are many considerations in ensuring confidentiality while using technology-driven social work practices (Groshong & Phillips, 2015). We recommend reviewing your field placement agency's Health Insurance Portability and Accountability Act (HIPAA) policies and procedures and that you review the federal HIPAA policies and guidelines at www.hhs.gov/hipaa/index.html.

CASE SUMMARY: "SOCIAL MEDIA BLUNDER"

PRACTICE SETTING DESCRIPTION

Newport Community Ministries is a small not-for-profit organization that strives to meet the needs of community members by providing resources such as food, clothing, and financial assistance to community members who are affected by poverty. In addition to supporting individuals and families directly, the organization works to engage members of the local business community. By engaging businesses, Newport Community Ministries strives to create opportunities such as jobs as well as educational and training opportunities that will assist individuals in becoming more employable in the future. Newport Community Ministries also connects with local politicians to advocate for poverty reform initiatives.

This semester, I have been placed at Newport Community Ministries as a BSW intern. There is only one social worker employed with this agency, Todd, and he serves as my field supervisor. Todd is excited to be working with me this semester because sometimes it gets overwhelming keeping up with everything he needs to do.

IDENTIFYING DATA

One of my learning objectives this semester is to create an online social media presence for Newport Community Ministries. Todd assigned me this task because it has been on his "to-do list" for a while. Since I am a lot younger than he, he thought that I would have the skills to develop these electronic resources. Because I do have a lot of experience on social media (not to brag, but I have more than a thousand followers on Instagram), I was excited to have this opportunity; I believe that I will really be able to use my creativity. Todd said that he wants to have a platform for Newport Community Ministries to be able to share their achievements (e.g., relationships with business partners, policy successes) and reach out for help (ask for donations from the community, request volunteers, and so on) online.

PRESENTING PROBLEM

A few weeks after I launched the Newport Community Ministries social media accounts (I created Twitter, Snapchat, and Facebook accounts), I started having some problems. First, to boost the followers on these platforms, I decided to share them on my social media sites, asking my followers to follow the Newport Community Ministries pages. That worked and got a lot of followers on the new page. The only problem is that because I connected my personal page with the Newport Community Ministries page, people now can access my personal accounts. I noticed that I was starting to get "likes" and "follows" from community business partners, current volunteers, and even a couple of individuals who have come to Newport Community Ministries for services.

At first, I did not think it was that big of a deal. Then one day this week, I posted a meme on my personal social media page that had a funny saying about having a tough day at work because of people who are clueless. A friend had posted it and the meme had my favorite actor in it, so I shared it on my page. Actually, I did not even have a bad day at work, so the content of the meme did not apply to me; I just thought that it was funny and liked the actor. I guess I shared it without thinking.

Within a couple of hours, I noticed that I had a ton of notifications. One client who I had worked with at Newport Community Ministries that day commented on my post, asking if it was him who ruined my day. He posted again saying that he hopes I do not quit working at Newport Community Ministries because I am really friendly and always help him when he comes in. He also sent me a few private direct messages about my post, asking about how I was feeling and saying that he was concerned about me. He said he was there if I needed someone to talk to about it. I did not respond to the messages from the client; I did not know what to say.

ASSESSMENT

The next day when I went to Newport Community Ministries, I knew I should talk to Todd about it—but to be honest, I was embarrassed and thought it would just go away on its own. I mean, I did not message the client back; that was the right thing to do, I think. Well, I was wrong.

That afternoon, the client who had messaged me on my personal social media came into Newport Community Ministries and demanded to see me. He was really agitated and visibly upset. When I went out to see him, he started yelling at me and he called me a "liar." He said that he thought we were friends and he could not believe that I ignored his messages online. I felt bad because I could see how upset he was; at the same time, I was a little scared because I was being yelled at by this client.

Thankfully, Todd was in his office near where the client and I were standing. When the client started getting loud, Todd quickly came out of his office to intervene. Todd asked the client if he would talk with him for a little bit, to which the client agreed. Todd and the client went into his office and talked for almost an hour!

After the client left, Todd came to my office and shut the door. I was nervous. Thankfully, Todd just wanted to talk to me about what happened. I came clean and shared what happened. I told Todd how I thought I was doing the right thing by ignoring the client online, but now I realized that ignoring the client made the situation worse. The client took my post personally and felt dismissed by me. Even if it was not my intention to offend anyone with what I posted, as a professional social worker, it is my responsibility to consider such things before I make such a post.

Todd and I were able to process the entire situation and explore how we were using social media professionally for Newport Community Ministries and how I was using it personally as well. Todd and I looked online and found copies of ethical standards set forth by NASW and other professional social work organizations.

CASE PROCESS SUMMARY

Through my supervision with Todd, I was able to see that I was not in compliance with social media standards set forth by NASW and as a result I risked the well-being of my clients. Now that I have a clearer understanding of what is required ethically by social workers when using technology, I am better able to manage my personal social media and distinguish between my personal and professional online identities. On the basis of my conversation with Todd, we both agreed that it would be a good idea to develop a social media policy for Newport Community Ministries to post on the social media pages. By posting our social media policy, it can serve to inform clients of how and why we have our online pages and what they can expect from us as professionals.

Holly, BSW Student Intern

CASE DISCUSSION QUESTIONS

1. *Based on this scenario, what steps could Holly have taken to avoid this problem in the first place? Once the problem occurred, what should Holly have done to address the situation?*

2. *How did Holly's personal social media interfere with her ability to be a professional social worker? How could she avoid such issues in the future?*

3. *How could developing a social media policy at the launch of the Newport Community Ministries social media pages have helped in this scenario?*

4. *As a social worker, working at an organization like the one described in this scenario, create a social media policy that could be included on the agency's social media site.*

END-OF-CHAPTER RESOURCES

 A robust set of instructor resources designed to supplement this text is located at http://connect.springerpub.com/content/book/978-0-8261-3753-1. Qualifying instructors may request access by emailing textbook@springerpub.com.

CRITICAL THINKING QUESTIONS

1. How would you define professionalism and being a professional? How is being a professional social worker different from being simply a professional?

2. In your field placement, how can you ensure that your communication is always professional? Are there differences in how you would professionally communicate with a client as opposed to with another professional? If so, what are they?

3. How can you ensure that you are using technology in an ethical way as a social work professional?

4. What would you do if a client sent you a friend request on a social media site? What would you say to the client during your next session about this request?

LEARNING ACTIVITIES

1. Consider your current online presence. Through a personal audit, reflect upon how you present yourself electronically and consider how it aligns with the

values and ethics of our profession. Consider potential areas for growth related to your use of email and social media. Develop two SMART goals related to how you can demonstrate a more professional online presence.

2. Review your resume and consider how you can illustrate your commitment to ethical and professional behavior through this document. Revise your resume to spotlight these commitments and share it with a social worker for feedback.

ELECTRONIC RESOURCES

WEBSITE LINKS

Telemental Health: Legal Considerations for Social Workers: www.socialworkers.org/About/Legal/HIPAA-Help-For -Social-Workers/Telemental-Health

8 Ethical Considerations for Starting a Telehealth Practice: https://naswcanews.org/8-ethical-considerations-for-starting -a-telehealth-practice

APA Bias-Free Language: https://apastyle.apa.org/style-grammar -guidelines/bias-free-language

NASW, ASWB, CSWE, and CSWA Standards for Technology in Social Work Practice (2017): www.socialworkers.org/includes/newIncludes/ homepage/PRA-BRO-33617.TechStandards_FINAL_POSTING.pdf

Infographic by University at Buffalo School of Social Work (n.d.)— Social Worker's Guide to Social Media: https://socialwork.buffalo .edu/resources/social-media-guide.html

VIDEO LINKS

 Ted Talk by Dale Atkins, "Being a Professional" (2013): www.youtube.com/watch?v=sLv7sdGJWPI

 Stanford Graduate School of Business presentation, "Think Fast, Talk Smart: Communication Techniques" (2014). This presentation provides tips and techniques to improve oral communication in spontaneous conversations. www.youtube.com/watch?v=HAnw168huqA

REFERENCES

American Psychological Association. (2020). *Publication manual of the American Psychological Association* (7th ed.).

Council on Social Work Education. (2022). *Educational policy and accreditation standards for baccalaureate and master's social work programs.* https://www.cswe.org/getmedia/94471c42-13b8-493b-9041-b30f48533d64/2022-EPAS.pdf

Curington, A. M., & Hitchcock, L. I. (2017, July 28). *The social media toolkit for social work field educators.* http://www.laureliversonhitchcock.org/2017/07/28/social-media-toolkit-for-social-work-field-educators-get-your-free-copy

Groshong, L., & Phillips, D. (2015). The impact of electronic communication on confidentiality in clinical social work practice. *Clinical Social Work Journal, 43,* 142–150. https://doi.org/10.1007/s10615-015-0527-4

Hepworth, D. H., Rooney, R. H., Rooney, G. D., & Strom-Gottfried, J. (2017). *Direct social work practice: Theory and skills* (10th ed.). Cengage.

Hitchcock, L. I., & Battista, A. (2013). Social media for professional practice: Integrating Twitter with social work pedagogy. *Journal of Baccalaureate Social Work, 18*(Suppl. 1), 33–45. https://doi.org/10.18084/basw.18.suppl-1.3751j3g390xx3g56

Khani, R., & Darabi, R. (2014). Flouting the netiquette rules in the academic correspondence in Iran. *Procedia: Social and Behavioral Sciences, 98*(6), 898–907. https://doi.org/10.1016/j.sbspro.2014.03.498

Loue, S. (2016). Ethical use of electronic media in social work practice. *Romanian Journal for Multidimensional Education, 8*(2), 21–30. https://doi.org/10.18662/rrem/2016.0802.02

McDonald, D., Boddy, J., O'Callaghan, K., & Chester, P. (2015). Ethical professional writing in social work and human services. *Ethics and Social Welfare, 9*(4), 359–374. https://doi.org/10.1080/17496535.2015.1009481

National Association of Social Workers. (2021). *Code of ethics.* https://www.socialworkers.org/About/Ethics/Code-of-Ethics/Code-of-Ethics-English

National Association of Social Workers, Association of Social Work Boards, Council on Social Work Education, & Clinical Social Work Association. (2017). *NASW, ASWB, CSWE, & CSWA standards for technology in social work practice.* https://www.socialworkers.org/includes/newIncludes/homepage/PRA-BRO-33617.TechStandards_FINAL_POSTING.pdf

Park, S., Na, E. Y., & Kim, E. (2014). The relationship between online activities, netiquette, and cyberbullying. *Children and Youth Services Review, 42,* 74–81. https://doi.org/10.1016/j.childyouth.2014.04.002

Rai, L., & Lillis, T. (2013). 'Getting it write' in social work: Exploring the value of writing in academia to writing for professional practice. *Teaching in Higher Education, 18*(4), 352–364. https://doi.org/10.1080/13562517.2012.719157

Westwood, J. (2014). *Social media in social work education.* Critical Publishing.

Advancing Human Rights and Social Justice in Your Field Placement

Kendall was a second-year MSW student doing her placement at an agency on an Indian Reservation in the midwestern United States. A few months into her placement, Kendall began to hear complaints from her clients about health issues that were cropping up within families and the community. Concerned about this trend emerging in her placement, Kendall decided to do a little research to gather recent health data from the community and found few resources available that could provide any information.

She began to ask service recipients at the agency about their experiences and documented that information. It was not long before she heard about community groups that had formed to identify the cause of the issues that her clients were reporting to her—with a main hypothesis that a local oil refinery is causing both air and water pollution. They struggled to find any definitive data, but similar symptoms among residents began popping up near another oil refinery a few states away. Kendall began to attend the community group meetings to assist in data collection and brainstorming potential action efforts.

However, Kendall has noticed some in the community have cooled off to her, and others have started to get openly hostile to all her work in the community—not just her efforts to stop the presumed pollution and poor health issues. Jobs are hard to come by on the reservation and in the nearby areas, and any position at the refinery—from janitorial to engineer—is extremely coveted. Plus, the wages of the refinery workers support local businesses. New restaurants have opened, and a new grocery store is planned to open soon. For the first time that many can recall, the flood of people away from the community has slowed, and anecdotal accounts suggest alcohol and drug abuse is also slowly declining.

- *What should Kendall do if her own values around environmental justice conflict with community leaders' steadfast support of the refinery and the economic benefits it has provided?*

- *How should Kendall approach her work in the community if the large majority of community members, including many of her own clients, want her to stop volunteering with the community agency that they see as radical?*

- *How does Kendall reconcile her desire to adhere to the National Association of Social Workers (NASW) Code of Ethics, which include advocating for environmental justice, economic justice, and upholding her clients' rights to self-determination?*

COMPETENCY 2: ADVANCE HUMAN RIGHTS AND SOCIAL, RACIAL, ECONOMIC, AND ENVIRONMENTAL JUSTICE

Social workers understand that every person, regardless of their position in society, has fundamental human rights. Social workers are knowledgeable about the global intersecting and ongoing injustices throughout history that result in oppression and racism, including social work's role and response. Social workers critically evaluate the distribution of power and privilege in society in order to promote social, racial, economic, and environmental justice by reducing inequities and ensuring dignity and respect for all. Social workers advocate for and engage in strategies to eliminate oppressive structural barriers to ensure that social resources, rights, and responsibilities are distributed equitably and that civil, political, economic, social, and cultural human rights are protected.

Social workers

- advocate for human rights at the individual, family, group, organizational, and community system levels; and
- engage in practices that advance human rights to promote social, racial, economic, and environmental justice. (Council on Social Work Education [CSWE], 2022, p. 9)

LEARNING OBJECTIVES

By the end of this chapter, you will be able to:

- Recognize the importance of advancing social, economic, and environmental justice.
- Understand the conceptual theories and frameworks for social justice work.
- Understand the facets of power and social aspects that contribute to injustices in these areas.
- Utilize change strategies to implement social justice strategies in your field placement and beyond.

CONCEPTUAL THEORIES AND FRAMEWORKS FOR SOCIAL JUSTICE

Social justice is a broad concept that encompasses fair and unbiased treatment of all individuals, eradication of discriminatory practices and institutionalized oppression, and establishment of equality for members of historically marginalized and oppressed groups—achieved through the establishment of truly equal opportunity and access to resources (Barsky, 2010; Reisch, 2002; Young, 2001). The meanings of social justice have wide implications, yet can be ambiguous, and interpretation into practice is challenging. It is important to remember that the concept of social justice is bound by context and history. Attempts to define the correct relationship between individuals, communities, states, and countries have been explored for centuries by philosophers, political theorists, and social workers (Finn & Jacobson, 2017).

The notion of social justice within the field of social work is generally based on Western ideologies and the Judeo–Christian religious tradition (Finn & Jacobson, 2017). Beliefs around social justice are generally abstract and are in line with what is moral and/or right—with a specific focus on the notion that all citizens are equal and have the right to meet their basic needs, the desire to share opportunities as equitably as possible, and the obligation to work toward eliminating unjustified inequalities. Caputo (2002) points out that while many notions of social justice within social work actually maintain the status quo, it still remains an important goal of social work.

Some scholars examine social justice through the always-present tension that exists between individual liberty and the common good. These scholars would argue that social justice is endorsed to the degree that we can promote collective good without violating basic individual freedoms (Finn & Jacobson, 2017). Others contend that social justice incorporates fairness within fundamental rights and duties, economic opportunities, and social conditions (Miller, 1976).

A perspective often utilized by social work is that of a distributive approach of social justice—advocating for an organization of societal institutions that assures human rights and access to meaningful social participation, as well as equitable distribution of resources. Distributive justice focuses on what society owes an individual. Other frameworks focus on what people owe society—legal justice—and what individuals owe one another—commutative justice (Reichert, 2003; Van Soest, 1992).

Social work generally addresses the conflicting philosophical frameworks used to explain choices in the realm of social justice using three dominant theories: utilitarian, libertarian, and egalitarian (Finn & Jacobson, 2017). Utilitarian theories consider decisions that result in greater good and less harm for the most people to be the appropriate course of action. The right of the individual is deemed less important than the needs of the community or society at large, and as such, those rights may be infringed upon if a particular decision results in assisting the greater good (McCormick, 2003).

Libertarian perspectives focus on individual freedom from external control or

> **Field Reflection Questions**
>
> In your current field placement, what human rights and social justice theoretical perspective(s) do you see in action?
>
> In what ways do those perspectives manifest (e.g., who is allowed to receive services)? What theoretical framework would that decision likely be classified as?
>
> How are the theoretical perspectives similar to your own? How are they different?

influence. This framework rejects the concept of equitable resource distribution, instead arguing that individuals have the right to any resources they acquire if no law is broken (Nozick, 1974). Clearly, this is in direct contrast to the utilitarian perspective as the obligation to society lies in the protection of individual freedoms.

Finally, egalitarian theoretical frameworks argue that everyone should be guaranteed the same rights, opportunities, and access to goods and resources (Rawls, 1971). This approach advocates for the redistribution of resources to the vulnerable, oppressed, or disadvantaged in society to guarantee that unmet needs are rectified (Rawls, 1971).

Political philosopher Rawls (2001) examines what would need to be present in a society that meets basic human needs, reduces excessive stress, encourages individuals' abilities, and reduces threats to well-being. Rawls advocates for an equal distribution of resources and burdens from tangible resources (good and services) and intangible resources (power and opportunity). Social justice comes down to two principles (Rawls, 2001, pp. 42–43)

- each person has the same indefeasible claim to a fully adequate scheme of equal basic liberties, which scheme is compatible with the same scheme of liberties for all; and

- social and economic inequalities are to satisfy two conditions: First, they are to be attached to offices and positions open to all under conditions of fair equality of opportunity, and second, they are to be to the greatest benefit of the least-advantaged members of society (the difference principle).

Distributive justice, as defined by Rawls, helps the field of social work to integrate social justice into both micro and macro practice settings (Wakefield, 1988). This theoretical framework focuses counteracting inequalities by advocating for unequal distribution of resources only if done to advance the least advantaged groups in society (Reisch, 1998).

TYPES AND SOURCES OF POWER

In this chapter, we will discuss forms of oppression that exist due to inequities in power that allow groups in power to act out their biases, prejudices, and stereotypes in ways that deprive those not in power full access to resources, self-actualization, and autonomy (Thomas & Schwartzbaum, 2017). This section will do a deeper dive into the types of power that exist, as well as social dimensions that contribute to these power differences.

While power is a complex term with multiple meanings depending on context, the type of power we are focused on in regard to social justice refers to power within social structure and systems. Legitimately or otherwise, certain individuals and groups have power, and with that power utilize force (of varying types) to exploit others for their own gain. The purpose of focusing on power within social relationship and societal structures is to better understand how we, as social workers, can better understand how social justice advocacy can attempt to address the connections between privilege and exploitation.

Three different types of power exist (Dobratz et al., 2012):

1. *Coercive and dominant power:* Likely the most obvious use of power, coercive power uses the command of resources to dominate others into submission. For example, coercive power in the form of physical force could include military strength, brute force, violence, and so forth.

2. *Authority and legitimate power:* Society creates order by acknowledging power based on tradition, norms, and laws. Authority and legitimate power is the form of power that arises from this acknowledgment. Members of society accept that specific individuals or groups have power based on a sense of legitimacy and obedience or duty. This type of power can be obtained because individuals believe that placing power in states offers protection to members of society and preserves community interests.

3. *Privileged and interdependent power:* This type of power tends to be subtler, but still holds dramatic implications for social interactions and distribution of power in society. This type of power focuses specifically on the power relationship between two actors. Often, the actors do not realize exactly how much influence they have in a given situation. Piven and Cloward (2005) point out that people have potential power when others depend on them for the contributions they make to interdependent relationships that make up society. Johnson (2006) also points out that privilege links to the ways society makes differences important or significant. These include unearned advantages (one specific group rewarded) and conferred dominance (when one group pressures another group, or groups, into conforming to that privilege) as ways that privilege is created in society.

Framing societal power within the field placement experience, it is important to recognize that power is the ability of individuals, groups, and/ or structures to attain a plan through authority, influence, or even force (Dobratz et al., 2012). This is important because it recognizes that power exists on the

> ### Field Reflection Questions
>
> In your current field placement, which of these types of power do you currently see play out?
>
> Can you think of an example of each of these types of power in your field placement? If so, what are they? If not, can you imagine an example that could potentially exist?

micro level as well as the macro level. When we are thinking about social justice and human rights, we are particularly concerned with the ways that dominant power, individually or collectively, is exploited by privileged individuals or groups. Often within the guise of preserving societal interests, certain groups end up marginalized, scapegoated, and exploited for the benefit of more powerful groups.

SOCIAL IDENTITES

Kirk and Okazawa-Rey (2010) define identity as how we define ourselves at any specific instance in time that is a process of growth, change, and renewal. Identity may seem fixed, but over the course of the life span, it is more fluid. An interplay of individual choices, particular life events, community recognition and expectations, societal categorization, classifications, and socialization all come into play in identity formation. Most definitions of identity point to the connections between us as individuals, how we are perceived by other people, and how we are classified by social institutions. You can conceptualize social identities through the lens of social work practice. The micro level is usually the level at which individuals are most comfortable with themselves and their social identities. At the mezzo level, individual identities and needs meet group standards, expectations, obligations, responsibilities, and demands. Comparisons are made and individuals have their identities affirmed or they may discover incongruities in who they believe they are and how they are viewed by others. "Classifying and labeling human beings, often according to real or assumed physical, biological, or genetic differences, is a way to distinguish who in included and who is excluded from a group, to ascribe particular characteristics" and to prescribe social locations (Kirk & Okazawa-Rey, 2010, p. 52).

SOCIAL LOCATIONS

Social location is a way of expressing the core of a person's existence in the social and political world. Social locations are the groups people are a part of because of their place or position in history and society. Individuals all have a social location that is based on the intersection of all their identities and group memberships. These identities include race, gender, ability, religion, sexual orientation, social class, age, actual geographic location, and more. How we see the world and how we can move through the world are greatly influenced by our group memberships. Specific roles, rules, power, and the existence or lack of privilege is a result of these memberships as well.

SOCIAL CONSTRUCTIONS

Social constructions are difficult to define because social construction scholars are generally averse to the limitations of definitions. When thinking about social constructions in regard to field placement, it is the understanding that the world we live in and the world our clients live in is not simply there, but is actually continually constructed in elements of everyday life (Holstein & Gubrium, 2008). Instead of viewing the world as something that exists and can be discovered, social constructions are the variety of social interchanges that make up the reality of the world. In essence, the clients you work with participate in the creation of their own world, just as you participate in the creation of your own world.

Additionally, social constructionists recognize that there is no reality, only descriptions, which lends an immense amount of importance to language. Everything about the world is mediated by language, and because of this, you as the social worker benefit from focused attention on how language functions for your clients, within your agency, and within society.

Important aspects of social construction, as described by Witkin (2011), include the understanding that knowledge is dependent on historical and cultural aspects; a recognition that language has the power to establish and give organized existence to something; a critical lens concerning any knowledge that is taken for granted (regularly seen in our dichotomous, categorical society); an understanding that knowledge is social action; and a belief that knowledge is sustained by social processes. The belief that human beings, in relation to one another, construct the world is often difficult for individuals to accept because it is antithetical to Western cultures' emphasis on individualism.

> **Field Reflection Questions**
>
> What social identities and social locations can you identify when thinking about the clients you work with within your field placement?
>
> Can you think of an example from your field placement in which social constructions would be a useful lens for you to utilize in your work? In what ways are realities socially constructed in your current work?

SOCIAL PROCESSES

Originating from sociology theories, social processes refer to the various patterns of social interactions in which individuals and groups interact and establish social relationships. Examples of different forms of social interaction include competition, cooperation, conflict, assimilation, exploitation, accommodation, and others (Ginsberg, 1953). While there are a large number of social processes (e.g., education, political, religious, economic), Ruhela (2005) argues that within the vast array of social processes there are really only two categories they can all fall under:

1. *Integrative, conjunctive, or associative processes*: Social processes which bring the individuals and groups together to produce unity among members of a group or society. These processes take the interests of all members into account. Examples of this are cooperation and accommodation.

2. *Disintegrative, disjunctive, or dissociative processes*: Social processes that produce hatred, tension, and bring disagreement among the members of a group or society. Competition, rivalry, and conflict are the main disintegrative processes.

Oppression and discrimination are embedded in the complexity of ever-changing and constant social processes.

CONFLICT

Conflict is an important social process that is a huge part of society as a whole. It is a codified form of struggle that is deliberate in its attempt to oppose or resist the will of others. Conflict is universal, ever-present, and personal. While there are a multitude of theories on the origin of conflict, we do know that social change can be a direct cause of conflict, and conflict can result in social change. Conflict may seem overwhelmingly negative, due to the fact that it resists cooperation and can cause chaos; however, conflict can perform positive functions as well. It can result in a redefinition of circumstances by the conflicting individuals or groups. Generally, the groups in conflict have to give up outdated value systems and accept new value systems at the end of the conflict—this may result in new efforts of cooperation and accommodation.

There is perhaps no better known example of using conflict in the pursuit of social justice than that documented in a passage from Martin Luther King, Jr.'s (1963, p. 5) *Letter from Birmingham Jail.* (1963, p. 5) in which King states: "[T]here are two types of laws: there are just laws, and there are unjust laws. I would agree with St. Augustine that 'An unjust law is no law at all.'"

FORMS OF OPPRESSION

As discussed earlier in the chapter, oppression is the result of inequities in power that allow groups in power to act out their biases, prejudices, and stereotypes in ways that deprive those not in power full access to resources, self-actualization, and autonomy (Thomas & Schwartzbaum, 2017).

There are many ways in which oppression, discrimination, and prejudice are seen in everyday life: prejudicial talk, avoidance of certain groups or individuals, segregation or exclusion in social systems (e.g., employment, education), violence to person or property, exploitation, marginalization (exclusion from social life), cultural imperialism (repressing the nondominant group's norms and values), and organized extermination of a group of people based on their membership (Allport as cited in Thomas & Schwartzbaum, 2017, p. 9; Young, 1990). Social workers will be able to identify the ways that these oppressive actions take place on micro, mezzo, and macro levels. Daily microaggressions (common, regularly occurring humiliations—intentional or not, based on stereotypes and prejudices as defined by Sue et al., 2007), imbalances of power within interpersonal relationships, and systemic institutional and cultural discrimination and exclusions deny individuals the ability to be seen, and see themselves, as spiritually, mentally, and emotionally whole.

The damaging effects of oppression reach their height when individuals begin to internalize the negative stereotypes about the group they have membership in (Sue & Sue, 2012). Internalization of oppression can manifest itself in a variety of ways that can include self-hatred, engaging in self-harming behaviors, and acting in ways that are in accordance with the stereotypical messages they have received, among others. Kagan and Burton (2005) argue that the helplessness that many oppressed individuals feel is also a form of internalized oppression—they have internalized the dominance of those in power, and are rendered incapable, helpless, and powerless. While some are able to prevent this internalization through the coping skills they have developed, other are overwhelmed by the ongoing assault on their sense of self. Because of this, social workers must remember to utilize an ever-present lens of culture and oppression when working with clients. The next section will define the ways in which individuals are often targets for oppression—this list is not exhaustive.

> **Field Reflection Questions**
>
> What are some instances of microaggressions or interpersonal acts of oppression you have heard from clients, or witnessed yourself in your field placement?
>
> What other ways, beyond the examples listed, can internalized oppression impact individuals?

RACISM

Racism is pervasive, rooted in assumptions of superiority based on race, deeply infused in the history of the United States, and requires the critical attention of all social workers (Rodgers, 2015). As overt racism (legalized segregation, lynching, etc.) became less acceptable during the civil rights era, the acting out of racist ideologies evolved into a more concealed form of racism that is persistent in the institutions of society. The resulting policies create unequal outcomes for people of color including higher rates of incarceration; unequal access to financial, employment, and educational resources; inequity in representation; disparities in health outcomes; and more (Rodgers, 2015). A very important and often confusing concept is color-blind racism (Bonilla-Silva, 2003). Perhaps some of you reading this passage were even coached as children to "see people, not color." While regularly well-intentioned, claiming to not see people with regard to their race is actually an exceptionally damaging approach—not acknowledging and celebrating the differences in culture imposes the dominant (White) culture on everyone, robs people of color of their cultural uniqueness and pride, and assumes that everyone has the privilege of moving through the world in the same way, with a total disregard for the impact of discrimination, oppression, and ongoing microaggression (Bonilla-Silva, 2003). Very recently, the United States has been experiencing a significant increase in the expression of overt forms of racism, including the use of brazenly racist slogans, aligned with belief systems of the Ku Klux Klan and Nazism, with the intention of inciting violence and discrimination toward people of color (Siddique & Laughland, 2017).

XENOPHOBIA AND ETHNOCENTRISM

Often fueled by racism, xenophobia is the fear or hatred of other countries and individuals from other countries. This is often seen in conjunction with ethnocentrism—the belief that one group (ethnic, religious, or specific culture) is superior to others—and often leads to prejudice and oppression based on ethnicity, religion, or country of origin (Sue & Sue, 2012). This greatly impacts beliefs and policies around immigration and globalization. Targeting immigrants as the cause of society's ills has long been a practice in the history of the United States. Which groups of immigrants are targeted and what those forms of discrimination look like fluctuates significantly based on political and economic factors (Thomas & Schwartzbaum, 2017). However, racism often plays a role in who is most often targeted, with people of color at a greater risk of discrimination due to racial profiling.

CLASSISM

Classism is the differential treatment based on (actual or perceived) social class. Lott and Bullock (2007) point out that classism occurs both individually and institutionally. Individual classism refers to the stereotypes and prejudices believed about individuals living in poverty, as well as working class individuals. Institutional classism refers the social institutions that enact policies and procedures that negatively impact, marginalize, and harm individuals living in poverty. This can be seen in the education system, legal system, political system, and beyond. Additionally, denying the fact that class difference has systemic roots and blaming the poor for their poverty are additional forms of classism (Thomas & Schwartzbaum, 2017).

RELIGIOUS OPPRESSION

The pervasive oppression based on minority religious status is the product of the intersection of the historical tradition of Christian hegemony in the United States, the unequal power relationships of minority religious groups with the Christian majority, and the often-held belief of "one true religion." Christian beliefs and norms are hegemonic in that they are an assumed status and are interwoven into society. Some examples are the adoption of "In God We Trust" as the national motto and the observance of Christian holidays by governmental agencies. Religious persecution based on these beliefs has resulted in violence and religious cleansing (systematic extermination of groups based on religious belief).

SEXISM

Sexism is the discrimination on the basis of gender, most commonly demonstrated by men toward women. This form of discrimination is often rooted in a belief that women should be subservient to men, and that men are superior to women intellectually (Thomas & Schwartzbaum, 2017). Traditional notions of gender link behavioral, cultural, and social characteristics to an individual's gender. Sexism and gender-based discrimination and inequality practices include violence; restricted access to education, economic, and governmental opportunities; resource restriction that results in health disparities; and others (Littlefield et al., 2015). Moral, religious, and cultural practices often reinforce traditional gender roles and attitudes. These beliefs are so strongly held that violence is perpetrated against those who violate them. Challenging traditional beliefs of gender and advocating for policies that decrease gender discrimination and sexual harassment are some of the ways that discrimination based on gender can be confronted (Littlefield et al., 2015).

HOMOPHOBIA, BIPHOBIA, AND HETEROSEXISM

Homophobia is the intense fear, hatred, or dread of homosexuals and homosexuality (Moses & Hawkins, 1982). Biphobia is an aversion to bisexuals and bisexuality. It is important to remember that individuals of any sexual orientation can hold homophobic and biphobic beliefs. Similar to other forms of oppression, homophobia and biphobia can manifest in a variety of ways, including violence, discrimination in education, employment, and housing. State-sponsored homophobia includes practices and policies that criminalize homosexuality; governmental figures engaging in hate speech toward gay, lesbian, and bisexual individuals; and withholding certain rights and privileges (e.g., marriage, healthcare decision-making capacity) from same-sex couples.

Often, many homophobic and biphobic beliefs are rooted in heterosexism (sometimes referred to as heterocentrism)—the systematic preferencing of opposite-sex sexuality and relationships (Jung & Smith, 1993). Heterosexism is pervasive in societal customs and institutions by keeping homosexuality and bisexuality invisible. Some examples include denial that bisexuality and homosexuality exist, the assumption that sexual orientation can and should be changed, hostility toward same-sex relationships (with same-sex marriage only recently becoming legally recognized nationally), the existence of sodomy laws in a third of states, and resistance to the addition of sexual orientation to nondiscrimination statutes resulting in a lack of legal protection from discrimination based on sexual orientation. Additionally, social workers often unintentionally utilize heterosexist language in service delivery to clients, such as asking a female client if she has a boyfriend or husband. Evaluating service delivery for inclusion and making changes, such as moving away from exclusive language, takes intention and practice for social workers.

TRANSGENDER OPPRESSION

Transgender oppressions refer to the devaluing, discrimination, stereotyping, and violence that individuals face when their appearance or identity does not conform to conventional beliefs of gender—namely, that only two genders exist, that they are fixed at birth, and are determined solely by the chromosomal and anatomical sex of an individual. Common beliefs tied to transgender oppression include that transgender individuals do not actually exist, that individuals presenting as gender nonconforming are doing so for an ulterior motive (e.g., attention, political motivation), that transgender individuals are defying nature, and/or that they are acting against the will of God. These beliefs are tied to transphobia—the disgust, fear, hatred, or disbelief in the existence of transgender and gender nonconforming individuals (Chakraborti & Garland, 2009). Transgender oppression includes bullying, physical violence, harassment, false arrest, and sexual assault. Transgender and gender nonconforming individuals are often discriminated against in employment, education, and healthcare settings, and lack of legal protection from discrimination based on the absence of gender identity in many nondiscrimination statutes. Data collected by the Federal Bureau of Investigation (FBI) concluded that lesbian, gay, bisexual, and transgender individuals are more likely to be targets of hate crimes than any other minority group—with transgender women of color being the most frequent targets of violence (Park & Mykhyalyshyn, 2016). Transgender oppression is further reinforced throughout the social systems in the United States, most notably through transgender and gender nonconforming invisibility. One obvious example is that most federal, state, institutional, organization, and agency forms only provide two options for gender or sex: male or female.

ABLEISM

Field Reflection Questions

What are some ways you may have unintentionally participated in discriminatory or exclusive behavior?

What are some ways you can change your practice to become more inclusive of nondominant groups?

Ableism is discrimination in favor of able-bodied people, the negative judgment about the capabilities of individuals with disabilities, the expression of hate for people with disabilities, and the denial of accessibility and resources (Smith et al., 2008; Thomas & Schwartzbaum, 2017). Discrimination against individuals with disabilities is often characterized by the belief that they are abnormal, have some sort of deficit, need to be fixed, and cannot fully function in society. This framing of disability as deficient as opposed to different has resulted in the ignoring of this dimension of cultural competence (Smith et al., 2008). Discrimination based on ableism manifests as discrimination in employment (most specifically the rejection of disabled applicants for housing and jobs), failing to provide accessibility at all or beyond wheelchair ramps, using ableist language, individuals without disabilities utilizing resources allocated for those with disabilities (e.g., parking spaces, restrooms), making assumptions about an individual's disability status based on the visibility (or invisibility) of their disability, and policies and systems that, intentionally or not, keep people with disabilities in poverty.

JUSTICE-INFORMED PRACTICE MODELS

Harrison et al. (2016) identify three strategies for implementing a social justice infused-practice framework even in micro-level social work practice. The first of these is, as discussed in Chapter 7, increased self-awareness. Bonnycastle (2011) provides a helpful continuum for examining this critical theme of the self-aware-ness needed for effective justice-focused micro practice. This includes moving from a simple recognition that discrimination is bad to a full confrontation of the privilege the social worker holds, and the impact of the social worker's practice in relation to the social locations of the clients served. This process involves overcom-ing the social worker's denial and struggle to change.

The second strategy discussed by Harrison et al. (2016) is justice-informed engagement, assessment, and intervention. Because of the person-in-environ-ment perspective, social workers are better prepared to infuse justice through their micro practice skills. This includes a focus on enhancing individuals' eco-nomic, psychological, and social conditions through collaborative approaches. The quest of social justice within micro practice can be infused into many the-oretical approaches and intervention models. Examples of this include client-centered and collaborative approaches; strengths-based and empowerment approaches; biopsychosocial assessment that include historical and political bases for social constructions; and a focus on the ways in which oppression, discrimination, and historical trauma can contribute in the development of indi-vidual difficulties.

The final strategy discussed by Harrison et al. (2016) is jus-tice-informed policy and sys-tems advocacy. As discussed in greater detail in Chapter 10, social workers must infuse social justice in their micro work by addressing social and orga-nizational policies that perpetu-ate inequities. Similarly, social workers work in concert with their client toward social and

> **Field Reflection Questions**
>
> In what ways do you infuse a justice-informed lens in your current field placement practice? What ways could you be more intentional about the infusion of the justice focus?
>
> What therapeutic approaches lend themselves to justice-informed micro practice? Which of these could you apply in your current field placement?

economic justice, as they may begin to strive to address inequities in their own lives as their awareness of such inequities arises in their therapeutic experience (Moradi, 2012).

Reisch and Garvin (2016) stress the importance of utilizing social justice-infused approaches especially in relation to processes and outcomes. While you are unable to deeply scrutinize every action you take, every facial expression, every word decision, and so on, it benefits you to critically self-reflect on the implica-tions of these social interactions with clients. You need to consider the social justice implications of such process, including how each part of the process reveals infor-mation about power differentials; how the actions reflect considerations for the empowerment of clients and oppressive social conditions; how you have informed your work through critical self-reflection on sources of injustice; what roles you are fulfilling in your social interactions with clients and whether those are reflective of the needs and rights of others; and finally, a critical self-reflection of the potential of abuse of power.

RIGHTS-BASED APPROACHES IN SOCIAL WORK PRACTICE

Androff (2018) explains that theoretically social work is clearly a human rights–based profession, yet many social workers in the United States rarely use human rights, and when they do, it is only on a superficial level. Beyond this point, social workers have violated the rights of their clients. Mapp et al. (2019) aptly describe social workers as gatekeepers to social benefits that have been used to oppress and preserve the status quo. A rights-based approach in practice in all arenas of social work can be achieved using the five principles of human rights declarations, which align with our field's *Code of Ethics* (Androff, 2018; Mapp et al., 2019):

- *Human dignity:* In line with the *Code*'s highlighting of dignity and worth of the person and right to self-determination, a rights-based approach in practice requires that every client and community has their dignity respected. Those we work with are not charity cases, in need of rescue, or broken. They are humans with strengths, rights, and expertise. Social workers must avoid dehumanization of those they work with and, just as important, must work to rehumanize people who are experiencing exclusion, discrimination, and stigma.

- *Nondiscrimination:* Rights-based practice recognizes that simply having a diverse environment and including all is not enough to actualize nondiscrimination. To do this, social workers must strive to provide culturally appropriate service to all historically excluded populations, and do so with cultural competence and humility. Social workers should break down inequities, reduce power differences, and work to emphasize more equal relationships.

- *Participation:* Rights-based practice ensures that those impacted by decisions get to contribute and have sway in the decision-making process. Simply asking potentially impacted individuals and communities for their opinion is not enough. An authentic commitment to increasing the impacted individual's access to power and decision-making is not only empowering for the client but results in a better decision-making process.

- *Transparency:* Rights-based practice approaches emphasize transparency as it works against corruption and is a key to trustworthiness. There are many realms in social work that require transparency, including organizational budgets and policies in the macro practice space, and assessment, evaluation, monitoring with micro-level practice. All social workers should utilize self-reflective practice to maximize transparency in their work.

- *Accountability:* Accountability in rights-based practice advocacy, promotion of justice, and taking action to protect rights can look like calling out violations of clients' rights or working to strengthen laws, policies, and norms that promote and respect human rights. Additionally, emphasizing the interdependence of all persons' human rights is an important advocacy focus.

IMPLICATIONS FOR FIELD AND STRATEGIES FOR CHANGE

The previous section invites you to reflect on what is, potentially, a new way of thinking about the world and your experience in your field placement. So often, social justice is considered something that a social worker simply carves time out for (for instance, on something like an advocacy day), as opposed to being a framework for practice. It can be challenging to envision a practice philosophy that infuses these theories in an effort to have a human rights and social justice focus in daily work in your field placement. For example, traditional assessments in clinical practice often focus on problems, which a social construction framework will remind you are culturally and relationally bound. This opens the possibility of seemingly endless interpretations with no one interpretation as the truth. However, the social worker can utilize collaborative approaches to seek to understand the client's theory of problem, which helps the social worker toward collaboration solutions.

Within practice, these lenses provide the social context necessary to recognize the impacts of oppression and economic disadvantages experienced by clients. Social justice requires practitioner transparency, collaboration, and respectful curiosity and humility in work with clients. Major (2012) emphasizes how social constructions are well-suited for practice with families in the child welfare system due to their emphasis on contextual meanings—so often families are judged according to the same standards as those with significantly more opportunities and resources.

In thinking about social justice implications in mezzo and macro levels of practice, it is important to relate the personal and the political. The concerns that clients bring in to their work with you are not due solely to individual shortcomings, but also to unjust policies and practices that occur within agencies and the larger society. The driving force for social justice–infused social work practice is the skill of challenging inequalities, which create opportunities for change. You must understand that not every mezzo and macro challenge you attempt will be successful, and the process of challenging oppressive practices and policies can be uncomfortable and tedious for you as you attempt to institute the challenge. The most effective and appropriate challenges need to be person-centered; use an egalitarian value approach; use empowerment approaches to assist individuals in reducing unjust policies; and, like micro work, focus on process and outcome.

As an example of challenging a potential abuse of power, consider this experience. In your placement with Child Protection Services, one of your clients, a 17-year-old foster youth, was denied a request to begin attending an after-school church youth group. The agency made this decision based upon some bullying experiences the client had experienced. Upon reflection, you recognize that the agency you are working within may have misused their power under the guise of "protecting" the client from harm. You decide to challenge this decision by approaching your supervisor and explaining that you appreciate the agency's concern for the client's safety, but you are concerned about the organization taking away the client's right to self-determination. You share with your supervisor the importance of this client, who is approaching the age of 18, having the opportunity to make his own decisions, and not be denied the opportunity to attend an activity that may benefit him greatly. Using the NASW (2021) *Code of Ethics* as your guide, you would be able to challenge this decision in a constructive way, and assert the client's right to self-determination and his right to nonoppressive service delivery from the agency.

CASE SUMMARY: "PUTTING ON A SHOW"

PRACTICE SETTING DESCRIPTION

My name is Sara and I am a senior BSW student completing an internship at a local family service agency in a small city on the West Coast. The agency provides individual and family counseling services on a sliding fee scale. The agency also works with Child Protection Services on reunification causes. I was assigned to work with J. for 6 months in an effort to reunify her with her three children.

IDENTIFYING DATA

J., a 28-year-old Latina female, has three children, Brenda, Tasha, and Darren. J.'s children were removed due to substantiated charges of neglect. The children are aged 12, 6 and 3. The children stayed with J.'s sister after they were removed from J.'s care. J. has been battling a drug addiction and she was unable to care for her children—their home was found to be squalid. After the removal of the children, J. began her third attempt at completing a drug treatment program. She was successful and was reunified with the children 2 months prior.

PRESENTING PROBLEM

J. comes to weekly sessions, and reports that she is doing well and maintaining her sobriety. We spend a significant amount of time in our work discussing coping strategies for her stressors. She reports that the majority of her stress includes the demands of parenting three children with little support and financial stressors.

In field seminar, one of my peers, who is placed at a local middle school, shared a situation from her field placement that she was conflicted about. My peer shared that a student named "Jane" was expressing concerns about the fact that her mother had begun using marijuana at home. The personal use of marijuana is legal in our state, but it is not allowed under the conditions of the reunification agreement. This concerned Jane because she and her younger siblings just barely moved back in with their mom. Jane also shared that her mother recently got a new boyfriend and he has been spending more and more time in the home. Her mom told Jane not to say anything about the marijuana because they could be split up again. Jane is very stressed that someone is going to find out and she and her siblings will be forced to move back in with her aunt. This is causing Jane a lot of stress and anxiety.

I recognized the similarities in the story, and I know that Brenda attends the same school that my peer is at for her field placement. It is clear that the young woman being described is my client's daughter.

ASSESSMENT

When assessing the situation only from my interactions with J., she appears to manage this transition fairly well. The most important aspect of our work together is the focus on coping strategies for her to utilize so she does not relapse. Additionally, J. is focused on finding a new job because her current job stocking shelves at a local grocery chain is only providing her 20 hours of work. J. has reported that while she is stressed and anxious, she has not had the urge to use drugs or alcohol to cope with the stress.

J. has many strengths. She is highly motivated to maintain custody of her children. She mentioned that the thought of losing custody of the children was what motivated her to finally complete a treatment program. While in treatment, she became aware of the myriad services that her family qualified for, and she is not receiving Supplemental Nutrition Assistance Program benefits, and her children are not covered by Medicaid.

My interactions with J.'s children indicate that they are much happier now that they are back with their mother. In talking with Brenda specifically, she noted that her aunt's house was "fine," but it wasn't the same as being with her mother. They were relieved that they were able to stay with their aunt, and not a "stranger," while J. worked on her sobriety.

J. has shown great resilience in achievement and the maintenance of abstinence from drugs, and her quest to be reunified with her children. She has identified ways that she can support her family, and took the initiative to access services they needed. She is also actively looking for a full-time job or a second part-time job.

CASE PROCESS SUMMARY

I was very surprised when I made the connection between my peer's story and my client. J. and I have worked together for 6 months and I believe that we have worked very well together. It seemed as though she was being very open with me, and now I am questioning if perhaps J. felt the need to put on a show with an overly happy face in our work together. While she has been honest with me about the ongoing stressors in her life, she has remained positive and open to collaborating on solutions and strategies for facing these stressors. During supervision I shared that I felt a simultaneous sense of betrayal and hurt, given that J. has possibly been lying about her sobriety to me. I began to self-reflect on how my actions may have encouraged J.'s actions.

Sara, BSW Student Intern

CASE DISCUSSION QUESTIONS

1. *Based upon the information provided, what issues related to human rights and social, economic, and environmental justice can you identify within this case?*

2. *Consider the case example in terms of social location. From the information provided, what are the different social identities that J. may inhabit? How might these locations be influencing J.'s construction of reality?*

3. *Similarly, think about Sara's social identities and social locations. How might they impact Sara's construction of reality?*

4. *What are some of the areas that Sara should focus her self-reflection on using a justice-infused lens? Identify which of the strategies discussed in the chapter that Sara may be able to use in her work with J.*

END-OF-CHAPTER RESOURCES

A robust set of instructor resources designed to supplement this text is located at http://connect.springerpub.com/content/book/978-0-8261-3753-1. Qualifying instructors may request access by emailing textbook@springerpub.com.

CRITICAL THINKING QUESTIONS

1. Charlotte is a BSW intern placed with a housing agency. Many of the clients in low-income housing face housing discrimination. Charlotte knows it is her duty to advocate for her clients both inside her agency and outside. Identify potential injustice-infused micro-level practice steps that Charlotte can take. Identify mezzo-level justice-infused practice steps Charlotte can take. Identify macro-level justice-infused practice steps Charlotte can take. Discuss how you would approach this scenario.

2. Consider some of the conflicts that Charlotte may encounter as she engages in the multilevel justice-infused practice you identified. How might she work through those conflicts? Is it Charlotte's role to bring justice-informed perspectives to her colleagues?

3. Concepts of social constructions encourage us to be critically self-reflective of our language usage with clients. Can you identify problematic language you have heard used with clients? Reflect and describe what was problematic about it, and how the situation could have been approached in a justice-informed way?

4. Advancing social justice requires practitioner transparency, collaboration, and respectful curiosity and humility in work with clients. It also requires that

you consider the social justice implications of your interactions with clients. In reflecting upon your work with clients in your field placement, describe an experience in which you identified a potential abuse of power, either by yourself, someone else, or the agency as a whole. Reflect on and describe your affective reaction to this experience. Describe how this situation could be approached if it were to happen in the future.

LEARNING ACTIVITIES

1. Choose one of the examples from the chapter. Identify what a charity-based approach (relief of immediate suffering of those who are disadvantaged) would look like, what a needs-based approach (identifying resources to address a deficit in an individual or community) would look like, and what a rights-based approach (fulfilling human rights to move toward more equitable distribution of resources and power) would look like.

2. Consider your field placement agency. Provide at least one example of a justice-informed practice model and/or human rights–based approach. Also identify the ways the agency's approach could be strengthened to be more justice and/or human rights oriented for the clients and community they serve.

ELECTRONIC RESOURCES

WEBSITE LINKS

Defining Economic Justice and Social Justice—Center for Economic and Social Justice: www.cesj.org/learn/definitions /defining-economic-justice-and-social-justice

Community Voices Heard: Engaging Constituents for Social, Economic and Racial Justice—Emerging Practitioners in Philanthropy: www.slideshare.net/EPIPNational/community -voices-heard-engaging-constituents-for-social-economic -and-racial-justice?qid=c6ee9dc7-4ff1-44f2-a19e-b38286c6 d6e3&v=&b=&from_search=31

Environmental Social Work: A Call to Action—Claudia Dewane: www.socialworkhelper.com/2017/10/09/ environmental-social-work-call-action

VIDEO LINKS

 Who Am I? Think Again—Hetain Patel & Yuyu Rau: www.ted
.com/talks/hetain_patel_who_am_i_think_again?language=en

 Developing a Human Rights Approach to Strengthen Practice—
Jane McPherson: www.youtube.com/watch?v=2PHTaqYeB1M

 Social Work Education: Environmental Justice—Sondra Fogel:
www.youtube.com/watch?v=TB_9fVGQNdI

 Social Constructionism—Sydney Brown: www.youtube.com/
watch?v=gVCkJ7jLnz0

REFERENCES

Allport, G. W. (1954). *The nature of prejudice*. Beacon Press.

Androff, D. (2018). Practicing human rights in social work: Reflections and rights-based approaches. *Journal of Human Rights and Social Work, 3*(4), 179–182. https://doi.org/10.1007/s41134-018-0056-5

Barsky, A. E. (2010). *Ethics and values in social work: An integrated approach for a comprehensive curriculum*. Oxford University Press.

Bonilla-Silva, E. (2003). "New racism," color-blind racism, and the future of whiteness in America. In A. W. Doane, & E. Bonilla-Silva (Eds.), *White out: The continuing significance of racism* (pp. 271–284). Routledge Taylor & Francis.

Bonnycastle, C. R. (2011). Social justice along a continuum: A relational illustrative model. *Social Service Review, 85*(2), 267–295. https://doi.org/10.1086/660703

Caputo, R. K. (2002). Social justice, the ethics of care, and market economies. *Families in Society: The Journal of Contemporary Social Services, 83*(4), 355–364. https://doi.org/10.1606/1044-3894.10

Chakraborti, N., & Garland, J. (2009). *Hate crime: Impact, causes and responses*. SAGE Publications.

Council on Social Work Education. (2022). *Educational policy and accreditation standards for baccalaureate and master's social work programs*. https://www.cswe.org/getmedia/94471c42-13b8-493b-9041-b30f48533d64/2022-EPAS.pdf

Dobratz, B., Waldner, L., & Buzzell, T. L. (2012). *Power, politics, and society: An introduction to political sociology*. Pearson.

Finn, J. L., & Jacobson, M. (2017, March 25). What is social justice? *OUPblog.* https://blog.oup.com/2017/03/what-is-social-justice

Ginsberg, M. (1953). On the diversity of morals. *The Journal of the Royal Anthropological Institute of Great Britain and Ireland, 83*(2), 117–135. https://doi.org/10.2307/2844026

Harrison, J., VanDeusen, K., & Way, I. (2016). Embedding social justice within micro social work curricula. *Smith College Studies in Social Work, 86*(3), 258–273. https://doi.org/10.1080/00377317.2016.1191802

Holstein, J. A., & Gubrium, J. F. (Eds.). (2008). *Handbook of constructionist research.* Guilford Press.

Johnson, A. (2006). *Privilege, power, and difference.* McGraw-Hill.

Jung, P. B., & Smith, R. F. (1993). *Heterosexism: An ethical challenge.* State University of New York Press.

Kagan, C., & Burton, M. (2005). Marginalization. In G. Nelson, & I. Prilleltensky (Eds.), *Community psychology: In pursuit of liberation and well-being* (pp. 292–308). Palgrave Macmillan.

King, M. L., Jr. (1963). Letter from Birmingham jail. *The Atlantic.* https://www.theatlantic.com/politics/archive/1963/08/martin-luther-kings-letter-from-birmingham-jail/274668

Kirk, G., & Okazawa-Rey, M. (2010). Living in a globalizing world. In G. Kirk, & M. Okazawa-Rey (Eds.), *Women's lives: Multicultural perspectives* (5th ed., pp. 371–392). McGraw-Hill.

Littlefield, M. B., McLane-Davison, D., & Vakalahi, H. F. (2015). Global gender inequality. In *Encyclopedia of social work.* NASW Press and Oxford University Press. https://doi.org/10.1093/acrefore/9780199975839.013.932

Lott, B., & Bullock, H. E. (2007). *Psychology and economic injustice: Personal, professional, and political intersections.* American Psychological Association. https://doi.org/10.1037/11501-000

Major, D. R. (2012). Mostly we played with whatever she chose. In S. L. Witkin (Ed.), *Social constructions and social work practice: Interpretations and innovations* (pp. 154–187). Columbia University Press.

Mapp, S., McPherson, J., Androff, D., & Gatenio Gabel, S. (2019). Social work is a human rights profession. *Social Work, 64*(3), 259–269. https://doi.org/10.1093/sw/swz023

McCormick, P. (2003). Whose justice? An examination of nine models of justice. *Journal of Religion & Spirituality in Social Work: Social Thought, 22*(2–3), 7–25. https://doi.org/10.1080/15426432.2003.9960338

Miller, D. (1976). *Social justice.* Clarendon Press.

Moradi, B. (2012). Feminist social justice orientation: An indicator of optimal functioning? *The Counseling Psychologist, 40*(8), 1133–1148. https://doi.org/10.1177/0011000012439612

Moses, A. E., & Hawkins, R. O., Jr. (1982). *Counseling lesbian women and gay men.* C. V. Mosby.

National Association of Social Workers. (2021). *Code of ethics.* https://www.socialworkers.org/About/Ethics/Code-of-Ethics/Code-of-Ethics-English

Nozick, R. (1974). *Anarchy, state, and utopia.* Basic Books.

Park, H., & Mykhyalyshyn, I. (2016, June 16). L.G.B.T. people are more likely to be targets of hate crimes than any other minority group. *The New York Times.* https://www.nytimes.com/interactive/2016/06/16/us/hate-crimes-against-lgbt.html

Piven, F. F., & Cloward, R. (2005). Rulemaking, rulebreaking, and power. In T. Janoski, R. Alford, A. Hicks, & M. Schwartz (Eds.), *Handbook of political sociology* (pp. 33–53). Cambridge University Press.

Rawls, J. (1971). *A theory of justice.* Harvard University Press.

Rawls, J. (2001). *Justice as fairness: A restatement.* Belknap Press of Harvard University Press.

Reichert, E. (2003). *Social work and human rights: A foundation for policy and practice.* Columbia University Press.

Reisch, M. (1998). *Economic globalization and the future of the welfare state.* University of Michigan School of Social Work.

Reisch, M. (2002). Defining social justice in a socially unjust world. *Families in Society: The Journal of Contemporary Social Services, 83*(4), 343–354. https://doi.org/10.1606/1044-3894.17

Reisch, M., & Garvin, C. D. (2016). *Social work and social justice: Concepts, challenges, and strategies.* Oxford University Press.

Rodgers, S. T. (2015). Racism. In *Encyclopedia of social work online.* NASW Press and Oxford University Press. https://doi.org/10.1093/acrefore/9780199975839.013.1009

Ruhela, S. P. (2005). *Introduction to sociology.* Shubhi Publications.

Siddique, H., & Laughland, O. (2017, August 23). Charlottesville: United Nations warns US over 'alarming' racism. *The Guardian*. https://www.theguardian.com/world/2017/aug/23/charlottesville-un-committee-warns-us-over-rise-of-racism

Smith, L., Foley, P. F., & Chaney, M. P. (2008). Addressing classism, ableism, and heterosexism in counselor education. *Journal of Counseling & Development*, *86*(3), 303–309. https://doi.org/10.1002/j.1556-6678.2008.tb00513.x

Sue, D. W., Capodilupo, C. M., Torino, G. C., Bucceri, J. M., Holder, A. M. B., Nadal, K. L., & Esquilin, M. (2007). Racial microaggressions in everyday life: Implications for clinical practice. *American Psychologist*, *62*, 271–286. https://doi.org/10.1037/0003-066x.62.4.271

Sue, D. W., & Sue, D. (2012). *Counseling the culturally diverse: Theory and practice*. Wiley.

Thomas, A. J., & Schwartzbaum, S. (2017). *Culture and identity: Life stories for counselors and therapists*. SAGE Publications.

Van Soest, D. (1992). *Incorporating peace and social justice into the social work curriculum*. National Association of Social Workers.

Wakefield, J. C. (1988). Psychotherapy, distributive justice, and social work. Part 2: Psychotherapy and the pursuit of justice. *Social Service Review*, *62*(3), 353–382. https://doi.org/10.1086/644555

Witkin, S. (2011). *Social constructions and social work practice: Interpretations and innovations*. Columbia University Press.

Young, I. M. (1990). *Justice and the politics of difference*. Princeton University Press.

Young, I. M. (2001). Equality of whom? Social groups and judgments of injustice. *The Journal of Political Philosophy*, *9*(1), 1–18. https://doi.org/10.1111/1467-9760.00115

Engaging Diversity and Difference in Practice

Chanté was a first-year MSW student doing her placement at a community-based counseling center that provided free and reduced cost counseling services. A few months into her placement, Chanté was starting to feel more confident in her abilities providing services to members of different populations. Chanté recently began working with a client who is gender nonconforming. While Chanté had learned some about the lesbian, gay, bisexual, and transgender population in her Diversity class, working with someone who is gender nonconforming was a new experience for her. In her personal life, she had not had much interaction with gender nonconforming individuals.

In her work with this client, Chanté has noticed that she feels uncomfortable and is unsure where these feelings are coming from. Chanté does recall getting the message from her parents that gender nonconforming individuals were abnormal, and perhaps confused. Thinking back to her Diversity class, Chanté consulted the National Association of Social Workers (NASW) Code of Ethics *in hopes that it would provide her some clarity.*

Unfortunately, Chanté's reading of the NASW Code of Ethics *only left her feeling more confused. Is she able to competently provide counseling services to her client when having these conflicting feelings? Is it more appropriate to refer her client to another counseling intern? What is in her client's best interest?*

COMPETENCY 3: ENGAGE ANTI-RACISM, DIVERSITY, EQUITY, AND INCLUSION IN PRACTICE

Social workers understand how racism and oppression shape human experiences and how these two constructs influence practice at the individual, family, group, organizational, and community levels and policy and research. Social workers understand the pervasive impact of White supremacy and privilege and use their knowledge, awareness, and skills to engage in anti-racist practice. Social workers understand how diversity and intersectionality shape human experiences and identity development and affect equity and inclusion. The dimensions of diversity are understood as the intersectionality of factors including but not limited to age, caste, class, color, culture, disability and ability, ethnicity, gender, gender identity and expression, generational status, immigration status, legal status, marital status, political ideology, race, nationality, religion and spirituality, sex, sexual orientation, and tribal sovereign status. Social workers understand that this intersectionality means that a person's life experiences may include oppression, poverty, marginalization, and alienation as well as privilege and power. Social workers understand the societal and historical roots of social and racial injustices and the forms and mechanisms of oppression and discrimination, and they recognize the extent to which a culture's structures and values, including social, economic, political, racial, technological, and cultural exclusions, may create privilege and power and systemically oppress, marginalize, and alienate.

Social workers

- demonstrate anti-racist and anti-oppressive social work practice at the individual, family, group, organizational, community, research, and policy levels; and

- demonstrate cultural humility by applying critical reflection, self-awareness, and self-regulation to manage the influence of bias, power, privilege, and values in working with clients and constituencies, acknowledging them as experts of their own lived experiences. (Council on Social Work Education [CSWE], 2022, p. 9)

LEARNING OBJECTIVES

By the end of this chapter, you will be able to:

- Recognize the role of oppression in your clients' lived experiences.

- Recognize the importance of self-awareness and personal biases in working with diverse clients.

- Engage in practices that are anti-oppressive by recognizing the myriad factors that are impacting client and client systems.

- Use ongoing supervision to do continual work on cultural awareness. (CSWE, 2022)

SOCIAL WORK VALUES AND ETHICS

Our personal identity is our cultural identity—it impacts how we see ourselves in the world and how we move through the world. Culture is the most influential determinant of identity (McGoldrick et al., 2005). When social workers do not address implications of culture in their work with their clients, they may, unintentionally, be further oppressing their clients instead of helping them. The field of social work is developing different ways of conceptualizing models of practice for students in social work programs regarding cultural competence (Hall & Lindsey, 2014). The field is moving away from focusing solely on knowledge about specific cultures as the means of reaching a level of cultural competence in practice (Locke, 1992; Rodgers & Potocky, 1998). There is now an acknowledgment that the competency level of social workers is narrowed when they do not, in conjunction, learn the skills necessary to recognize how their own identity greatly impacts the work that is done with diverse individuals, groups, and communities.

The foundation of social work is based on practices that advocate for social, environmental, and economic justice in a culturally sensitive way. The NASW *Code of Ethics* explains to social workers their responsibility to "obtain education about and seek to understand the nature of social diversity and oppression" (NASW, 2021, Standard 1.05(c), para. 3). NASW "promotes and supports the implementation of cultural and linguistic competence at three intersecting levels: the individual, institutional, and societal. Cultural competence requires social workers to examine their own cultural backgrounds and identities while seeking out the necessary knowledge, skills, and values that can enhance the delivery of services to people with varying cultural experiences associated with their race, ethnicity, gender, class, sexual orientation, religion, age, or disability [or other cultural factors]" (NASW, 2015, p. 65).

As future social workers join the field, the importance of identity in practice will continue to further nurture a "more comprehensive view of cultural competence" (Garran & Rozas, 2013, p. 99). However, this emphasis will also promote concepts of effectiveness and well-being within the profession. Focusing on continual growth in the skills related to cultural sensitivity will only help the incoming generation of social workers to be mindful of the ways in which their identity can benefit or hinder the work they do with the clients. Ignoring issues related to race, ethnicity, sexuality, religion, and other factors will result in poor service delivery to the client (Seipel & Way, 2006).

> **Field Reflection Questions**
>
> In your current field placement, what skillsets do you need to strengthen in regard to your cultural competence and humility?
>
> In what ways can you, as a new social worker, integrate ongoing learning around cultural competence and cultural humility as part of your continued growth?

CONCEPTUAL FRAMEWORKS FOR DIVERSITY, BIAS, AND CULTURAL COMPETENCE

This section of the chapter is devoted to defining important concepts that play a role in engaging diversity in practice in culturally competent and culturally humble ways. Diversity, intersectionality, bias, culture, competence, and culturally competent practice are explored.

DIVERSITY AND BIAS

Diversity is considered to reference difference, and more specifically, human difference, and refers to every individual, given that all individuals are unique (Lum, 2000). Ridlen and Dane (1992) point out that discussions around diversity often originate when individuals or groups in power have defined certain behaviors as problematic. Often, those in power determine the values, negative or positive, assigned to behaviors in a way that preferences those with fewer differences. This predisposition to favor those with fewer differences is considered a bias that can impede an individual or group's ability to be impartial (American Heritage Dictionary, 2017). This preference extends to justify the exploitation of others for the benefit of those in power. As van Dijk (1997) explains, this process, coined "othering," stifles the development of people who do not conform to the norms and expectations of the majority group, which has been White Anglo-Saxon Protestants with Eurocentric worldviews throughout the entire history of the United States.

The field of social work has had a difficult time defining the depth of human experience based on dual concern for both "person and environment." Intersectionality examines how multiple social constructions of oppression or privilege can intersect to shape an individual's lived experiences (Battle-Walters, 2004). Intersectionality acknowledges that identities are not separate from one another, and discrimination and oppression of marginalized individuals and groups have interactive effects. For example, Kornblum and Julian (2007) point out that African-American women over the age of 70 are among the poorest population group, which highlights the ways in which race, gender, and age can intersect to layer oppression.

CULTURE

The worldview of social workers and the clients they serve is based in large part on their culture. Because culture is such a vital component of worldview, it also greatly impacts the ways in which social workers deliver services. Pinderhughes (1989) states that social workers who acquire positive self-identities show more ability to respect their client's identity. Social work has defined culture differently over time. In the past, scholars limited what component of an individuals' identity and experience constituted their culture. Early definitions used by social workers did not always acknowledge the impact of race, religion, gender, and other cultural components on the lived experiences of individuals (Mitchell, 1999). Culture is a multidimensional concept that includes life experiences, behavioral patterns, and intergenerational messages (Lum, 2000).

COMPETENCE

Aponte (1995) aptly defines competence as a term that encompasses ways of moving through the world that are acquired by individuals as a way to survive and includes the skills and abilities they acquire to complete necessary functions in a successful manner. Competence suggests one is capable to complete a task, has the sufficient skillset, and will achieve an adequate outcome (Lum, 2000). When thinking about competence in terms of social workers, competence is referring to the acquisition of skills in order to provide services that are therapeutic, not oppressive, to all clients.

CULTURAL COMPETENCE

CSWE (2008) defines cultural competence as the ability of professionals to effectively interact with individuals of all cultures based on curiosity and respect about difference related but not limited to race, ethnicity, culture, class, gender, sexual orientation, religion, physical or mental ability, age, and national origin. Unlike the linear acquisition of skills, cultural competence is an ongoing process that involves attentiveness to one's own biases and is built on a framework of respect and validation of difference. The ongoing work of cultural competence often begins with self-reflection to fully understand how our own cultural beliefs and practices result in different truths than others may have. It also includes the humility to understand that our way may not be the only "right" way.

STANDARDS FOR CULTURAL COMPETENCE

The NASW (2015) revised the Standards for Cultural Competence in Social Work Practice in conjunction with the National Committee on Racial and Ethnic Diversity. That revision highlights the importance of an intersectional approach to social work practice, the acknowledgment of one's own position of power in their work, and the recognition that cultural competence is an ongoing process. The revision also reinforces the importance of these standards within all levels of social work practice (micro, mezzo, macro) and emphasizes the expectation of continual learning and growth within these standards. This section provides a brief overview of the standards with some examples taken from the NASW Standards of Cultural Competence in Social Work. Social workers are encouraged to review the document in its entirety—it can be found on NASW's website (see www.socialwork ers.org/LinkClick.aspx?fileticket=7dVckZAYUmk%3d&portalid=0).

Regarding cultural competence, social workers must understand the significant role that culture holds in effective practice, while also acknowledging that all cultures have strengths. It is the responsibility of the social worker to seek out knowledge about their clients' cultures and to infuse that knowledge into their service delivery with clients. Social workers also need to acknowledge and engage in continued education about the nature of oppression and discrimination.

STANDARD 1: ETHICS AND VALUES

Social workers practice within the standards of our *Code of Ethics* (NASW, 2021), which directly communicates expectations around cultural competence and ethical behaviors. The commitments set forth in the *Code of Ethics* include the importance of sensitivity to cultural and ethnic diversity and a commitment to service for those who are vulnerable and oppressed for any reason, including those oppressed due to their cultural and ethnic identities. Culture has a significant impact on who we are and how we move through the world. It can impact how we cope with problems, how we interact with others, and what we believe to be acceptable or unacceptable behavior as well as an individual's help-seeking behavior. The practice of social workers must be both designed and effected in culturally sensitive and responsive ways. Social workers must address the struggle with ethical dilemmas arising from cultural differences and value conflicts.

STANDARD 2: SELF-AWARENESS

All social workers must continually assess their assumptions and biases and identify how those beliefs impact their attitudes, worldview, and behaviors, which directly impact their service delivery. Simply identifying information about one's cultural heritage is not sufficient. Social workers must also take the time to learn and celebrate other cultural heritages and identify how their own cultural heritage may encourage damaging beliefs. Once identified, social workers must work in community with others to identify strategies to change detrimental beliefs and acknowledge and correct when they are impacting service delivery. Self-reflection is the basis for professional development in social work, and that process is never completed.

STANDARD 3: CROSS-CULTURAL KNOWLEDGE

It is the responsibility of social workers to obtain a grounded sense of their own identity, and then move on to learning and valuing other identities. Cultural competence is an ongoing activity that requires continual learning, unlearning, and relearning of a multitude of different topics related to diversity. Examples include religious traditions, historical experiences, communication styles, help-seeking behaviors, and other cultural traditions. To be effective in our service delivery, we must expand our knowledge and understanding of these topics to better accommodate the needs of clients we are working with. Additionally, understanding the applicability of practice models to specific client populations is vital to ensure effective service delivery.

STANDARD 4: CROSS-CULTURAL SKILLS

This standard applies specifically to the obtainment of skills to work with individuals and groups of different cultures, as well as the broad range of skills necessary to advocate for clients at the micro, macro, and mezzo levels. This includes sharpening one's ability to convey authenticity and warmth, assessing policies for cultural inclusiveness, selecting and developing the appropriate service interventions that take into account the clients' cultural experiences, and effectively identifying resources in the client's life—including those that you may be unfamiliar with (e.g., healers, spiritual guides, families of choice).

STANDARD 5: SERVICE DELIVERY

Social workers are responsible for making culturally appropriate referrals, identifying service gaps that impact specific groups, evaluating service delivery models for cultural sensitivity and inclusiveness, assessing the cultural competence among other social work agencies, and including clients in the development of service delivery plans. Agencies should actively recruit and work to retain multicultural staff and include cultural competence skills as requirements in social work positions.

STANDARD 6: EMPOWERMENT AND ADVOCACY

Social policies, programs, and systems greatly impact client populations, especially those that are vulnerable and oppressed. Social workers should advocate on behalf of their clients and participate in the development and implementation of policies that empower marginalized and oppressed populations. Social workers should be socially aware and confront stereotyping, discrimination, and other oppression of their clients and their clients' communities. This includes advocacy and action that works toward the empowerment of communities.

STANDARD 7: DIVERSE WORKFORCE

Social workers should encourage recruitment, admissions, hiring, and retention efforts that ensure diversity in social work programs and organizations. Recruiting and retaining multicultural students and staff naturally increases cultural competence through the expertise of those social workers. Statistics show that while social work aspires to be a diverse and inclusive field, U.S. social workers are predominantly White females, making up 86% of the social workers (NASW, 2006). Given that social work client populations are significantly more diverse than the profession, an intentional push toward aligning these demographics would help the field of social work bridge cultural differences. This intentional push should be evident within all levels in social work organizations, and social workers who possess unique knowledge or a specific skillset, such as bilingual speaking abilities, should be compensated appropriately.

STANDARD 8: PROFESSIONAL EDUCATION

As mentioned in previous parts of the chapter, it is imperative that social workers embrace a culture of lifelong learning around topics related to cultural competence.

Just as social workers continue to improve their skills through the use of continuing education credits to learn cutting-edge therapeutic techniques, they must also utilize those and other avenues to participate in education and training that provide a continued focus on the current and changing needs of diverse client populations.

STANDARD 9: LANGUAGE AND COMMUNICATION

As the NASW standards (2015, pp. 43–44) point out, "language is a source and extension of personal identity and culture and, therefore, is one way that individuals interact with outs in their families and communities and across different cultural groups." Given that language is a part of an individual's identity, it is a part of our client that we must accept without judgment or agenda. It is the client's right to utilize the language they are must comfortable using, and as such, it is the social worker's responsibility to ensure access to services in their preferred language. Social work professionals should promote diversity in language and confront discrimination based on linguistic abilities. They should also seek out opportunities to be trained in how to work effectively with interpreters and translators.

STANDARD 10: LEADERSHIP TO ADVANCE CULTURAL COMPETENCE

The field of social work is committed to advancing cultural competence within and beyond the profession, and has a responsibility to confront oppressive systems and promote a diverse and inclusive environment for the communities we work in. Part of leadership is a skillset that includes the ability to facilitate challenging conversation that promote growth and understanding in areas related to diversity and cultural competence. Social workers should recognize and utilize their formal and informal positions of power and privilege and utilize those to advance cultural competence and challenge problematic practices.

Field Reflection Questions

After reviewing the cultural competency standards, which standard do you feel you have the most difficulty applying in your field placement work?

Which standard is the easiest for you to apply? What makes one harder to incorporate into your practice than the other?

EMPATHY AND HUMILITY

Engaging diversity in practice requires cultural humility. According to Tervalon and Murray-Garcia (1998),

> Cultural humility incorporates a lifelong commitment to self-evaluation and self-critique, to redressing the power imbalances in the patient–physician

dynamic, and to developing mutually beneficial and nonpaternalistic clinical and advocacy partnerships with communities on behalf of individuals and defined populations. (p. 117)

Incorporating a lifelong commitment to self-critique in practice requires both empathy and humility in practice. Based on the work of Carl Rogers, the person-centered approach of working with clients with unconditional positive regard, congruence, and empathy has been the foundation of clinical social work practice (Holosko et al., 2008; Rothery & Tutty, 2001).

EMPATHY

Sinclair and Monk (2005) identified empathy as the most productive therapeutic condition, even across varying treatment modalities. Empathetic therapeutic relationships have been identified as an agent of change among multiple outcome evaluations (King, 2011). Vanaerschot (2007) explains the use of empathy in the therapeutic relationship as the helping professional seeking to understand the unique experience of the client and the personal meaning they ascribe to it. This approach is incomplete without acknowledgment of the client's cultural identities and experiences.

One of the ways empathy plays a role in the helping relationships is through the social worker's desire to understand the meanings a client has attributed to the events in their life. This requires the social worker to encourage the client to explore different explanations, and to be open to different explanations themselves. For example, often an individual who experienced childhood abuse will attribute that experience to something they themselves did to prompt the violent outburst of the abuser, as opposed to attributing that experience to deficiencies in the abuser's coping mechanisms. When a social worker uses the therapeutic relationship to direct the client toward healing alternative attribution of that experience, they become what Vanaerschot (2007) calls a "surrogate experiencer" (p. 317).

Gerdes and Segal (2011) have identified three different components of empathy that contribute to the surrogate experiencer concept. The first component is affective sharing with other—a mainly automatic process of the brain. Neuroscience research suggests that when human beings hear another individual express their feelings or see their nonverbal communication (e.g., gestures, facial expressions), the neural pathways in the brain simulate a "shared representation" and generate mirrored feelings. While important, affective sharing can be detrimental without the second component, self–other awareness. This allows human beings to separate their own feelings from the feelings of others, allowing the social worker to make inferences about the information being provided. This "brake" allows social workers to avoid emotional overloading from the experiences shared by clients. The third component described by Gerdes and Segal (2011) is mental flexibility. An important skill for social workers, it allows humans to receive the perspective of the client, and also turn it off, in rotation as necessary to move forward with accomplishing the goals of the working relationship.

Specific to empathy and cultural competence in social work is the critique of the absence of an emphasis on cultural context. Buckman et al. (2001) aptly point out that much of the empathy literature fails to recognize that client self-actualization is not available to all because of the power of cultural forces such as racism, sexism, economic disparities, and others. Ignoring cultural context emphasizes damaging dominant discourses and can contribute to further harm of the client (King, 2011; Sinclair & Monk, 2005). The lived experiences of clients is in direct relation to the biased experiences forced upon them by the dominant groups, which results in severe consequences for vulnerable and oppressed populations, including lower placement in the hierarchy of social structure (Buckman et al., 2001; Sinclair & Monk, 2005).

Humility and empathy are vital within service to clients, as they allow the privileged social worker to acknowledge how the harmful societal systems function to oppress the client and cause, or at the very least contribute to, the problems they are facing within the work they hope to do. The social worker must use the surrogate experience to assist the client in moving past attributions that may be paralyzing them in feelings of fault, and assist them in viewing their struggle in light of oppressive cultural contexts (Sinclair & Monk, 2005).

HUMILITY

Tervalon and Murray-Garcia (1998) coined the term cultural humility to recognize the fact that culture is central to all human interactions, and that competence is never truly achieved as the needs of groups and dynamics oppressive social systems continually shift. The need for humility is vital in the context of cultural competence because engaging diversity in practice requires that the social worker learn with and from the client. This requires the vulnerability to admit to self and others that you do not have all of the answers, and the readiness to acknowledge that education, licensing, and other credentials do not solely qualify one to fully address the many ways that inequality pervades society. Not only are we limited through lack of knowledge, we are also limited by our unconscious biases and stereotyping to explain client behaviors (Ortega & Faller, 2011).

While at first this focus on humility and vulnerability may feel intimidating to the new social worker, it actually liberates the social worker from the pressure of being the expert on everything their clients have and will experience. The social worker is a collaborator with the client in the helping relationship. Collaboration allows the client to teach the social worker about the uniqueness of their intersectionality. This allows for a mutually beneficial relationship and helps to reduce the harmful effects of power dynamics within the helping relationship.

Considering cultural humility in mezzo and macro terms, it is easy to recognize how agencies and organizations can easily go astray. Decisions about

Field Reflection Questions

What does empathy and cultural humility look like to you in direct practice? What about in mezzo and macro practice?

What aspect of cultural humility do you feel most comfortable with? What aspect are you least comfortable with?

programming are often made in a vacuum—with respect to funding requirements or guidelines, but without input from the experts: the individuals who will be using the services. Cultural humility charges social workers to advocate for client and community voice in decision-making.

CULTURAL SAFETY

Another concept related to culture in social work practice is that of cultural safety, a concept that originated in Aotearoa/New Zealand by Maori nurses but that is getting more attention from social workers (Danso, 2016; Hammell, 2013; Mlcek, 2014). This concept builds on the concept of competence by focusing on the risks associated with the absence of cultural competence, awareness, and sensitivity (Brascoupé & Waters, 2009, p. 8). Cultural safety centers the historical effects and inequities that shape the lives of historically excluded, marginalized, and oppressed groups and requires that social workers work to confirm that the services provided by the social worker and the agency suit cultural context, develop knowledge about the particular barriers that clients endure, and utilize (and develop, if necessary) intervention strategies that recognize each client's uniqueness (Danso, 2016).

CASE SUMMARY: "HOW DO I HELP?"

PRACTICE SETTING DESCRIPTION

My name is Makayla and I am a first-year MSW student completing an internship at a family service agency in a medium-sized city in the Midwest. The agency provides individual and family counseling services on a sliding fee scale. The agency also runs a number of educational and treatment groups. I was assigned to work with T., who is seeking assistance in finding resources for herself and her two children and in managing stress.

IDENTIFYING DATA

T. has two children, Maria and Luisa. T. fled to the area to escape her abusive husband. T. is 30 years old, her children are ages 8 and 6. T. and her daughters are undocumented. T. works, cleaning houses, while her children are at school. T. and her children have temporary shelter.

PRESENTING PROBLEM

T. and her children are facing multiple obstacles. They need to find permanent, affordable housing and also find ways to supplement T.'s income, as she is currently not making enough to pay rent and other bills and feed her children.

Additionally, T. is experiencing an immense amount of stress and anxiety, and has described an instance when she could not calm down her breathing, and she felt lightheaded. She is concerned about meeting her children's needs and finding a permanent housing situation, and is always concerned that either her ex-husband or the government will locate her.

ASSESSMENT

While there are many stressors facing T. and her family, the most immediate and pressing need is to find a permanent housing situation for them. T. was reluctant to even come in to the agency for counseling services out of fear of service refusal and fear of being turned in due to her undocumented status. The majority of the housing services in the area require applicants to be citizens or permanent residents.

Additionally, T.'s anxiety is causing her to have potential panic attack symptoms. While T. reports that this has only occurred one time, her increased levels of stress are certainly impacting her physical well-being. She reports difficulty sleeping at night, and exhaustion during the day.

T. is extremely reluctant to sign up for any federally funded services, even those that she and her children are entitled to receiving. Upon the suggestion that we connect them with Supplemental Nutrition Assistance Program (SNAP) services, T. became nervous and refused as she has heard that participation in SNAP services, and others like them, would draw the attention of Immigration Enforcement, and she had heard stories on the news of individuals being deported after signing up for such programs.

T. and her daughters have many strengths. They are all happier after relocating away from their abusive family member. While they moved away from family and friends, they moved to this specific location because of a small support system that already lived here. It is this support system that is providing them food and shelter until T. can establish permanent arrangements. Additionally, T. already is already employed, and her hours are increasing. All of them fluently speak and read English.

Another obvious strength is the determination and resilience that she has already shown. Their support network is growing further in part because of their new church community. Additionally, T. is highly motivated to find her own accommodations and support her children.

CASE PROCESS SUMMARY

I feel I have built significant rapport with T. She is very open with me, which took quite a bit of time. In discussion with my field supervisor, I shared that T.'s unwillingness to sign up for certain services that she and her daughters are allowed to use, even with their undocumented status, was a big challenge, and I was unsure why T. was being so resistant to most of the options I share. Because resources are so limited here, we don't really have the option of turning down what is available. In many ways, I find myself wondering "How do I help?" Upon reflection, my field instructor shared that she sensed my frustration with the situation, and she wondered if perhaps T. could sense my frustration as well.

Makayla, MSW Student Intern

CASE DISCUSSION QUESTIONS

1. *Based upon the information provided, how would you, as Makayla's field supervisor, encourage her to work through this apparent frustration? Would you encourage her to bring this topic up with T.? Why or why not?*

2. *Evaluate and critique Makayla's assessment of T. through the lens of engaging diversity and difference in practice. What are the strengths of the assessment? What areas need to be strengthened?*

3. *Consider the case example in terms of intersectionality. From the information provided, what are the different identities that T. may inhabit? How does that change her situation when compared to others? What additional information do you wish you had?*

4. *Thinking about cultural competence and cultural humility, what is something you would want to focus on with T. if you were working with her?*

END-OF-CHAPTER RESOURCES

A robust set of instructor resources designed to supplement this text is located at http://connect.springerpub.com/content/book/978-0-8261-3753-1. Qualifying instructors may request access by emailing textbook@springerpub.com.

CRITICAL THINKING QUESTIONS

Ella, a White, straight woman, has had three sessions with her client, who is Black and bisexual. Ella has been using active listening and empathetic reflection as she learns more about her client and the experiences that brought her in to receive services. Sometimes, after she reflects back on what she's heard, her client will respond with "Yeah, but I'm sure you have no idea what I'm talking about." While Ella agrees with her client that she cannot truly understand what those experiences have been like, she knows that she should appropriately respond with a statement or question that allows her and the client to explore cultural differences that exist between them. She is not completely sure how she could bring this up. Identify the potential for misstep on Ella's behalf. Describe how would you avoid or minimize the potential for these missteps. Discuss how you would approach this scenario. Reflect on and describe your affective reaction to this scenario.

1. Think back to earlier chapters—identify what engagement and assessment skills you would utilize during this conversation. What skills are you less confident about using in this scenario? Identify how you may be able to strengthen

those skills to be able to more effectively approach this conversation with the client.

2. You must be able to engage your clients in a helping relationship beyond difference. In reflecting upon your work with clients in your field placement, describe a situation in which you were unable to fully grasp an experience your client attempted to share with you. Upon reflection, was this due to cultural or linguistic difference? How did you deal with this situation? Reflect and describe how you would approach a similar situation in the future.

3. Engaging diversity and difference in practice involves humility, curiosity, and ongoing self-reflection on your automatic stereotypical and biased assumptions about your clients. Everyone holds implicit biases. In reflecting upon your work with clients in your field placement, describe an experience in which you recognized yourself having a stereotypical or biased assumption about a client you were working with. Reflect on and describe your affective reaction to this experience. Describe how you handled this experience. Reflect and describe how you could improve your reaction when it happens in the future.

LEARNING ACTIVITIES

1. Consider your field placement agency. Identify an example (real or fictitious) of how a social worker might behave if they held an individual implicit bias (an unconscious attitude or belief) about a certain group. How might a social worker behave if they held an individual explicit bias (behaving in a discriminatory way)? What is an example of an institutional implicit bias (unintentional positive or negative impacts for specific groups)? Identify an example of institutional explicit bias (explicit discrimination on an institutional level).

2. Identify what cultural safety looks like in practice at your field placement agency. What particular barriers do your clients deal with in their lives? What types of intervention strategies might be most useful for specific clients, and why? Can you identify a gap in cultural appropriate interventions for clients who utilize your agency, and if so, what are those gaps?

ELECTRONIC RESOURCES

WEBSITE LINKS

Standard and Indicators for Cultural Competence in Social Work Practice—National Association of Social Workers: www .socialworkers.org/LinkClick.aspx?fileticket=PonPTDEBrn4%3D &portalid=0

Cultural Humility, Part I—What Is 'Cultural Humility'?—The Social Work Practitioner: https://thesocialworkpractitioner .com/2013/08/19/cultural-humility-part-i-what-is-cultural-humility

Intersectional Theory—Dustin Kidd: www.slideshare.net/ dustinkidd1/intersectional-theory

VIDEO LINKS

Race and Racism—Camera Jones: www.youtube.com/ watch?v=GNhcY6fTyBM

Power of Vulnerability—Brené Brown: www.ted.com/talks/ brene_brown_on_vulnerability

Unconscious Bias—J. Renee Navarro: https://diversity.ucsf.edu/ resources/unconscious-bias

The Urgency of Intersectionality—Kimberlé Crenshaw: www.ted .com/talks/kimberle_crenshaw_the_urgency_of_intersectionality

REFERENCES

American Heritage Dictionary. (2017). *Bias*. HarperCollins. https://ahdictionary.com/word/search .html?q=bias

Aponte, H. (1995). *Bread and spirit: Therapy with the new poor*. Morton Press.

Battle-Walters, K. (2004). *Sheila's shop: Working-class African American women talk about life, love, race, and hair*. Rowman & Littlefield.

Brascoupé, S., & Waters, C. (2009). Cultural safety: Exploring the applicability of the concept of cultural safety to aboriginal health and community wellness. *International Journal of Aboriginal Health, 5*(2), 6–41. https://doi.org/10.3138/ijih.v5i2.28981

Buckman, R., Reese, A., & Kinney, D. (2001). Narrative therapies. In P. Lehmann, & N. Coady (Eds.), *Theoretical perspectives for direct social work practice: A generalist-eclectic approach* (pp. 279–302). Springer Publishing Company.

Council on Social Work Education. (2008). *Council on social work education curriculum policy statements.* Council on Social Work Education.

Council on Social Work Education. (2022). *Educational policy and accreditation standards for baccalaureate and master's social work programs.* https://www.cswe.org/getmedia/94471c42-13b8-493b-9041 -b30f48533d64/2022-EPAS.pdf

Danso, R. (2016). Cultural competence and cultural humility: A critical reflection on key cultural diversity concepts. *Journal of Social Work, 18*(4), 410–430. https://doi.org/10.1177/1468017316654341

Garran, A., & Rozas, L. (2013). Cultural competence revisited. *Journal of Ethnic and Cultural Diversity in Social Work, 22*(2), 97–111. https://doi.org/10.1080/15313204.2013.785337

Gerdes, K. E., & Segal, E. (2011). Importance of empathy for social work practice: Integrating new science. *Social Work, 56*(2), 141–148. https://doi.org/10.1093/sw/56.2.141

Hall, E., & Lindsey, S. (2014). Teaching Hall cultural competence: A closer look at racial and ethnic identity formation. *The New Social Worker.* http://www.socialworker.com/feature-articles/ethics-articles/ teaching-cultural-competence

Hammell, K. R. W. (2013). Occupation, well-being, and culture: Theory and cultural humility. *Canadian Journal of Occupational Therapy, 80*(4), 224–234. https://doi.org/10.1177/0008417413500465

Holosko, M. J., Skinner, J., & Robinson, R. S. (2008). Person-centered theory. In B. Thyer (Ed.), *Comprehensive handbook of social work and social welfare: Human behavior in the social environment* (Vol. 2, pp. 297–326). John Wiley & Sons.

King, S. H. (2011). The structure of empathy in social work practice. *Journal of Human Behavior in the Social Environment, 21*(6), 679–695. https://doi.org/10.1080/10911359.2011.583516

Kornblum, W., & Julian, J. (2007). *Social problems* (10th ed.). Prentice Hall.

Locke, D. C. (1992). *Increasing multicultural understanding: A comprehensive model.* Sage Publications.

Lum, D. (2000). *Social work practice and people of color: A process stage approach.* Wadsworth.

McGoldrick, M., Giodarno, J., & Garcia-Preto, N. (2005). *Ethnicity and family therapy* (3rd ed.). Guilford Press.

Mitchell, E. R. (1999). Assessment and development of cultural competence. *Dissertation Abstracts International, 61*(03B), 1699.

Mlcek, S. (2014). Are we doing enough to develop cross-cultural competencies for social work? *British Journal of Social Work, 44*(7), 1984–2003. https://doi.org/10.1093/bjsw/bct044

National Association of Social Workers, Center for Workforce Studies. (2006). *2004 National study of licensed social workers: Demographic factsheet—Female social workers.* National Association of Social Workers.

National Association of Social Workers. (2021). *Code of ethics.* https://www.socialworkers.org/About/ Ethics/Code-of-Ethics/Code-of-Ethics-English

National Association of Social Workers. (2015). *Standards and indicators for cultural competence in social work practice.* https://www.socialworkers.org/LinkClick.aspx?fileticket=7dVckZAYUmk%3d&portalid=0

Ortega, R. M., & Faller, K. C. (2011). Training child welfare workers from an intersectional cultural humility perspective: A paradigm shift. *Child Welfare, 90*(5), 27–49.

Pinderhughes, E. (1989). *Understanding race, ethnicity, and power.* The Free Press.

Ridlen, S., & Dane, E. (1992). Individual and social implications of human differences. *Journal of Multicultural Social Work, 2*(2), 25–41. https://doi.org/10.1300/J285v02n02_03

Rodgers, A., & Potocky, M. (1998). Preparing students to work with culturally diverse clients. *Social Work Education, 17*(1), 95–100. https://doi.org/10.1080/02615479811220081

Rothery, M., & Tutty, L. (2001). Client-centered theory. In P. Lehmann, & N. Coady (Eds.), *Theoretical perspectives for direct social work practice: A generalist-eclectic approach* (pp. 223–239). Springer Publishing Company.

Seipel, A., & Way, I. (2006). Culturally competent social work practice with Latino clients. *The New Social Worker*, *13*(4), 4–7. https://www.socialworker.com/feature-articles/ethics-articles/Culturally_Competent_Social_Work_Practice_With_Latino_Clients

Sinclair, S. L., & Monk, G. (2005). Discursive empathy: A new foundation for therapeutic practice. *British Journal of Guidance & Counseling*, *33*(3), 333–349. https://doi.org/10.1080/03069880500179517

Tervalon, M., & Murray-Garcia, J. (1998). Cultural humility versus cultural competence: A critical distinction in defining physician training outcomes in multicultural education. *Journal of Health Care for the Poor and Underserved*, *9*(2), 117–125. https://doi.org/10.1353/hpu.2010.0233

van Dijk, T. A. (1997). Political discourse and racism: Describing others in western parliaments. In S. H. Riggins (Ed.), *The language and politics of exclusion: Others in discourse* (pp. 31–64). Sage Publications.

Vanaerschot, G. (2007). Empathic resonance and differential experiential processing: An experiential process-directive approach. *American Journal of Psychotherapy*, *61*(3), 313–331. https://doi.org/10.1176/appi.psychotherapy.2007.61.3.313

Research-Informed Practice in Your Field Placement

Irene is completing her MSW field placement at an elementary school with a school social worker. She is really enjoying her work and all the things she is exposed to at this placement. She spends most of her time working with students, either individually or in a group setting. She works with the children on a variety of concerns, including behavioral issues, upsetting or strong feelings, and social skills issues. Recently, Irene thought that it might be beneficial if the students who were coming to see her for social skills issues would come at the same time and play an interactive game together during part of the session.

During her weekly supervision, Irene shared with her field supervisor that she had an idea to help students with social skills issues. The supervisor listened to what Irene wanted to do related to introducing a game in the group so that the children could practice their social skills in a play activity. The supervisor was intrigued by Irene's enthusiasm. The field supervisor asked Irene to research her idea—that is, her belief that having the students play interactive games helps build social skills.

At the next supervision, Irene came prepared with copies of the scholarly research articles she found that supported the use of a variety of play therapy techniques, including interactive games, to promote social skills with children in a group setting. Irene felt confident in her ability to find research articles because she had a research methods course last semester.

After the field supervisor and Irene reviewed the research together, they started planning a social skills group session to meet twice a week. After a couple of weeks of running the group, the field supervisor asked Irene to bring some data on her social skills groups to their next supervision to discuss how the group was working out.

Irene reviewed the student records to get actual data, looking at length of stay in treatment with the school social worker as well as severity of symptoms (using a checklist that was completed routinely while the kids were seeing the social worker) to compare students who had been participating in Irene's group with students who were coming only to meet with Irene individually. After reviewing the data, Irene found that the students who participated in the group showed much more progress than the children with social skills deficits who were coming to the social work office individually. Irene was proud of her ability to use research to inform her decision to add games to her social skills groups and to evaluate the effectiveness of her group sessions.

- *How is Irene using research to inform her professional practice as a social worker?*

- *How could Irene use her practice to inform research?*

COMPETENCY 4: ENGAGE IN PRACTICE-INFORMED RESEARCH AND RESEARCH-INFORMED PRACTICE

Social workers use ethical, culturally informed, and anti-racist and anti-oppressive approaches in conducting research and building knowledge. Social workers use research to inform their practice decision-making and articulate how their practice experience informs research and evaluation decisions. Social workers critically evaluate and critique current, empirically sound research to inform decisions pertaining to practice, policy, and programs. Social workers understand the inherent bias in research and evaluate design, analysis, and interpretation using an anti-racist and anti-oppressive perspective. Social workers know how to access, critique, and synthesize the current literature to develop appropriate research questions and hypotheses. Social workers demonstrate knowledge and skills regarding qualitative and quantitative research methods and analysis, and they interpret data derived from these methods. Social workers demonstrate knowledge about methods to assess reliability and validity in social work research. Social workers can articulate and share research findings in ways that are usable to a variety of clients and constituencies. Social workers understand the value of evidence derived from interprofessional and diverse research methods, approaches, and sources.

Social workers

- apply research findings to inform and improve practice, policy, and programs; and

- identify ethical, culturally informed, anti-racist, and anti-oppressive strategies that address inherent biases for use in quantitative and qualitative research methods to advance the purposes of social work. (Council on Social Work Education, 2022, p. 8)

LEARNING OBJECTIVES

By the end of this chapter, you will be able to:

- Describe the steps involved in critical thinking.

- Identify barriers to research-informed practice.

- Critically evaluate existing research.

- Evaluate online sources.

- Describe the components of evidence-based practice.

- Conduce literature searches.

NATIONAL ASSOCIATION OF SOCIAL WORKERS *CODE OF ETHICS*

Social workers need to understand and be able to apply research to their practice. They need to use research to inform clinical decisions and select best practices when working with clients. Our clients deserve the best services available. The National Association of Social Workers (NASW) *Code of Ethics* sets forth ethical standards regarding research and evaluation for social workers that have 17 standards. Of relevance to this chapter is Ethical Standard 5.02c—"social workers should critically examine and keep current with emerging knowledge relevant to social work and fully use evaluation and research evidence in their professional practice" (NASW, 2021, para. 3).

CRITICAL THINKING

The focus of this chapter is on using research to inform your social work practice. A fundamental component of every aspect of research-informed practice is critical thinking. Critical thinking should come into play at every decision point in your generalist social work practice with your clients and in your field placement setting. Do not accept anything at face value. Be curious, ask questions, and assess possible choices every step of the way. A challenge of being a social worker is trying to figure out what is really going on with your clients and then choosing the best possible course of action to address the situation. This requires the development of critical thinking skills and your willingness to think critically before you act.

Critical thinking is more than a rational step-by-step problem-solving process (Gibbons & Gray, 2004). It involves an intuitive process as well as disciplined evaluation and analysis. "Thinking critically includes the synthesis, comparison and evaluation of ideas from a variety of sources, such as texts, direct observation and experience and social dialogue" (Gibbons & Gray, 2004, p. 21). A critical thinking social worker attempts to understand the client systems' perception of their reality and how their perceptions inform their work together. Critical thinking in social work practice is "the process of figuring out what to believe or not about a situation, phenomenon, problem or controversy for which no single definitive answer exists" (Mumm & Kersting, 1997, p. 75). Social work practice is a process in which there is no definitive answer. Effective social work practice requires critical thinking. A key component of generalist social work practice is formulating hypotheses and critically assessing them to better understand the client system. Practice interventions and/or strategies flow out of our understanding of the client's perception of their situation and social reality. Critical thinking is the open-minded search for "understanding, rather than the discovery of a necessary conclusion" (Mumm & Kersting, 1997, p. 75).

Heron (2006) identified key features of critical thinking: "Instead of viewing critical thinking as having separate features, it may be more useful to present them as being linked and cyclical in nature" (p. 221). Critical thinking is a process with the center of the cycle focused on explaining the why. Heron's (2006) conceptualization focuses on an explanation of why a phenomenon is significant. The process includes "providing evidence, examining the implications of the evidence, recognizing any potential contradictions and examining alternative explanations" (p. 221).

Although critical thinking is a nonlinear process going back and forth there are several steps that you will need to incorporate into your decision-making. Critical thinking can be applied to any problem or type of decision-making. There are several websites that describe critical thinking skills, or the steps used in critical thinking. For example, see https://zety.com/blog/critical-thinking-skills or www .rasmussen.edu/student-experience/college-life/critical-thinking -skills-to-master-now.

The following describes the steps you might take in your work with clients in your field placement. These steps can also be applied to nonclient decisions you make in your field placement. We recommend that you review your critical thinking processes with your field instructor before making any major decisions regarding your clients or any field placement activities. In fact, all your supervision sessions should involve critical thinking, which we believe is a fundamental component of being a competent professional social worker.

Typically, the first step is to identify the problem. What is the problem your client is facing? Identify the specific problem you are trying to address. We recommend that you write it out and that you be as specific as possible. Ask yourself several questions. Who is doing what? What are the possible causes or reasons for the problem? What factors are contributing to the problem? How serious is the problem? What are the consequences of the problem and for whom? Your task at this point in the process is to clearly identify the problem and to develop possible assumptions as to the underlying factors that might be contributing to the problem. This process is a critical first step.

The next step in your critical thinking process is to identify possible sources of data on the factors that contribute to the identified problem. What evidence would support each of your assumptions? What evidence would not support your assumptions? What are the possible sources of data that can help you assess your assumptions about the problem being addressed? What information do you need to verify or dismiss your assumptions about the underlying causes to the identified problem? The key here is to think through possible sources of data that will help you test your questions about the causes of the identified problem. Be inclusive. Identify multiple potential sources of data including the client perceptions, perceptions of others in the client's support network, your own practice experiences, your colleagues' perceptions and experiences, theories of human behavior, and available research evidence.

Having identified potential data sources, you then need to gather and assess the data. Examine the data for possible answers to your questions or assumptions. Rarely will you find definitive answers. What you are looking for are the answers with the highest probability. You will have to use inference. You will need to assess the information and draw conclusions based upon the available data. An important part of your data assessment is identifying bias. Do your best to evaluate the data objectively. Look at both sides and try to identify any possible biases. Who does this benefit? Does the source of this information appear to have an agenda? Is the source leaving out information that does not support its position?

You will also need to use personal reflection to identify your own personal biases that may influence your judgment. Ask yourself: Do I have any value conflicts with the client or their situation? Am I being objective? Do I have a preferred explanation? Am I more comfortable with one assumption over others? If possible, recognize your biases and do your best not to let them influence your critical thinking process. The conclusions you reach based upon your data assessment will guide your professional judgment and ultimate decision-making on how to best proceed in addressing the identified problem or client situation.

Based upon assessment conclusions you are now in the position to develop and implement your plan of action. Weigh the strengths and limitations of all possible options. It is at this point that you would research the literature on possible interventions or approaches and engage in research-informed practice. However, critical thinking does not end here. It is ongoing. You continue to critically examine every practice decision and professional judgment you make as a professional social worker. Question everything and accept nothing at face value.

Field Reflection Questions

In thinking about your field placement experience to date, to what extent have you used critical thinking in making your case decisions? Would you say "almost all the time," "occasionally," or "not at all"? If your answer was "occasionally" or "not at all," what do you need to do to increase your use of critical thinking in your case decision-making process? What has been holding you back?

RESEARCH-INFORMED PRACTICE

As we have discussed, social workers should include research evidence to inform their practice. What we know is constantly evolving as we learn more and find better ways to address social problems. As social workers we must be ready and willing to continually reflect on and go to the research evidence to determine if there are new, better ways to address client conditions.

Some social workers cite barriers to incorporating research into their professional practice. Often cited is being too busy. Increasingly, social workers are being called upon to do more with less. Social workers may find it difficult to find time to seek out relevant research that can inform their practice. Furthermore, some social workers may worry that if they are seen looking for research during their workday, others may think that they are not busy enough and in turn give them more duties or cases.

A second barrier is lack of access. It can, at times, be difficult to locate relevant, reliable, valid research that is related to a specific area of practice. While in college, social work students often have access to library resources including sophisticated search engines that identify pertinent research. Social workers must know where to look to find the appropriate information that is required to inform their practice. Thankfully, there are increasingly more and more avenues to find good quality research through domains such as Google Scholar as well as other portals designed to specifically disseminate information to professionals targeted by type of practice.

A third barrier is difficulty in interpreting the findings. For some, interpreting research can feel daunting. When a social worker is insecure in their ability to read, interpret, and infer from the research they have found, it is difficult to integrate research into practice. Sometimes statistics can be quite complicated and overwhelming. For this reason, some avoid looking for scholarly research (McLaughlin, 2012).

> **Field Reflection Questions**
>
> Think about the barriers to research-informed practice. What barriers are impacting your use of research to inform your practice decisions?
>
> What strategies could you use to address each barrier?

CRITIQUING EXISTING RESEARCH

It is not enough that social workers find research that relates to their area of practice; they must be sure that the research they are finding is valuable. Not all research is created equal, and social workers must recognize this before they begin fusing research into their practice. Before allowing research to inform one's professional practice, they should critically analyze and critique the source. Unfortunately, bad research is out there. It is the duty and obligation of the professional social worker to ensure that this research does not infiltrate their practice. One way that social workers can be sure they are not incorporating bad research into their practice is by applying critical thinking skills to the analysis of research. Critical thinking is a necessary piece of professional practice. As it relates to integrating research into social work practice, it is necessary that social workers are critical thinkers and able to critique existing research. It is important to not simply accept information without first considering several factors. First, where is this information coming from? It is important to consider who is authoring or supporting this research. At times groups that have a vested interest in a particular outcome will share research that supports their position. An example of this would be research on the effectiveness of products that are put forth by pharmaceutical companies. It is not that these studies cannot be trusted, but it is important to consider the source of the information. Another important consideration when critiquing existing research is to examine where the information was found. Information from peer-reviewed journals is typically held to a higher degree of scrutiny and thus can be relatively trustworthy. Not all journals are equal. It is important to consider the source.

Another crucial component of critically analyzing research is to apply anti-oppressive lens to your critique (Rogers, 2012). This entails an assessment of power and the values of equity and social justice (Lukes, 2005). Anti-oppressive researchers:

1. focus on social justice and resistance in process and outcome,

2. recognize that all knowledge is socially constructed and political, and

3. understand that process is all about power and relationships. (Potts & Brown, 2005)

In critiquing existing research through an anti-oppressive lens ask yourself if the study participants were involved in the design and implementation of the research. What are the underlying values of the research and is there evidence of equity and social justice values? Does the research take into consideration organizational issues or is it just focusing on service users? Did the research use empowering research methodologies? What is the power relationship between researcher and participants (Rogers, 2012)?

Another place where social workers must use good critical judgment is when finding research online. The internet can provide exceptionally valuable research. Unfortunately, it can also provide useless research. It is important to critique where the information is found. We live in an age where information is more readily available than ever before. We are lucky that with a few clicks of the mouse, we can peruse a myriad of source material. Additionally, we can connect with other professionals more rapidly than ever before. These benefits are truly astounding and can assist us and enhance our professional practice. However, we must be mindful that, as with most great advancements, there are potential drawbacks.

There are numerous websites with guidelines on how to evaluate online sources and websites. Many are maintained by university libraries. Widener University's librarians recommend that students use the C.R.A.A.P test (Wolfgram Memorial Library, 2018). The acronym stands for currency, relevance, authority, accuracy, and purpose. Exhibit 9.1 briefly lists questions that can help you begin to apply the C.R.A.A.P test to evaluate online sources. We recommend that students visit the C.R.A.A.P web pages or other university web pages for a more detailed information on how to evaluate online sources.

Field Reflection Questions

How well have you incorporated existing research into your social work practice with your clients in your field placement?

To what extent have you critically evaluated the research you have identified?

How can you strengthen your ability to critically evaluate existing research?

EVIDENCE-BASED PRACTICE

Evidence is a collection of facts that demonstrate a position to be true. Evidence-based practices (EBPs), which began flourishing in the late 20th century, are professional practices and strategies that have a basis of research that indicates the

EXHIBIT 9.1

EVALUATING ONLINE SOURCES USING THE C.R.A.A.P TEST

When evaluating resources consider the following five criteria:

1. Currency—How current is the information posted? When was it published? Has it been updated? How old are the sources upon which the information is based?

2. Relevance—How important is the information to the topic you are researching? Who is the intended audience? Is it written at the appropriate level?

3. Authority—What is the source of the information? Who is the author? What are the author's credentials? What is the URL domain (com, gov, edu, org)?

4. Accuracy—How reliable is the information? Is the language used biased or objective? Has the information been reviewed or refereed? Are there spelling, grammar, or typographical errors?

5. Purpose—Why does the information exist? What is its purpose? To inform? To educate? To sell something?

Source: Adapted from Wolfgram Memorial Library. (2018). *Evaluating web pages.* Widener University. https://widener.libguides.com/EvalWebPages/CRAAP

method is successful to address a specific condition or use with a particular population. EBPs are utilized by helping professions to provide the best practices.

EBP serves to ground the social work profession in empiricism (Okpych & Yu, 2014). There is a generally accepted process of EBP, which begins with identifying the need for information. That need for information must then be translated into a question. Evidence to answer this question is then sought. After finding evidence, it is then critically analyzed or critiqued to determine its validity. If the evidence if valid and applicable for the current need, it is then incorporated with the clinician's expertise. The clinician should also be mindful of how well the evidence fits with the client system. If it is a good fit, the evidence is integrated into the social worker's practice with the client. The social worker monitors this implementation and seeks out additional evidence as necessary.

Haynes et al. (2002) developed a four-part EBP model. The four components are (1) client circumstances, (2) research evidence, (3) client's values and preferences, and (4) expertise of the professional. In this model the clinical expertise is the key in bringing the other three components into the decision-making process (Drisko & Grady, 2019). You as the professional social worker combine and integrate all the elements of the EBP model. However, this is not done in isolation. Your client plays an active role in the decision-making process. While research evidence is important it does not take precedence over the client's values, preferences, or circumstances (Drisko & Grady, 2019). It is a collaborative process. You and your client need to come together in agreement about the best possible course of action given the research evidence, the client's circumstances and preferences, and your clinical judgment. Case 9.1 illustrates a social worker going through the process of EBP.

CASE EXAMPLE 9.1: THE EBP PROCESS

Melody is a social worker at a child welfare organization. She very much enjoys her job and supporting families. Melody was recently transferred to a new unit within the organization. As Melody was familiarizing herself with the new requirements of this position, she began to notice that many of the children on her new caseload have had multiple disrupted placements. Disrupted placement occurs when an out-of-home placement must be terminated, and the child must be placed in a new home. Melody thought that this must be difficult for the children. Melody wondered what she could do to support placements to avoid multiple disruptive placements.

Melody began searching scholarly material to find research on how to best support placements to avoid disruption. Melody found several articles and reports that address this issue. The practices that were found to be beneficial included providing additional support for foster families as well as respite care. Melody spoke with her supervisor about these recommendations to possibly improve placements. Both supports and respite were something that the organization already had available but were often underutilized. Melody and her supervisor discussed ways to share this information with families including having the caseworkers speak with the family members about resources available to them. Melody began incorporating this into her practice. Over time, Melody noticed fewer and fewer disrupted placements.

EBP encourages social workers to be considerate of the importance of outcomes in practice, whether client situations are improving, staying the same, or worsening. Good assessment is ongoing assessment. Social workers must be particularly thoughtful in recognizing changes in the client system when incorporating an EBP. Furthermore, social workers must be cautious in assuming causation between their EBP and client changes. This underscores the importance of a thorough assessment to determine if there are other changes occurring that could account for the change in client presentation.

The process of EBP involves finding the "best available evidence to support clinical decision-making that also considers a social worker's clinical judgment and professional ethics and the client's personal and cultural preferences" (Langer & Lietz, 2015, p. 14). Social workers must be aware that clients are not "passive recipients of social work practice" and therefore, EBP should be selected in consideration of the clients' rights to self-determination (McLaughlin, 2012). We must continuously be aware that clients come to us with their own unique histories and experiences and we as professionals must meet the clients where they are. It is our job to begin where the client is.

MULTIPLE WAYS OF KNOWING

How do you know what you know? This may seem like quite a philosophical question, but it is an important one to consider. There are multiple ways of knowing, each coming with benefits and limitations. It is important that social workers are critical thinkers. To be a critical thinker, one must consider where the information they are receiving originates. It is important for social workers to consider such things because social workers are often called upon to make many decisions every day that have implications for clients, communities, and the profession itself.

Social workers must be aware that it is easy to make errors in logic. Common errors in reasoning include overgeneralization, selective observation, illogical reasoning, resistance to change, and adherence to authority (Engel & Schutt, 2014). Overgeneralization refers to the tendency of individuals to take what they know to be true in one case and apply it in all situations. This is a simplistic error that does not allow for individual experiences. As we know, most issues that social workers deal with are quite complex and multifaceted. Overgeneralizations do not consider individual differences or experiences. Social workers must be cautious to avoid this error in logic. Selective observation occurs when an individual seeks out only information that is confirmatory to already held beliefs. For example, if a person believes that boys are more aggressive than girls, they may only notice situations in which boys are engaging in aggression as that fits their predetermined belief. Illogical reasoning happens when an individual holds to untrue assumptions or jumps to conclusions without support. At times, individuals have always thought a certain way about something, and as a result, they may be resistant to changing their beliefs. This is an error in logic as the person is not open to new information. This error in logic is sometimes referred to as tradition. Social workers must recognize that at times people hold tightly onto traditionally held beliefs even when presented with evidence to the contrary. Adherence to authority refers to a person believing something simply because they were told it by a person in a (real or perceived) place of authority.

Social workers must also be on the lookout for pseudoscience. Thyer and Pignotti (2015) put forth that "pseudoscientific practices are practices that give the superficial appearance of being derived from science and yet lack an actual scientific basis" (p. 6). Believing pseudoscience can be an additional error in logic. For social workers to distinguish between true science and pseudoscience, they must have a basic understanding of good research methods in order to detect issues with a research design. Social workers must have a critical eye when evaluating research to determine if it is truly good science.

Practice wisdom is something that is valued in many professions, including social work. The capstone of the social work educational experience is a field experience where social work students are placed with competent social work professionals who guide students, many times with practice wisdom, into becoming competent professionals themselves. Practice wisdom is complex and requires reflection and analysis that brings together various learning sources and contexts in order to encapsulate or understand better how things work (Shaw, 2016). Though practice wisdom is an integral part of our profession, we encourage social workers to not solely rely on practice wisdom. Practice wisdom based in best practices and sciences is best. As a result, social workers must be critical thinkers and evaluate and not just blindly accept or conform to faulty logic (Rubin & Bellamy, 2012).

Various forms of research knowledge are available for social workers. Three types of research knowledge include descriptive, predictive, and prescriptive knowledge (Yegidis et al., 2018). Descriptive knowledge, as its name implies, seeks to describe how things are. This type of knowledge may describe things as they are currently and as they change over time. Predictive knowledge attempts to predict what will happen in the future. This type of knowledge is possible when we have enough descriptive knowledge to be able to make reasonable inferences about possible future occurrences. Prescriptive knowledge provides insights into the intervention to address a current condition. Yegidis et al. (2018) set forth that "in EBP, social workers use prescriptive knowledge, along with their experience, client preferences, and so forth, to decide what intervention should be used to address an existing problem or to prevent one that they predict will occur" (p. 14).

TRANSLATING FINDINGS INTO PRACTICE

Research findings are only beneficial if they can be used and applied to practice. As we discussed at the start of this chapter, it is unreasonable to separate research and practice from one another. Research must be integrated into practice to be of any value or use. When thinking about integrating research findings into professional practice, social workers should learn copiously about the proposed methods. Furthermore, social workers must be critical thinkers to determine if these new methods would be a good fit for their client population. Social workers must be considerate of cultural limitations regarding some findings. For example, some EBPs have only been researched on specific populations (age, gender, race/ethnicity, etc.). Also, it is necessary that social workers only implement EBP and other findings in their practice that they have been sufficiently trained on and competent in. If a social worker is not trained in a specific EBP, it would be unethical to administer that EBP. Social workers should also be mindful of their limits of competence and seek out ongoing learning opportunities to enhance their practice skills related to innovative methods.

USE OF SELF-REFLECTION

In the field, how do you make decisions regarding what to do with the people you are working with? Ideally, you are calling upon your foundation of knowledge from your social work courses regarding building relationships, interviewing, assessing, and intervening. In the field, you also have the advantage of having a field supervisor to help guide you through your learning process in addition to your faculty liaison. It is important that you are aware of what you are doing and why you are doing it. In field education, supervisors will often pass along their practice wisdom to you, which can be a very valuable thing. However, professional social workers cannot rely solely on the practice wisdom of others. Good, competent, professional social workers must actively seek out information that is relevant, trustworthy, and sound to make practice decisions. McLaughlin (2012) suggests that social workers should "be in a continuous reflective relationship with their practice seeking to find evidence and answers that help them to identify whether their intervention is effective or more interference" (p. 1). It is important that you engage with research to improve your practice skills. Also, as discussed earlier in this chapter, as a competent social worker, you must continually be learning, knowing, and growing to provide the best services possible to your clients. To be able to engage with research, you must first be able to find (good) research.

LITERATURE SEARCHES

Research is available from a variety of sources. Yes, you can go to a library for information, but often more resources are available online. As a student, you most likely have access to online search tools such as EBSCO, but there are a variety of other sources, including the popular Google Scholar and other publicly hosted database sites. For example, the Child Welfare Information Gateway is a great public resource where you can find a wealth of research related to children and families (see www.childwelfare.gov).

ONLINE SEARCHING

Computers are amazing machines that can provide us with access to a lot of great information. However, we must know how to access the quality information, because sometimes there is not-so-great information online as well. As the old phrase suggests, "Garbage in, garbage out." This cliché is very true regarding online searching. To improve your search results, we urge you to consider how you are searching.

BOOLEAN LOGIC

Boolean logic is a simple yet powerful tool that allows you to refine your search results using three simple words: "and," "or," and "not." By using these three words, you can expand or narrow your search based on what you need. The term "and" will narrow your search by requiring that both concepts you joined by this word be present in your results. The term "not" will also narrow your results by eliminating specific concepts. Finally, your search can be expanded by using the term "or," which allows for another concept to be included in your results.

EVALUATING YOUR SEARCH RESULTS

Now that you have found the research, you must evaluate it. In a perfect world, all the information available for public consumption would be sound, empirically based research that has high levels of validity and reliability, is collected with good sampling procedures, and is obtained through an ethically sound design. Sadly, that is not always the case. As a result, we must be cautious and careful consumers of research. An adage says, "Numbers never lie." In evaluating your search results, you need to understand that numbers can, in fact, lie. People can manipulate numbers to tell the narrative they desire. This is unethical, but it does occur.

The internet has a wealth of information ready for you to explore, but not all that information is created equal. A quick and easy way to evaluate the quality and integrity of a website and its information is to consider the following questions:

- Does it list an author?
- Is there a reference list?
- Is there a date of publication?
- What is the website URL? Generally, websites that end in .edu, .org, or .gov are more likely to contain scholarly material than .com sites.

Positive responses to these questions suggest that the website and the information are probably legitimate and okay for your use. If you are unsure, however, we strongly urge you to take a closer look and conduct a more comprehensive assessment. Most guidelines list five criteria we discussed earlier: accuracy, authority, objectivity, currency, and coverage. Examining the five criteria will give you a reliable assessment of the quality and integrity of the website.

CASE SUMMARY: "ALL YOU NEED IS LOVE"

PRACTICE SETTING DESCRIPTION

Social Work Counseling Services (SWCS) is a pro bono clinic that is run by a school of social work. It is in a predominantly low-income community that has a high percentage of minority residents of whom the majority are African American. The community has high unemployment, drug use, single parent families, crime rates, and school failures. It also has a very poor housing stock and several environment issues such as toxic waste and high lead-paint and air pollution levels. By every conceivable measure, the community is disadvantaged and has limited social services and employment opportunities.

SWCS is primarily staffed by MSW and BSW student interns. The interns are placed on service teams comprised of four to six students and a full-time MSW field instructor. Students are placed on an elderly service team, an individual and family counseling team, an after-school enrichment team, or a job training–life skills team. Social work faculty provide monthly workshops and trainings and a faculty member also facilitates a weekly case conference.

During the case conferences two student interns present one of their cases to the group for discussion. The case conferences are intended to help the student critically evaluate their work on the case, identify potential underlying issues or factors contributing to the client's problem or concerns, and to identify possible strategies for the student to pursue with the client.

IDENTIFYING DATA

I am a second-year MSW student assigned to the SWCS individual and family counseling team. My client, Tom, is a 14-year-old Caucasian boy who was brought to the counseling service by Gabe, his mother. Gabe stated at admission that Tom was failing in school, was not doing his homework, and that he consistently disobeyed her at home—not doing his chores or cleaning his room. She stated that he has no real friends and that he is often agitated and aggressive. He is not physically aggressive with her, but he frequently has angry outbursts with lots of screaming and swearing. Their family doctor diagnosed Tom as having attention deficit hyperactivity disorder (ADHD) and prescribed Ritalin, which he has been on since he was 8 years old.

Tom's mother, Gabe, is a single parent with a high school education. She has a retail job at a shopping mall in a nearby community and struggles financially. She was raised in a very strict household with a very authoritarian father and stay-at-home mother. Her husband left her when Tom was 3 years old.

PRESENTING PROBLEM

Tom was referred to SWCS because of his school performance and behavior problems around the house. His mother states that he does not obey her in terms of doing his chores, cleaning his room, and generally helping out. She also states that he has frequent angry outbursts when she tries to make him do his work.

ASSESSMENT

I have seen Tom four times for counseling sessions, and I have had one follow-up session with his mother. At first, he was very closed off, but he quickly began to open up. Tom stated that he does not like the way his medication makes him feel. When he takes it he feels all jumpy and in a bad mood. He tries not to take it, but his mother closely monitors him and makes sure he does. He also confided that he does not think his mother loves him and that she blames him for his father leaving. "She seems angry all the time and is always bossing me around." As far as school goes, he stated that "it is hard" and that he has stopped trying.

Based upon his interactions with me I did not see any indications of distractibility or attention deficits. With his mother's permission Tom has tested for ADHD by PsyD intern at SWCS. Her assessment was that he did not have ADHD. I researched possible side effects of Ritalin and found that irritability and aggressive behaviors are common.

My assessment is that Tom does not have ADHD and should stop taking Ritalin, which might be the cause of his behavior problems. I am also hypothesizing that Tom feels unloved and unappreciated by his mother. Her behavior toward him reinforces these feelings. I also believe that his school problems will improve if progress is made strengthening his relationship with his mother. Even if he is motivated to do better in school, he will probably need extra support to catch up and succeed.

CASE PROCESS SUMMARY

During my follow-up meeting with Tom's mother, I shared with her my assessment. She completely rejected everything I told her. She insisted that Tom had ADHD and that he needed to continue taking Ritalin. Her doctor said he had it and that he needed to be on medication. She was unwilling to accept the ADHD assessment performed by our PsyD intern. She also rejected my recommendations for engaging with her son. I had suggested that she listen to his feeling and that she try a more supporting and encouraging approach. She stated that "his job was to do what she says and that coddling him would encourage his laziness." She stated that her parents were strict task masters and that worked for her as a child. I did not feel a lot of warmth or genuine concern about Tom's welfare from his mother. Her focus seemed to be solely on getting him to obey her and do what he is told to do.

John, MSW Student Intern

CASE DISCUSSION QUESTIONS

1. *What type of attachment does Tom have with his mother? How is their attachment affecting how she parents Tom? How is it affecting Tom's interactions with his mother?*

2. *What additional underlying factors might be contributing to Tom's behavior and/or his mother's behavior?*

3. *What are the consequences to Tom staying on Ritalin? Are there any long-term effects of taking Ritalin if it is not medically needed?*

4. *Gabe sees Tom as the client and is unwilling to make any changes in her behavior. How would you engage her in the helping process?*

5. *What suggestions do you have for possible interventions going forward? What EBP interventions would be appropriate for the issue John is having with Tom's mother?*

END-OF-CHAPTER RESOURCES

A robust set of instructor resources designed to supplement this text is located at http://connect.springerpub.com/content/book/978-0-8261-3753-1. Qualifying instructors may request access by emailing textbook@springerpub.com.

CRITICAL THINKING QUESTIONS

1. Why is it important for social workers to remain aware of research related to their area of practice? What does it mean to you to be a competent social worker?

2. In your field placement, how do you use research to inform your practice decisions? How do you gather the research you need to be an effective social work professional in field?

3. How can you ensure that you are following the standards set forth by the NASW's *Code of Ethics* related to research and evaluation at your field placement? Provide three specific examples.

4. How does EBP fit with the way you approach your work with your clients? What do you need to do differently to incorporate EBP into your work? What are the obstacles to implementing EBP in your field placement? What are the benefits?

LEARNING ACTIVITIES

The following lists several possible field placement learning activities that could be undertaken to help develop your research-informed practice competency. Competency in using research findings to inform your practice is part of Competency 4: Engage in Research-Informed Practice and Practice-Informed Research. We have found that students often have difficulty implementing this competency in their field placements. The activities listed below are some of the possible ways the research-informed practice component of Competency 4 can be addressed as part of your field placement experience. If you did not include any research-informed practice activities in your initial learning contract, we suggest that you add some to your learning contract to be addressed during your second semester of field.

1. Conduct a literature search for scholarly research related to your field placement population. Present your findings to your field instructor and provide a critical evaluation of one of the research articles you identified.

2. Research and identify an EBP intervention appropriate to an issue or problem you are addressing with one of your clients. Discuss with your field instructor the results of your research and present the strengths and challenges of implementing the identified EBP intervention.

3. Create a case note that describes your critical thinking around a decision that you made with a client. Critically evaluate the critical thinking pro-

cess you used and discuss how you might improve your critical thinking skills.

4. Conduct an online search on a problem or issue faced by one of your clients. Prepare a summary of three sources of information that also includes a critical evaluation of each online source. Share your results with your field instructor and discuss the usefulness of your search information for your work with your clients.

ELECTRONIC RESOURCES

WEBSITE LINKS

 Critical Thinking: www.skillsyouneed.com/learn/critical-thinking .html

 Evidence-Based Practice (EBP): www.asha.org/research/ebp

 Critically Evaluating Research Articles: www.omicsonline.org/ open-access/critical-analysis-of-clinical-research-articles-a-guide -for-evaluation-2471-9919-1000e116.php?aid=80078

 Critically Evaluating Literature Search Sources: https://libguides .msvu.ca/help/evaluation

VIDEO LINKS

How to Find Social Work Research: www.youtube.com/
watch?v=yoJH75DCxEc

How to Review a Research Paper: www.youtube.com/
watch?v=7lf3Q5BlNWo

Evaluating Journal Articles With the CRAAP Test: www.youtube
.com/watch?v=Q5Se7lxSANM

REFERENCES

Council on Social Work Education. (2022). *Educational policy and accreditation standards for baccalaure-ate and master's social work programs.* https://www.cswe.org/getmedia/94471c42-13b8-493b-9041-b30f48533d64/2022-EPAS.pdf

Drisko, J. W., & Grady, M. D. (2019). *Evidence-based practice in clinical social work* (2nd ed.). Springer.

Engel, R. J., & Schutt, R. K. (2014). *Fundamentals of social work research* (2nd ed.). SAGE.

Gibbons, J., & Gray, M. (2004). Critical thinking as integral to social work practice. *Journal of Teaching in Social Work, 24,* 19–38. https://doi.org/10.1300/J067v24n01_02

Haynes, R. B., Devereaux, P., & Guyatt, G. (2002). Physicians' and patients' choices in evidence-based practice. *BMJ: British Medical Journal, 324*(7350), 1350. https://doi.org/10.1136/bmj.324.7350.1350

Heron, G. (2006). Critical thinking in social care and social work: Searching student assignments for the evidence. *Social Work Education, 25*(3), 209–224. https://doi.org/10.1080/02615470600564965

Langer, C., & Lietz, C. (2015). *Applying theory to generalist social work practice.* Wiley.

Lukes, S. (2005). *Power: A radical view* (2nd ed.). Palgrave Macmillan.

McLaughlin, H. (2012). *Understanding social work research* (2nd ed.). SAGE.

Mumm, A., & Kersting, R. (1997). Teaching critical thinking in social work practice courses. *Journal of Social Work Education, 33*(1), 75–84. https://doi.org/10.1080/10437797.1997.10778854

National Association of Social Workers. (2021). *Code of ethics.* https://www.socialworkers.org/About/Ethics/Code-of-Ethics/Code-of-Ethics-English

Okpych, N., & Yu, J. (2014). A historical analysis of evidence-based practice in social work: The unfinished journey toward an empirically-grounded profession. *Social Service Review, 88*(1), 3–58. https://doi.org/10.1086/674969

Potts, K., & Brown, L. (2005). Becoming an anti-oppressive researcher. In L. Brown, & S. Strega (Eds.), *Research as resistance: Critical, indigenous, and anti-oppressive approaches* (pp. 255–286). Canadian Scholars Press.

Rogers, J. (2012). Anti-oppressive social work research: Reflections on power in the creation of knowledge. *Social Work Education, 31*(7), 866–879. https://doi.org/10.1080/02615479.2011.602965

Rubin, A., & Bellamy, J. (2012). *Practitioner's guide to using research for evidence-based practice* (2nd ed.). John Wiley & Sons.

Shaw, I. (2016). *Social work science*. Columbia University Press.

Thyer, B., & Pignotti, M. (2015). *Science and pseudoscience in social work*. Springer Publishing Company.

Wolfgram Memorial Library. (2018). *Evaluating web pages*. Widener University. https://widener.libguides.com/EvalWebPages/CRAAP

Yegidis, B. L., Weinbach, R. W., & Myers, L. L. (2018). *Research methods for social workers* (8th ed.). Pearson.

Engaging in Policy Practice in Your Field Placement

Reggie was a first-year MSW student doing his placement at a homeless shelter. He typically had a caseload of approximately 20 to 25 clients. Reggie assisted clients with going through their orientation to the shelter, scheduling medical and dental appointments, obtaining referrals to other community resources providers, and transportation to those providers.

After about 2 months at the shelter, Reggie began to notice some themes in his work within his caseload. First, he noticed that within the field of social work, individuals who are experiencing homelessness are often "lumped together." However, his experience indicates that the needs of his clients range significantly. Some only need connection to resources to be self-sufficient again. Others are lacking important skills needed for employment, are facing addiction or mental health problems, or are facing other serious challenges.

This reflection left Reggie with some questions. How do we get community members, agencies, funders, and others to see that approaches cannot be one size fits all? How can we develop a new model of service? Once developed, what needs to happen next? Community support, political will, and funding initiatives were all ideas Reggie had to move forward.

COMPETENCY 5: ENGAGE IN POLICY PRACTICE

Social workers identify social policy at the local, state, federal, and global level that affects well-being, human rights and justice, service delivery, and access to social services. Social workers recognize the historical, social, racial, cultural, economic, organizational, environmental, and global influences that affect social policy. Social workers understand and critique the history and current structures of social policies and services and the role of policy in service delivery through rights-based, anti-oppressive, and anti-racist lenses. Social workers influence policy formulation, analysis, implementation, and evaluation within their practice settings with individuals, families, groups, organizations, and communities. Social workers actively engage in and advocate for anti-racist and anti-oppressive policy practice to effect change in those settings.

Social workers

- use social justice, anti-racist, and anti-oppressive lenses to assess how social welfare policies affect the delivery of and access to social services; and
- apply critical thinking to analyze, formulate, and advocate for policies that advance human rights and social, racial, economic, and environmental justice. (Council on Social Work Education [CSWE], 2022, p. 10)

LEARNING OBJECTIVES

By the end of this chapter, you will be able to:

- Recognize the importance of policy practice to the field of social work.
- Recognize the ways in which social work and political work are intertwined through the lens of the National Association of Social Workers (NASW) *Code of Ethics.*
- Engage in organizational policy field practice.
- Engage in advocacy practices.

CONNECTION TO NATIONAL ASSOCIATION OF SOCIAL WORKERS *CODE OF ETHICS*

No other helping profession includes what Section 6.04 of the NASW *Code of Ethics* calls for social and political action (NASW, 2021a). The *Code* states that social workers should

> engage in social and political action that seeks to ensure that all people have equal access to the resources, employment, services, and opportunities they require to meet their basic human needs and to develop fully. Social workers should be aware of the impact of the political arena on practice and should advocate for changes in policy and legislation to improve social conditions to meet basic human needs and promote social justice. (p. 30)

The *Code* makes very clear the importance of engaging in social and political action. Unique and essential to the field of social work is the dual emphasis on not only individuals but also their corresponding environments. An important distinction to the social work lens is the understanding that, within the helping relationship, it is sometimes necessary to focus on social conditions and oppression within the individual's environment, which may be the root cause or be intensifying the individual's problems. This dual focus is emphasized within in the NASW *Code of Ethics* (2021a).

When people think of social work, what often comes to mind is the micro-level roles that social workers fill—often lost is the knowledge around social work's emphasis on working in the political arena to promote a variety of important social causes and to champion disadvantaged client populations. In fact, this has been engrained in the fabric of social work since the beginning of the profession. As Ritter (2013) details, social workers have been working to improve living conditions and their efforts were involved in the movements around settlement houses, child labor, women's suffrage, occupational safety, immigrant rights, the development of policies to address poverty during the Great Depression, and the fight for welfare rights and civil rights.

You may be feeling discomfort, or even fear, about being political within in your work. You would not be alone in this discomfort (Harding, 2004). However, social workers must come to terms with the fact that the work we do is fundamentally political—one cannot claim ownership in the pursuit of social justice without recognizing the ways in which policies, on all levels, disenfranchise and marginalize. If a social worker's mission is to simply help their clients adjust to their separate, disenfranchised, unequal living conditions— which take the form of environmental hazards, subpar educational opportunities, lack of access to healthcare, and more—without any concern for assisting in organizing and advocating for social change, is the social worker not, in some way, complicit in the maintenance of the status quo?

> **Field Reflection Questions**
>
> What does the responsibility to social and political action, detailed in the NASW *Code of Ethics*, mean to you for your future practice?
>
> What do you need to change to meet this obligation?
>
> In your current field placement, have you had the opportunity to meet this responsibility? If not, how can you begin to implement this part of your role as a social worker?

POLICY PRACTICE

The Council on Social Work Education (2022) explains that one of the main components of policy practice is the ability to "analyze, formulate, and advocate for policies that advance human rights and social, racial, economic, and environmental justice" (p. 11). While often conceptualized as something that occurs within federal, state, and local political systems, policy practice occurs at multiple levels. Micro-level policy practice is the translation of mezzo- and macro-level policies into actual services for clients (Ritter, 2013). It is important to point out that micro-level workers are often the first to recognize patterns that call for change in policy, as was true in the case example that opened this chapter. In this way, the direct service social worker has the obligation to initiate change in organizations and communities by calling attention to these patterns.

Mezzo-level policy practice is the work done on administrative policy within organizations (Ritter, 2013). Organizational policy is integral to what actually happens on the ground. Who is allowed access to the services the organization provides? What services are provided? What interventions are utilized? The list of ways in which organizational policies impact service providers and clients is endless. This fact highlights why a practice orientation that recognizes how certain problems necessitate action to effect change at the organizational level is imperative.

Macro-level policy practice is focused on impacting policies at all levels of government and within the judicial system (Ritter, 2013). There are, again, endless ways in which legislation and policy impact the ways in which individuals and groups can go about their lives. These include foreign policy, labor policy, environmental policy, tax policy, healthcare policy, transportation policy, education policy, agriculture policy, energy policy, and the policy most often focused on within the field of social work and discussed later in this chapter—social welfare policy. These policies have such a drastic impact because they have the ability to create and improve social programming, determine and alter funding levels, determine the goals of specific policies, provide protection to vulnerable populations, and cause significant harm (Ritter, 2013).

Field Reflection Questions

Do you believe that all social work is inherently political? Why or why not? Can you give examples from your field placement to help articulate your stance?

Can you think of examples of policy that has helped vulnerable populations on the micro, mezzo, and/or macro levels? What about policy that has caused harm on those levels? Can you point to a policy within your field placement that you think does one or the other, or potentially both?

HOW CAN SOCIAL WORKERS ENGAGE IN POLICY PRACTICE?

As indicated, policy can be practiced at various levels: local government, city councils, at the agency or organizational level, or at higher levels such as state, national, or international government of governing bodies (Pawar, 2019). Every level is vital to the success of policy practice and is dependent on the practitioner's identity, position, power, resources, and other varying contexts. Jansson (2018) and Pawar (2019) argue that to effectively practice in the policy realm as a social worker, one must engage in critical introspection, enhance social awareness and commitment to social work values, develop vision, seek opportunities for policy practice instead of waiting for them to appear, and learn to be assertive, be persistent, tolerate uncertainty and ambiguity, and engage in sensible risk-taking. Second, social workers must reject the current climate that prioritizes micro-level engagement and work to adapt to other levels of engagement as well. This can be done by engaging at the organizational, community, political, and bureaucratic level. Often the skills utilized in micro-level work are the same that are used to engage with individuals in an effort to mobilize and organize. Additionally, policy analysis is a vital comment of policy practice for social workers. This can take the form of evaluating existing policy or examining existing information to create new policy or new advocacy opportunities. Both involve identifying concerns and barriers, consequences, and solutions.

ORGANIZATIONAL POLICIES

Organizations, public and private, must continually obtain pertinent information and adjust accordingly if they are going to continually provide effective service delivery in constantly changing circumstances. This ability to adapt will allow the organization to assess current client needs, project forward to predict future needs, and brainstorm possible alternative service delivery strategies. These processes often result in a ripple effect of change, intentional or not. In practice, the result of this adaptability could look a variety of ways: designing new programs, expansion of services offered, change in client population served, obtaining new funding sources, implementing cutting-edge training programs for service providers, or developing new collaborators, to name a few. As discussed earlier in the chapter, organizations are required to develop and implement their own policies—with said policies often greatly impacted by funding providers that specify certain guidelines on service delivery and population. Because of the contextual nature of the social problems social workers are working against, they must continually examine and engage in organizational policy adjustment. Think of the complexities faced by the clients in your field placement—some may be experiencing substance use, violence, poverty, lack of healthcare, homelessness, and more. Regardless of the situation they are in, a labyrinth of organizations has been established for the purpose of providing services that attempts to address the needs of individuals in their communities. If you think about it, you can really identify the major impacts that organizations have on people's lives. This section will acquaint you with the practice of assessing policies, the process of updating policies, and dissemination of organization policies in your work.

ASSESSING POLICIES

During the assessment process, it is important that the social worker identify if the phenomenon they are focused on has been formally recognized as a problem or unmet need by the organization, as this recognition impacts the how the social worker will need to begin in their efforts. In the assessment process, one of the main goals is the acknowledgment of the problem or unmet need, if it has not already happened, in order to advocate for formal resources to be dedicated to updating problematic policies or gaps (Netting et al., 2017).

The assessment of policies often requires substantial information gathering, which can take many forms. Familiarizing oneself with the policies that are connected to the issue, conducting interviews with people within the organization, researching the professional knowledge base, locating data and information about the problem or unmet need, and obtaining information about the organization's receptiveness to policy change are some of the ways that social workers engage in the assessment of organizational policies. After gathering as much information as possible to gain a better understanding of the problem or unmet need and the specific population, both through the existing knowledge base and the information collected for sources within the organization, a profile should begin to emerge.

EXHIBIT 10.1

STEPS FOR ASSESSING ORGANIZATIONAL POLICIES

Step 1: Identify problem or unmet need	• Continually evaluate work for themes around problematic policies and/or unmet needs.
Step 2: Gather information	Gather information about: • the organization's recognition that the problem exists • organizational history and receptiveness to policy change • experience of individuals within the organization • data and information about the problem or unmet need • population served • policies that may be impacting the problem or unmet need
Step 3: Develop hypothesis for policy change	• State the problem or unmet need. • Share profile that emerged through the research. • Develop a hypothesis for policy change.

This profile will assist in better understanding potential responses to the problem or need, and allow the social worker to develop a hypothesis on how the policy or policies need to be updated to address the problem or unmet need. Exhibit 10.1 lists the three major steps for assessing organizational policies.

UPDATING AND DISSEMINATING POLICIES

The updating of policies often indicates the hand-off of responsibility from the social worker to those with decision-making authority within the organization. Kirst-Ashman and Hull (2001) developed an organizational assessment called "PREPARE: An Assessment of Organization Change Potential." While designed specifically for macro practitioners, its usefulness applies also to the steps necessary in the process of updating problematic or outdated organizational policies. Following is the seven-step process of PREPARE.

- Step 1: Identify problems to be addressed.
- Step 2: Review your macro and personal reality.
- Step 3: Establish primary goals.
- Step 4: Identify relevant people of influence.
- Step 5: Assess potential financial costs and potential benefits to consumers and the organization.
- Step 6: Review professional and personal risks.
- Step 7: Evaluate the potential success of the macro change process.

Steps 1 through 3 were completed in the assessment process covered in the previous section. Step 4 focuses on identifying key change agents within the organization. The social worker who originally identified the problem or need would need to answer the following questions: Who has decision-making power in this process? Who may be able to assist in moving this policy change forward? Who may be potentially resistant to this policy update, and why? How will you address the concerns for those who are resistant?

Step 5 is the process by which the organization evaluates the financial costs and benefits. This often happens after the social worker has presented their assessment, and it has been recognized formally or informally as a problem or gap. Important to note, this is often one of the first steps in policy updating if the potential problem or service gap was identified by those with decision-making authority. Also reviewed by the organization are the risks in implementing the policy change— step 6. Will implementing this policy update place the organization in violation of any funding agreements? How will the policy update be perceived by recipients of services, collaborating organizations, current and potential funders, employees, community members, and others? What stakeholders have not been consulted that may be impacted by this change? Finally, those with decision-making authority will decide if this policy change is worth the resources it will take to implement it, and if so, when that should take place. Additionally, organizations should also decide upon how they will evaluate if this policy change resulted in the intended outcome of solving the identified problem or service gap—all components of step 7.

What the dissemination of organizational policies will look like will depend on the scope of the policy change. Minor policy changes may only need to be disseminated to those internal to the organization that are impacted by that particular change. An example may be a change in intake procedure that will save both organization and client time. This policy change may only impact intake staff. Something as small as a memo, or more involved, such as a training, would suffice. However, for further-reaching policy changes, wider dissemination may be necessary. Some examples of dissemination methods include publishing program or policy briefs via news release; presentations of the policy change to local community groups, agencies, and other local stakeholders; creating and distributing program materials, such as flyers or pamphlets that detail how the policy change impacts programming; creating training materials and curricula for internal and external stakeholders; sharing vital information through social media or on an organization's website; hosting informational events at community functions; and publicizing new or altered services.

SOCIAL WELFARE POLICY

The social welfare system of the United States is made up of a highly complex set of programs, services, and agencies that are designed to address the multitude of needs that citizen have. These include, but are not limited to, healthcare needs, economic needs, educational needs, and others. Examples of social welfare programs include Temporary Assistance for Needy Families (TANF), Medicare, Medicaid, public education, Social Security, Supplemental Nutrition Assistance Program (SNAP), Head Start, unemployment compensation, college financial aid, public housing, and others. Nonprofit organizations, for-profit organizations, and faith-based organizations are private entities that are also designed to meet individual and community needs around social welfare, some of which also receive government funding to deliver services through grants and other funding sources.

The legislation, laws, rules, and regulations that direct social welfare systems in the United States make up social welfare policy. DiNitto (2011) points out that social welfare policy includes whatever the U.S. government decides to do or not do that has an impact on its citizens' quality of life. This is an important viewpoint because it highlights that quality of life can be greatly impacted by governmental inaction, not only governmental action. In the United States, we have an ongoing debate about how much of a role, if any, and in what capacity, government should play in providing for the general welfare of its citizens (Ritter, 2013).

The ways in which the field of social work are impacted by social welfare policy are endless. Policy related to mental health, poverty, homelessness, child welfare, criminal justice, and many, many more all impact clients' and communities' quality of life through access—or lack thereof—of services and resources, experiences of discrimination, unequal application of policy (e.g., sentencing of individuals convicted of a crime), and in other ways. This is why social workers should be involved in political advocacy on behalf of the clients and communities they serve, as without that role, they are missing out on the potential for immense positive changes in those clients' lives.

Throughout the previous section, we have focused on social welfare policy as an agent for positive change. We would be remiss not to also focus on those ways in which social welfare policy has been used throughout U.S. history to further harm groups of people. The United States has a long history of using policy as a way to alienate, discriminate, marginalize, and inflict violence upon oppressed communities. Some examples include the Indian Removal Act, Jim Crow laws, legalized slavery, executive order 9,066—forcing Japanese Americans into internment camps, withholding the right to vote from all except White men, laws that made same-sex marriage illegal and barred same-sex couples from adopting children, and a number of other harmful policies.

RECENT DEVELOPMENTS

Every year, the NASW puts out the Blueprint of Federal Social Policy Priorities with recommendations to the administration on policies that "enhance human well-being and help meet the basic needs of all people, especially those who are vulnerable, oppressed, and/or living in poverty" (NASW, 2021b, para. 1). These priorities can be found on the Advocacy page of the NASW website, linked in the electronic resources section of this chapter. The priorities for the most recent Blueprint include the following (NASW, 2021b, para. 5):

- Support Our Essential Social Work Workforce
- Continue COVID-19 Recovery
- Improve Access to Mental and Behavioral Health and Social Care Services
- Provide High-Quality Healthcare for All
- Build Healthy Relationships to End Violence
- Advance Long and Productive Lives
- Eradicate Social Isolation
- End Homelessness
- Create Social Responses to Climate Change
- Harness Technology for Social Good
- Eliminate Racism
- Build Financial Capability for All
- Reduce Extreme Economic Inequality
- Achieve Equal Opportunity and Justice
- Advance Political Justice
- Reform Immigration Policy
- Protect and Provide for Maltreated Children
- Serve America's Veterans and Their Families
- Advance Lesbian, Gay, Bisexual, Transgender, and Queer Rights
- Promote the Rights of People With Disabilities

ADVOCACY

Schneider and Lester (2001) analyzed the literature and found more than 90 distinct definitions of advocacy. Schneider et al. (2013) point out that due to the multiple meanings and lack of common understanding, the field of social work neglected to refine its skill set around advocacy practice. Herbert and Mould (1992) felt this neglect prompted many social workers to believe that advocacy was something done primarily individually with a client by arranging services, not by partisan intervention when necessary.

Schneider and Lester (2001) defined social work advocacy as "the exclusive and mutual representation of a client(s) or a cause in a forum, attempting to systematically influence decision-making in an unjust or unresponsive system(s)" (p. 64). The benefit of this specific definition is that it explains the action piece of advocacy, not only the outcome piece of advocacy. Also, this definition is useful as it can be applied to micro, mezzo, and macro social work roles in a variety of settings. Schneider et al. (2013) hone in on specific language within the definition to explain some of the ways in which social workers act out advocacy. These include communicating concerns of the client, standing up for another person or group, and/or serving as an agent or proxy for another.

As Ritter (2013) points out, advocacy allows social workers to impact the lives of vulnerable populations by effecting large-scale social or political change. Social workers have unique, direct experience working with individuals, communities, and families, and as such, should use that expertise to weigh in on proposed legislation through advocacy efforts.

PROMOTING SOCIAL JUSTICE

Advocacy and the promotion of social justice are linked by the Preamble of the NASW *Code of Ethics* (2021a). Social justice is a broad concept that encompasses fair and unbiased treatment of all individuals, eradication of discriminatory practices and institutionalized oppression, and establishment of equality for members of historically marginalized and oppressed groups—achieved through the establishment of truly equal opportunity and access to resources (Barsky, 2010; Reisch, 2002; Young, 2001). The CSWE addresses the social justice mandate by stating that "the purpose of social work is actualized through its quest for social, racial, economic, and environmental justice; the creation of conditions that facilitate the realization of human rights; the elimination of poverty; and the enhancement of life for all people, locally and globally" (CSWE, 2022, p. 14) and specifically call upon all social workers to "recognize the historical, social, racial, cultural, economic, organizational, environmental, and global influences that affect social policy and critique the history and current structures of social policies and services and the role of policy in service delivery through rights-based, anti-oppressive, and anti-racist lenses … and engage in and advocate for anti-racist and anti-oppressive policy practice to effect change in those settings" (CSWE, 2022, p. 10–11).

What does promoting social justice look like in practice? While often thought of by social workers as a mezzo- or macro-level intervention only, the knowledge base of the field has theorized the promotion of social justice in all levels of social work—clinical social workers need not feel disempowered to incorporate social justice practices in to their daily work (Aldarondo, 2007; Johnson, 1999; Mitchell & Lynch, 2003; Parker, 2003; Stuart, 1999; Van Wormer, 2004). It can take many forms (Birkenmaier, 2003; Finn & Jacobson, 2008):

- advocacy
- empowerment of clients through consciousness-raising, skill-building, and resource development
- community education and organizing
- legislative and media activism

- social movement participation
- policy analysis and development
- violence intervention
- diversity promotion
- program development and evaluation

Social workers must be prepared to become part of a values-driven and applied profession (Havig, 2013). For many social workers in the field, there is a lack of specific attention to social justice practices—this is a disservice to the social worker's efforts in building their efficacy in this realm (De Maria, 1992). As Havig (2013) aptly points out, to move toward the promotion of social justice within social work education, and specifically in field placements, the social work student must be purposeful and proactive in seeking out opportunities to engage in order to obtain those skills. Seeking out these opportunities is truly parallel to the challenging of social injustices and oppression in society, as they will require intentional effort on behalf of the social worker (Havig, 2013).

ENGAGING IN ADVOCACY EFFORTS

Most agree that being actively engaged in issues of public concerns leads to stronger communities; however, most Americans feel that civic engagement is a choice, not a responsibility (Ritter, 2013). While that may be the opinion of many Americans, social workers know that we are truly obligated, as was discussed earlier in this chapter. Our profession is the only one in the United States that has a mission of social justice (Ritter, 2013). And indeed, social workers are uniquely positioned to be working toward social justice through advocacy efforts. Much like the clinical skills needed in social work direct practice, advocacy requires commitment, determination, patience, energy, support, the use of research, and evaluation and assessment skills. Also useful are political skills and knowledge of government and those involved in it (Schneider & Lester, 2001).

The ultimate goal of advocacy is to influence the modification, change, initiation, or altering of decisions by individuals or groups with authority or power over policies or resources that, in some way, impact others (Schneider et al., 2013). Some advocacy activities include establishing coalitions; forming client groups; educating community members and groups; reaching out to legislators or other decision-makers through letters, emails, phone calls, or individual meetings; providing testimony; and petitioning review boards (Hepworth et al., 2006). Similar to policy practice in organizations, there are steps to the process that allow for a more effective advocacy process (Schneider & Lester, 2001, pp. 116–147)

1. identify the issues and set goals;

2. get the facts;

3. plan strategies and tactics;

4. supply leadership;

5. get to know decision-makers and their staff;

6. broaden the base of support;

7. be persistent; and

8. evaluate your advocacy effort.

Ritter (2013) encourages social workers to advocate on issues they are already passionate about, reach out to those already working in that arena, and find out how you can be helpful to the cause. Ritter (2013) suggests multiple ways that social workers can become engaged in advocacy efforts

- joining an organization that is focused on your passion issue or issues, such as the National Alliance on Mental Illness (NAMI) or Court Appointed Special Advocates (CASA);

- joining in on electoral work, either on behalf of a specific issue (e.g., Medicaid expansion) or candidate(s) that support your issue(s); fundraising on behalf of a specific organization;

- influencing legislation by speaking directly with legislators, especially on local issues impacting clients;

- grassroots lobbying—this is lobbying that occurs on behalf of an organization or campaign to inform decision-makers, such as legislators, about specific legislation that you and the organization either support or oppose;

- obtaining media coverage about the importance of the specific issue you are focused on—this can be achieved by writing an opinion editorial (op-ed) or writing letters to the editor of local newspapers, using social media, or participating in action-oriented activities (rallies, protests, marches, etc.) with the intent to bringing media attention to the cause;

- bringing together groups of people that are focused on the same issue to gain power in numbers and the pooling of resources, also known as coalition building (e.g., environmentalist groups and outdoor sporting groups joining forces on protecting public lands);

- providing testimony in legislative committee hearings to share powerful stories that are related to specific issues (always remember to obtain client consent before sharing their story when testifying, and always protect the client's confidentiality even when permission is granted);

- providing education outreach about your specific issue; and

- utilizing civil disobedience or political dissent—this is considered going "outside" the system to participate in sit-ins, pickets, and other forms of protests that attract visibility. Civil disobedience takes special consideration and a full understanding of potential ramifications (e.g., arrest, ticketing).

EMPOWERING CLIENTS TO ADVOCATE FOR THEMSELVES

In micro practice, we focus on the strengths perspective and the empowerment approach—this focus goes beyond the individual work with clients. Social workers are asked to involve clients and community members in evaluating collective strengths and identifying opportunities for change (Long et al., 2006). The social worker does this by assisting in the formation of community-based groups. These groups are

> **Field Reflection Questions**
>
> What is an issue you are passionate about? What are you already doing in this arena? Which of the listed ways would you be more comfortable doing to advocate for that issue? What would be the one you would be least comfortable doing?
>
> What organizations are associated with the issue that you identified as being passionate about? Would you want to join forces with an organization, or advocate on your own?

designed to fulfill multiple roles: provide support for community members, assess the collective's resources, and find ways to advocate for policies and practices designed to improve the community's collective condition. Social workers should seek to establish spaces, electronic and in-person, that encourage open and productive dialogue among members.

Social workers need to be careful not to restrict the empowerment of community members, and to ensure others do not as well. Action, intentional or not, that compromises the community members' ability to be active participants in advocating for specific policies and programs is to be avoided. Including community members in the advocacy process is vital. When working with others that are not community members, but perhaps leaders or professionals that are also passionate about the issue, the social worker may have to encourage a reorientation of how community members are perceived. These individuals must acknowledge community members as rightful stakeholders and decision-makers during the advocacy process (Long et al., 2006).

Principles have been identified to help ensure that inclusion of community members is successful and beneficial for the community members. It is the social worker's responsibility to create opportunities for nonintrusive collaboration; establish mutual trust and respect; encourage a common analysis of strengths and issues; promote a commitment to solidarity; emphasize equality in relationships; focus on the process; recognize the importance of promoting inclusive and collegial language; and set a foundation that allows strengths to emerge. Thinking back to Chapter 7, we know the importance of honoring the community members' role as the experts on themselves and their communities—it is our role to also remind others of this fact when working together to advocate for common interests.

When possible, clients and community members should be encouraged to engage in any of the advocacy practices listed in the previous section—from joining organizations, to lobbying, to using media, and more. However, we as social workers know that the ability to carry out these tasks requires a substantial amount of resources. As such, there are a multitude of reasons why this may not be possible—the client may be intimidated to testify in front of professionals or legislators, they may be unwilling to share their marginalized status out of fear of retribution (e.g., violence, discrimination, deportation), they may be unable to attend such activities due to transportation issues or work responsibilities, and so on. These circumstances are when it is appropriate to advocate on behalf of the client or community member—working in close concert with them to carefully craft the message, only sharing the information that they have granted you permission to share, and always doing so anonymously.

APPLICATION TO FIELD PLACEMENT

The CSWE (2018) has instituted the "Policy Practice in Field Initiative" to create opportunities for social work students to develop skills around policy practice and deepen their knowledge around the intersection of race, ethnicity, and poverty. It is safe to assume that this initiative is the response to an identified gap in the skill building of social workers around policy practice within their field placements. This probably is not a surprise to many of you reading this chapter. While reading the different ways in which to engage in policy practice, it may feel as though you do not have the time or authority to engage in policy practice within your current placement.

Policy practice can occur at any level and can occur regardless of placement. Some ways that you can engage in policy practice in your field placement include identifying relevant existing policies to your agency or client population, identifying publicly available data sources, identifying legislators that are involved in advocacy pertaining to your field area or client population, and identifying federal, state, and local organizations that are working on key issues related to your work. Similarly, getting involved in legislative advocacy that pertains to your work in your field placement—including contacting legislators to address key barriers your clients are facing—is an exceptionally useful way of applying policy practice to your work. Also, signing up for Listservs and Clearinghouses to keep you up to date on pertinent information pertaining to your field placement is a very easy and helpful way to stay involved and get ongoing invitations to different advocacy events. Share the information you obtain through these activities with your field supervisor. Perhaps the two of you can brainstorm ways of further engaging in policy within your practice and mobilize others within the agency to get involved as well.

CASE SUMMARY: "BUT I AM CLINICAL"

PRACTICE SETTING DESCRIPTION

My name is Rita and I am a second-year MSW student completing an internship at a community counseling center in the northwest. The agency provides individual and family counseling services on a sliding fee scale to members of the surrounding community, most of whom are refugees from African countries, as our community is a resettlement area for incoming refugees. I work with clients on a variety of issues—mostly depression, anxiety, and posttraumatic stress disorder. My role at the agency has thus far been entirely clinical, which I am fine with because I want to become a licensed clinical social worker (LCSW).

PRESENTING PROBLEM

A new law has been proposed in my state with a stated goal of saving taxpayer money. This proposed law does two different things:

1. *Address a perceived problem of encouraging dependency on the government by reducing the amount of time refugees would qualify for specific social welfare services. Currently, the state augments federal funding to allow refugees access to certain social welfare services such as cash assistance, subsidized housing, day care, Medicaid, counseling services, and translation and interpretation services for 8 months to 1 year. The proposed bill would take away all state funding and drastically reduce refugees' ability to receive support while adjusting to the expectations of living in the United States and looking for employment.*

2. *Additionally, the proposed legislation would deny the children of refugees access to state-funded social services.*

This issue has been receiving an increased amount of media attention in recent years. People in our community are highly polarized over the issue. Racial tensions are also rising as a result of the increased attention and the proposed legislation. Recently, an anti-refugee group has begun a social media campaign stoking racial tensions and spreading inaccurate information about the cost of these services to taxpayers, unemployment rates in the area, and incidences of violence perpetrated by refugees. This campaign is implying that refugees are increasing the crime rate and "stealing" jobs, neither of which have been shown to be true in the crime or employment data.

My clients are sharing increased incidences of hate-filled and racist interactions in the community, and many are scared for their safety and the safety of their children. They are stressing about what they will do if their cash assistance and child care are cut off before the original termination date, and most are too afraid to reach out to the legislators in our area, as they are the ones that proposed the legislation.

CASE PROCESS SUMMARY

I am very upset about the proposed legislation, the anti-refugee campaign, and how many people in the community are falling for their lies. My clients are already experiencing the negative ramifications of this legislation and it hasn't even been passed in to a law. The thought of going to speak to my legislator is terrifying to me, because I know he and I are in disagreement on these issues. And somewhat selfishly, I am wondering if it is appropriate for me to be utilizing field placement time to be looking into how to potentially do something about this bill when my title is clinical social work intern.

Rita, Clinical MSW Student Intern

CASE DISCUSSION QUESTIONS

1. *Think about your own values. Think about the values of the profession of social work. How does this legislation fit within those values? Do you agree with the proposed legislation personally? What about professionally?*

2. *Evaluate what you know about the proposed legislation through the lens of the NASW* Code of Ethics. *Do you believe that this legislation would be harmful to Rita's clients? If so, what aspects of the NASW* Code of Ethics *would come into play?*

3. *What actions should Rita take? If you were in the same situation as Rita, how would you feel about the potential for taking on the actions you detailed for her?*

4. *Do you believe that action on this legislation is Rita's role as a clinical social work intern? Why or why not?*

END-OF-CHAPTER RESOURCES

 A robust set of instructor resources designed to supplement this text is located at http://connect.springerpub.com/content/book/978-0-8261-3753-1. Qualifying instructors may request access by emailing textbook@springerpub.com.

CRITICAL THINKING QUESTIONS

1. Elizabeth is a social worker who is working with the National Coalition Against Domestic Violence. Elizabeth has been discussing with a long-term client the potential of testifying in favor of legislation that provides additional resources for victims of domestic violence. Elizabeth had been working with the client for several weeks crafting her testimony—it was a powerful and heartbreaking account of her experience with domestic violence, and how much she would have benefited from the additional resources that may become available through this legislation. Two days before testimony was set to begin, the client called Elizabeth to say she just could not go through with a public testimony. The pain of recounting her story in front of so many would be more than she could handle. What are some potential options for Elizabeth and the client? Discuss how you would approach this scenario. Reflect on and describe your affective reaction to this scenario.

2. Think about your current field placement. What issue would you be able to advocate for on behalf of the clients you serve in your field placement? How could you envision yourself doing so within the agency? How would you envision advocating for your clients outside the organization? Identify what skills you possess that would help you during your advocacy effort. What skills would you like to improve?

3. Engaging in advocacy efforts requires an attention to diversity and inclusion, Competency 3. You must recognize the client and community members as the experts on their experience about the social issue targeted, much like you do while engaging in a helping relationship beyond difference. What skills do you utilize to be able to engage your clients in a helping relationship beyond difference that would also be useful in advocacy work?

4. In reflecting upon your work with clients in your field placement, identify a time when a client discussed an issue that reflected a social issue more than a personal issue. Reflect on and describe what social issue came up. Describe how you could potentially empower the client to advocate toward improving this specific social issue. If you are unsure, how might you go about finding out potential options?

LEARNING ACTIVITIES

1. Identify a policy at your agency that could use updating or is potentially problematic. Utilize the PREPARE organizational assessment of change potential to address the chosen policy concern at your agency.

2. Earlier in this chapter there was a discussion of the importance of seeking out opportunities for policy practice as it pertains to those you serve. Identify two or three policy practice opportunities at your field placement, and assess what a micro-, mezzo-, or macro-level policy practice approach might look like for each opportunity identified.

3. Examine recent local and state government legislative developments that impact the clients you work with at your agency. These bills may positively or negatively impact your clients or your field placement agency. Work with your supervisor to determine an appropriate policy practice approach to address this legislation. This may take the form of a meeting with a representative, testifying at a committee hearing, writing a letter to representatives or an op-ed in a local newspaper, and more.

ELECTRONIC RESOURCES

WEBSITE LINKS

Advocacy—National Association of Social Workers:
www.socialworkers.org/Advocacy

NASW Social Work Talks Podcast: www.socialworkers.org/news/nasw-social-work-talks-podcast

 Education Resources—Council on Social Work Education: https://www.cswe.org/education-resources/?

 Advocacy Handbook for Social Workers—Dan Beerman, ACSW, LCSW: https://cdn.ymaws.com/sites/naswnc.site-ym.com/resource/resmgr/Advocacy/Advocacyhandbook.pdf

VIDEO LINKS

 Labor Movement Leader—Delores Huerta: www.youtube.com/watch?v=eyEkOzYFf20

 The Role of the Social Worker—Steve Perry: www.c-span.org/video/?320179-1/discussion-role-social-workers

 David Sant Testimony in Support of HB 2,307—NASW Oregon: www.youtube.com/watch?v=mg_Zcb27tR8

 Community Organizers Share Experiences—Silberman School of Social Work at Hunter College: www.youtube.com/watch?v=fmKFSjp9CI0

Environmental Justice—Peggy Shepard at TEDxHarlem: www.youtube.com/watch?v=zJX_MXaXbJA

A Brief History of Social Work—Maria Beatriz Alvarez, LCSW-R & Michael Bettencourt, MFA: www.youtube.com/watch?v=CxctzJg-p-g

REFERENCES

Aldarondo, E. (Ed.). (2007). *Advancing social justice through clinical practice*. Routledge.

Barsky, A. E. (2010). *Ethics and values in social work: An integrated approach for a comprehensive curriculum*. Oxford University Press.

Birkenmaier, J. (2003). On becoming a social justice practitioner. *Journal of Religion and Spirituality in Social Work: Social Thought, 22*(2–3), 41–54. https://doi.org/10.1080/15426432.2003.9960340

Council on Social Work Education. (2018). *Policy practice in field education initiative*. https://www.cswe.org/Centers-Initiatives/Initiatives/Policy-Practice-in-Field-Education-Initiative

Council on Social Work Education. (2022). *Educational policy and accreditation standards for baccalaureate and master's social work programs*. https://www.cswe.org/getmedia/94471c42-13b8-493b-9041-b30f48533d64/2022-EPAS.pdf

De Maria, W. (1992). Alive on the street, dead in the classroom: The return of radical social work and the manufacture of activism. *Journal of Sociology and Social Welfare, 19*(3), 137–158.

DiNitto, D. M. (2011). *Social welfare: Politics and public policy* (7th ed.). Pearson.

Finn, J. L., & Jacobson, M. (2008). *Just practice: A social justice approach to social work* (2nd ed.). Eddie Bowers Publishing.

Harding, S. (2004). The sound of silence: Social work, the academy, and Iraq. *Journal of Sociology & Social Welfare, 31*(2), 179–197.

Havig, K. (2013). Empowering students to promote social justice: A qualitative study of field instructors' perceptions and strategies. *Field Educator, 3*(2), 1–24.

Hepworth, D. H., Rooney, R. H., Dewberry-Rooney, G., Strom-Gottfried, K., & Larsen, J. A. (2006). *Direct social work practice: Theory and skills* (7th ed.). Brooks/Cole.

Herbert, M. D., & Mould, J. W. (1992). The advocacy role in public child welfare. *Child Welfare, 71*(2), 114–130.

Jansson, B. (2018). *Becoming an effective policy advocate: From policy practice to social justice*. Brooks/Cole.

Johnson, Y. M. (1999). Indirect work: Social work's uncelebrated strength. *Social Work, 44*(4), 323–334. https://doi.org/10.1093/sw/44.4.323

Kirst-Ashman, K. K., & Hull, G. H., Jr. (2001). *Macro skills workbook: A generalist approach*. Brooks/Cole.

Long, D. D., Tice, C. J., & Morrison, J. D. (2006). *Macro social work practice: A strengths perspective*. Brooks/Cole.

Mitchell, J., & Lynch, R. S. (2003). Beyond the rhetoric of social and economic justice: Redeeming the social work advocacy role. *Race, Gender, and Class, 10*(2), 8–26.

National Association of Social Workers. (2021a). *Code of ethics*. https://www.socialworkers.org/About/Ethics/Code-of-Ethics/Code-of-Ethics-English

National Association of Social Workers. (2021b). *2021 blueprint of federal social policy priorities*. https://www
.socialworkers.org/Advocacy/Policy-Issues/2021-Blueprint-of-Federal-Social-Policy-Priorities

Netting, F. E., Kettner, P. M., McMurtry, S. L., & Thomas, L. (2017). *Social work macro practice* (6th ed.).
Pearson.

Parker, L. (2003). A social justice model for clinical social work practice. *Affilia, 18*(3), 272–288. https://doi
.org/10.1177/0886109903254586

Pawar, M. (2019). Social work and social policy practice: Imperatives for political engagement. *The International
Journal of Community and Social Development, 1*(1) 15–27. https://doi.org/10.1177/2516602619833219

Reisch, M. (2002). Defining social justice in a socially unjust world. *Families in Society: The Journal of
Contemporary Social Services, 83*(4), 343–354. https://doi.org/10.1606/1044-3894.17

Ritter, J. A. (2013). *Social work policy practice: Changing our community, our nation, and the world*. Pearson.

Schneider, R. L., & Lester, L. (2001). *Social work advocacy: A new framework for action*. Wadsworth/Thomson
Learning.

Schneider, R. L., Lester, L., & Ochieng, J. (2013). Advocacy. In *Encyclopedia of social work*. NASW Press and
Oxford University Press. https://doi.org/10.1093/acrefore/9780199975839.013.623

Stuart, P. H. (1999). Linking clients and policy: Social work's distinctive contribution. *Social Work, 44*(4),
335–347. https://doi.org/10.1093/sw/44.4.335

Van Wormer, K. (2004). *Confronting oppression, restoring justice: From policy analysis to social action*. CSWE
Press.

Young, I. M. (2001). Equality of whom? Social groups and judgments of injustice. *Journal of Political
Philosophy, 9*(1), 1–18. https://doi.org/10.1111/1467-9760.00115

Engaging With Individuals, Families, Groups, Organizations, and Communities

Josh is a senior BSW field placement student interning as a client advocate at a county-based resource center for individuals with disabilities. Josh participated in a care plan meeting to discuss his client, Scott, and review his treatment plans. Scott, 57 years old, had received a variety of services most of his life, as he was diagnosed with autism and learning disabilities at the age of 4. Each of Scott's service providers explained the issues they had encountered in providing him care. His service providers from the respite program, his adult day care center, and his in-home care provider shared their concerns. Scott was expressing frustration and confusion about his care plan, stating that he was hearing different things from different people. After attending the meeting, it became clear that everyone on the team was giving Scott the same information, but the differences in how they described the information made it challenging for Scott to understand. Josh met with Scott's social worker and debriefed her. After reviewing the information, the social worker suggested that each of the care providers brainstorm a potential alternative approach for Scott's care and regroup for another interprofessional meeting in 2 weeks' time. The meeting was attended by Scott's social worker, all of his care providers, and Josh. After sharing potential approaches, the interprofessional team decided to utilize the suggestion Scott's in-home care provider had: identify one member of the team as Scott's go-to person for clarification about his treatment plan. All questions that any member of the team received from Scott would be routed to that go-to person ensuring that Scott would know who to go to with his questions and that he would not get differently worded answers from multiple people essentially saying the same thing. A second meeting was set for 4 weeks later to review the effectiveness of the new approach.

What relationship qualities need to be present among all members of Scott's care team for the interprofessional approach to be effective? What are some of the strengths of the work the team did in this case example? What are some of the potential pitfalls? Suppose one of the care team members becomes hostile or resistant to continued meetings. What would be Josh's next steps? What would be the potential downside to not having all of Scott's care providers at the meeting?

COMPETENCY 6: ENGAGE WITH INDIVIDUALS, FAMILIES, GROUPS, ORGANIZATIONS, AND COMMUNITIES

Social workers understand that engagement is an ongoing component of the dynamic and interactive process of social work practice with and on behalf of individuals, families, groups, organizations, and communities.

Social workers value the importance of human relationships. Social workers understand theories of human behavior and person-in-environment and critically evaluate and apply this knowledge to facilitate engagement with clients and constituencies, including individuals, families, groups, organizations, and communities. Social workers are self-reflective and understand how bias, power, and privilege as well as their personal values and personal experiences may affect their ability to engage effectively with diverse clients and constituencies. Social workers use the principles of interprofessional collaboration to facilitate engagement with clients, constituencies, and other professionals as appropriate.

Social workers

- apply knowledge of human behavior and person-in-environment, as well as interprofessional conceptual frameworks, to engage with clients and constituencies; and

- use empathy, reflection, and interpersonal skills to engage in culturally responsive practice with clients and constituencies. (Council on Social Work Education, 2022, p. 11)

LEARNING OBJECTIVES

By the end of this chapter, you will be able to:

- Describe the role engagement plays in the helping relationship and the change process.

- Understand the importance of collaboration and trust building across all levels of social work practice.

- Understand the importance of interprofessional collaboration.

- Use skills that will make you more effective in collaboration with clients, colleagues, and interprofessional teammates.

- Identify potential pitfalls that may arise in the interpersonal and interprofessional collaborative relationship.

THE HELPING RELATIONSHIP

Sinai-Glazer (2020, p. 1) referred to the helping relationship between the social worker and the client as "the heart and soul in social work." When reading about the helping relationships, the term *client* is used to describe individual clients, as well as families, groups, communities, and organizations. The quality of the helping relationship between the social worker and the client is vital to the outcome the client experiences. Indeed, this phenomenon has been consistently cited within the empirical research (Glicken, 2009; Norcross, 2011; Warren, 2001). Saleebey (2008) discusses the importance of nonjudgment, trust, care, and competence as necessary, regardless of the issue that the client is focused on. Many scholars and clinicians believe that the actual helping relationship does not commence until all parties have established confidence in the others' competence and care. Glicken (2009) believes that the helping relationship is the trust that all parties put into the belief that their collaboration will lead to a positive outcome.

Authenticity has also been identified as a necessity for the helping relationship. Approaching the client with genuine concern, empathy, and warmth improves the relationships (Glicken, 2009). Empathy is the "act of perceiving, understanding, experiencing, and responding to the emotional state and ideas of another person" (Barker, 2014, p. 149). This means that you as a social worker must allow yourself to be genuinely concerned for the client, and respond, with warmth, to what your clients say. Given that most individuals seeking services have experienced trauma, loss, poverty, discrimination, and injustices, it is our responsibilities as social workers to provide them a helping relationship with the highest potential for meaningful, positive outcomes. We must lay the foundation to set clients up to thrive in the helping relationship by utilizing the skills of nonjudgmental care, competence, and empathy. The social work practice elaboration and empathy practice skills also contribute significantly to the development of a positive helping relationship. Recent qualititative research out of Israel identified seven different elements of a positive helping relationship: love (with varied meanings) and support; trust and feeling safe; listening and feeling understood; making an effort to help; humanness, compassion, and sensitivity; availability, continuity, and being there when needed; and chemistry (Sinai-Glazer, 2020).

ELABORATION SKILLS

Elaboration skills are micro-intervention techniques that encourage clients to tell their stories in detail. They help build trust and client engagement in the helping relationship. To understand a client's situation and perspective, we need to have their stories told in detail. The power of the story is in the specifics. Most people tend to avoid specifics and begin discussing their situation in very general terms. The social worker's job is to help the client tell a detailed story rich in facts and feelings. There are seven elaboration skills—using open-ended questions, using minimal prompts, seeking concreteness, summarizing, containment, exploring silences, and reframing.

Using Open-Ended Questions

There are basically two types of questions: those with predefined responses and those without predefined responses. The former is usually referred to as closed-ended questions. They do not encourage a detailed and elaborate response, and generally should be avoided. An example of a closed-ended question is, "Do you get along well with the other kids at school?" If the client responds at all, the answer will be yes or no. This is the only answer called for. Not much information is obtained from this type of question.

Alternatively, one should ask open-ended questions that elicit more information from the client. For example, the social worker could ask, "How do you get along with the other kids at school?" This cannot be answered with just a yes or no response. The client has to formulate a more detailed or elaborate response to answer the question. Although the questions are similar, the open-ended one encourages elaboration, whereas the closed-ended one does not.

Limit your use of closed-ended questions. If a question is warranted, ask an open-ended one.

Using Minimal Prompts

As the term implies, minimal prompts are brief nonverbal or verbal indications of encouragement. Nonverbal minimal prompts include "nodding the head, using facial expressions, or employing gestures that convey receptivity, interest, and commitment to understanding" (Hepworth et al., 2017, p. 140). These nonverbal prompts can be very effective in encouraging elaboration. They communicate in an attentive and nonintrusive way that you would like the client to tell you more and that you are interested in hearing their story.

Verbal minimal prompts are brief utterances such as "Mm-mmm" or "Ah-ha" or other short phrases such as "Tell me more" or "I see." As with the nonverbal prompts, the verbal ones encourage the client to go on without interrupting or asking a series of questions.

Another type of minimal prompt is an **accent response** in which the worker repeats a client's word or short phrase in the form of a question. The word or phrase selected should be the core component of the client's message. For example, if the client says, "I just hate all the kids at school," the social worker might say "Hate?" or "The kids?" to prompt the client to give more information about the client's feelings about the kids at school. Accent responses are easy to use, do not interrupt the flow of communication, and are very effective in getting clients to explore their feelings and concerns in depth.

Seeking Concreteness

As noted earlier, clients tend to introduce their concerns and describe their experiences in vague, general terms. Beginning social workers often do not probe for specifics and may allow clients to keep the conversation at a general level. Hepworth et al. (2017) point out that communicating one's feelings and experiences requires specificity. They call the process of helping clients to respond in specific terms "seeking concreteness"; Shulman (2009) refers to it as moving from the general to the specific.

Often clients begin their stories in general terms because they have never put their feelings and experiences into words. They need help in exploring their feelings and experiences. Asking for specifics helps clients articulate their stories. Thus, seeking concreteness not only deepens your understanding of clients' stories but also helps clients understand and articulate their feelings and experiences.

Seeking concreteness is easy to do. The key is to recognize and respond to vague and overly general comments. For example, a community member might say, "The neighborhood is falling apart. It is just not the same anymore." This is a fairly vague statement. At this point, the social worker really does not know what is causing the frustration. The worker could seek more concrete information by asking an open-ended follow-up question, such as, "How has it changed?" or "What do you mean by falling apart?" Both responses invite the client to elaborate on their concerns.

Summarizing

Summarizing is a basic interviewing skill that is often used to highlight key points in a conversation with a client. When used this way, summarizing can help the client and worker make the transition to a different topic. Summarizing, however, can also be used as an elaboration technique. This entails making connections between relevant aspects of a client's story. Summarizing can help clients explore in depth feelings and experiences that they might not recognize as being connected. This can be a powerful tool in helping them gain insight and understanding.

Summarizing is a more difficult skill to use than the other elaborating skills discussed earlier. It is a filtering and feedback process. It requires the ability to identify the key components of the story, pull them together, and repeat them back to the client in a combination statement–question form. The statement–question form prevents the social worker from taking the position of knowing or presuming to know that the different points are connected for the client. Typically, a summary statement is concluded with a question to see if the worker's perception or summary is consistent with the client's view of the situation.

Using Containment

Shulman (2009) defines containment as the skill of not acting. Many beginning social workers, in their desire to be helpful, rush in with solutions before the client has told their story. Containment is the ability to hold back on this impulse. It also is an important skill for those who tend to finish a client's sentences or to focus on identified outcomes very early in the helping process.

Exploring Silences

This skill involves attempting to explore the meaning of the silence. It is hard to understand the meaning of silences. The client might be processing a thought, struggling with powerful emotions, feeling bored, or any number of things. Beginning social workers are often uncomfortable with silence and rush in to fill it up. Doing so ensures that the meaning of the silence will be lost as the worker moves on to something else. The social worker needs to actively explore the silence. A clue to its meaning is the worker's own feelings (Shulman, 2009). Understanding one's own feelings at a particular moment helps one to make an educated guess about the meaning of the client's silence and actively explore the meaning of the silence.

The first strategy for dealing with silence is containment. Give the client some time and stay with the silence. A simple probing question, such as, "You are quiet right now. What's going on?" is often sufficient to get the client to open up. You have acknowledged the silence and encouraged the client to elaborate. If your feelings suggest that the client is feeling *(hurt)* then you could ask an open-ended question, such as, "Are you struggling with the *(hurt)* you feel?" The client needs to be encouraged to let the worker know if the guess is wrong. Even if the worker is off base, there is little harm done. The client can correct the misperception. Either way, the silence has been acknowledged and its meaning explored. Rather than feeling uncomfortable during periods of silence, view them as opportunities to better understand your client and their story.

Reframing

Reframing is a technique that is used often in family therapy. It is sometimes referred to as relabeling. Reframing is the process of giving a positive interpretation to what the client sees as a negative or concern. It is reframing a negative into a positive. In strengths-based social work, this is an important technique. It provides the worker with a way to highlight positives and help clients view their concerns from a different, more positive, perspective. It helps the identification of strengths and coping abilities. Reframing is an elaboration skill in that it invites clients to explore their stories from a different perspective. For example, a mother might say she is a bad parent because her daughter was suspended from school. A social worker might reframe this negative comment by pointing how well she had done raising her other children and that her daughter up to this point has done well in school and that they have a strong mother/daughter relationship.

EMPATHY SKILLS

Conveying understanding and empathy are critical to the development of trust and a positive helping relationship. The skilled use of empathy in your interactions with your clients will enable you to help your clients engage in the change process. The key empathy skills are focused listening, reflective empathy, and additive empathy.

Focused Listening

Focused listening (Shulman, 2009) or active listening (Chang et al., 2018) is the process of concentrating on a specific part of the client's message. The worker tries to identify the primary themes in the client's story and be sensitive to clues the client may give regarding the underlying feeling content of the message. With additive empathy, the worker tries to reach for the client's underlying feelings.

Focused listening requires the social worker to tune in to the meaning behind the client's words. This involves listening to the client's words, nonverbal communication, and affect as well as what is not being said. Listening and understanding the client's message is the first component of empathy. The second component is communicating your understanding back to the client.

Reflective Empathy

Conveying empathy and understanding is vital in developing a helping relationship. Clients need to feel understood. Those who do not feel understood are unlikely to share personal thoughts and feelings. Why risk vulnerability with someone who does not understand you? Disadvantaged and oppressed clients' experiences of discrimination, abuse, or exploitation have left many feeling profoundly misunderstood (Cournoyer, 2017). The ability to respond empathetically is a critical social work practice skill, particularly when one has to overcome mistrust and reluctance.

In its simplest form, empathetic responding is "reflecting" back to clients their message. At this level, the empathetic response accurately captures the factual content and feelings expressed by the client. The response communicates an equivalent message. Reflective empathy is more effective if you paraphrase the client's words rather than just "parrot back" the same words.

The use of empathetic responding is vital to the development of trust and the building of a strong helping relationship. Respond empathetically whenever your client is dealing with or expressing affective content. If there is an emotional component in the message, either on the surface or below it, an empathetic response is needed. The power of the relationship is in helping clients deal with and manage feelings. Understanding the facts is important, but understanding the feelings is essential. Doing so will communicate that you are listening, that you care about the client, and that you understand or, at the very least, are trying to understand.

Responding to the affective component is beneficial even if you have incorrectly described the client's feelings or their intensity. An incorrect empathetic response gives clients an opportunity to clarify their feelings.

Additive Empathy

This level of empathetic responding occurs when the social worker accurately identifies implicit underlying feelings. Not only does the social worker respond to the surface and underlying feelings, but the response connects the message to other themes of feelings expressed by the client. The use of additive empathy communicates a deeper level of understanding than the more basic reflective empathy. Both require the social worker to "risk" responding to the affective component of the client's message. Many beginning social workers shy away from dealing with clients' feelings directly. It is easier to stick to the facts and ignore the feelings. If one wants to build trust, then responding to the feeling content is necessary. This example is an additive empathetic response to the individual's statement. In this response, the worker tries to reach for the client's underlying feelings.

TRUST BUILDING

Trust, as it is in the supervisory relationship, is an important aspect of the helping relationship. Establishing trust between the social worker and the client has an impact on the collaborative decision-making process, improves communication, and increases the likelihood that clients with follow through with the plans developed with the social worker (Gamble, 2006).

Behnia (2008) defines trust as the ability and will to allow oneself to be vulnerable with others due to one's belief in other individuals' intentions and competence. This means that individuals have confidence that others will behave in a way that is nonharmful or even potentially beneficial (Levin et al., 2006).

At the start of the helping relationship, the only trust that exists is on a surface level. The client may trust the approach more than the individual social worker. They may be willing to try to work with the social worker due to training or expertise or reputation (Behnia, 2008). They enter into the helping relationship with the expectation that the social worker's intentions are positive. However, once the helping relationship is initiated the client begins to assess your trustworthiness and your competence.

Clients utilize a host of tactics to obtain information to arrive at their definition about the social worker. Especially in the beginning of the helping relationship, the clients are gathering information about the social worker's competence (Behnia, 2008). Questions going through the client's head can include: Does the social worker know what they're doing? Do they know enough about my specific issue? Do they actually care? What do they think of me? As a social worker, you must recognize that the client is intensely attuned to your verbal and nonverbal cues to come to their determinations about all the preceding questions and more. An example would be a social worker breaking eye contact or attempting to change the subject when a client attempts to share a trauma experience. With these cues, the client may come to the conclusion that the social worker is unable to handle the topic emotionally or lacks the expertise to help them work through their trauma (Behnia, 2008).

Clients may ask direct questions about your training and/or intentions, they may make assumptions based on your office presentation, they may test your knowledge about a multitude of topics, including a specific diagnosis to your understanding of oppression and racism, and they may ask personal questions to see if you may have had personal experience with the topic they want to discuss. Clients may also try to gather information to inform their perception of you as a worthwhile individual. Behnia (2008) shares that this is often done by disclosing potentially jarring information to be able to observe the social worker's reaction.

If you react negatively, showing signs of disgust, disapproval, or discomfort, the client may perceive you as judgmental and unsafe.

Building trust with clients is an interactional process. Trust cannot be built in the absence of interpersonal interactions between the client and the social worker. It is built upon a sequence of trusting and trustworthy interactions. Your client must act in a trusting manner by taking some level of risk and you the social worker must respond with trustworthy actions. Building a positive helping relationship is a process. Trust is earned by your behavior and trustworthy responses, and it is not given freely, especially if your clients have experienced oppression, discrimination, poverty, abuse, and/or trauma in their lives.

> **Field Reflection Questions**
>
> Consider your current field placement. How did you begin to lay the foundation for trust with your clients?
>
> Can you think of a time when you utilized empathetic listening skills? How did you convey that you perceived and understood the client's experience? How did you respond?

ENGAGEMENT IN THE TELEHEALTH SETTING

While telehealth did not come about because of the COVID-19 pandemic, many social workers (and social work students in placement) were required to utilize it in order to provide services to their clients. Telehealth is "remote provision of healthcare services using technology to exchange information for the diagnosis, treatment, and prevention of disease" (Weigel et al., 2020, para 2). Telehealth, regarded as an innovative, vital provision technology to support marginalized and underserved populations (Craig et al., 2021), is not without its challenges. Distractions are more common, the directness can cause some discomfort, and, of course, some social work services simply cannot be delivered remotely (e.g., violence, homelessness). Craig et al. (2021) developed a list of both practical and clinical skills considerations and adaptations to take into account when engaging in the online setting. These practical considerations include developing competency with the platforms; allowing time for technology checks with clients (and being willing to troubleshoot and provide instructions); reminding clients about privacy and removing sensitive information from the platform; establishing technology norms; ensuring accessibility needs are addressed; assigning roles with any cofacilitators (e.g., chat monitor, support person in online group settings) ahead of time; and ensuring clients have emergency and crisis information. The engagement considerations include transparency and use of self around awkwardness or discomfort with online modalities; utilizing additional transparency and vulnerability when appropriate; normalizing additional levels of stress or anxiety; adapting activities for the online environment; increasing use of check-in engagement techniques; increasing reminders about sessions; utilizing visual aids to deliver information (e.g., PowerPoint slides, Google Docs); utilizing grounding strategies at the beginning and conclusion of sessions; in groups, utilizing more visual aids and gradually reducing them to enhance comfort with other participants; asking clients to utilize chat function to alert the social worker of break needs, or other concerns; regularly clarifying and repeating; reporting technology issues with the client(s); and highlighting the importance of online community and activities during isolation.

INTERPROFESSIONAL COLLABORATION

As previously touched upon, interprofessional collaboration can be varied and diverse (Kvarnström, 2008). Collaborative care requires providers from different disciplines to work together to provide services to clients in an effective and caring way (Craven & Bland, 2013). Ambrose-Miller and Ashcroft (2016) discuss the factors that facilitate and enhance interprofessional collaborative practice:

- adopting values/ethics for interprofessional practice
- understanding interprofessional roles/responsibilities
- enhancing interprofessional communication
- facilitating teams and teamwork
- understanding organizational structure
- understanding professional identity
- knowing scope of practice
- understanding and addressing problematic power differentials

As social workers, it may be easiest to conceptualize interprofessional collaboration through systems theory (Crawford, 2011). Imagine if you were asked to make a list all of people you interact with in your daily life. It would be extensive, and you could potentially categorize all of the individuals on the list into different groups. You may even be able to map the groups, as a way to visualize the connections and interrelationships between them all. That is essentially how systems theory helps us to describe interprofessional collaboration.

Whittington's (2003) two-stage model of collaboration explains interrelationships between collaborative systems. In the first stage, you identify the main systems that are participating in the collaborative process. In the second stage, you describe the relationship and interchanges between all of the systems in the process. This nonhierarchical model helps to clearly define the boundaries of each system in the collaborative process.

Field Reflection Questions

Consider your current field placement. How might Whittington's (2003) two-stage model be applied to your own experience? What examples from field can you identify?

Using one of the preceding examples, who were the key participants? What were the interactions that took place?

BUILDING PROFESSIONAL RELATIONSHIPS

Understanding your own professional identity is vital to your effective collaboration with other professionals (Ambrose-Miller & Ashcroft, 2016). In order to have this understanding, you must first understand what it means to be a professional in the field of social work. Is it being recognized as part of the field, perhaps by the licensure that is bestowed on you through your state board? Is it adherence to the National Association of Social Workers (NASW) *Code of Ethics* (2021)? Is it something else entirely? Once you have identified what the key elements of professional social work are, you can then apply those standards to your own practice as a social worker (Crawford, 2011). You will develop your professional identity through the interactions you have within your field placement, your educational experiences, and your other environments. Crawford (2011) also points out that professional identity can also be tied to professional contributions, achieved status, uniqueness, power and authority, and self-interest.

Your professional identity comes into play in interprofessional collaboration because many of the aspects of professionalism are required to be an effective member of an interprofessional collaborative team. This can include a commitment to service recipients, explicit values, agreed-upon standards, code of ethics, recognition of the specific disciplinary contribution, and more (Crawford, 2011). One could also argue that it is more challenging to resist protectiveness of territorial expertise if the social worker is not confident in their professional identity, and thus not trying to "prove themselves" to other members of the collaborative process.

> **Field Reflection Questions**
>
> Reflect on yourself in your field placement.
>
> What does it mean to you to be a professional? Do you consider yourself to be a professional? Why or why not?
>
> Can you give examples from your field placement that explain your answer? How might this inform your professional identity?

Also vital is the need for all interprofessional collaborators to recognize the benefits of the collaborating. Crawford (2011) highlights the following benefits: knowledge of professional roles; trust and mutual respect; skillful communication; ability to recognize which member of the team is best suited to meet the needs of the client; and most importantly, having a shared set of values that includes the beliefs, ideas, and assumptions about the service recipients, the goals, and the approach. Clearly, this can be a challenge given that different professions adhere to different professional values.

Even though this is the case, Hammick et al. (2009) identified several core values for interprofessional collaboration:

● respect for everyone in the collaborative team

● confidence in what you know and what you don't know, and in what others know

● a willingness to engage with others rather than take a detached view of proceedings

- a caring disposition toward your colleagues

- an approachable attitude

- showing a willingness to share what you know as a means to the best possible outcome for the user of your service (p. 23)

Crawford (2011) also identified the following skills as necessary for interprofessional collaboration: interpersonal skills such as negotiating, listening, articulating, dealing with conflict, empathy, person-centered practice skills, and the ability to demonstrate trust and respect; and personal skills that include self-awareness, reflexivity, confidence in practice, emotional awareness, problem-solving skills critical thinking skills, and a sense of responsibility.

ROLE AND RESPONSIBILITIES

Having an awareness of one's own role, and the role of others, within the interprofessional collaboration has been noted as being important to the effectiveness of the process. Social workers should be able to clearly and accurately describe their own role and the roles of others in the collaborative process. You should be able to recognize and respect that there are a myriad of roles, responsibilities, and competencies across disciplines. You must consider the impact that performing your role may have on other professionals within the interprofessional group, and recognize that other professions may view the world differently. Although the task may seem easy, understanding one's own and other professionals' roles and responsibilities can be complicated—boundaries between professional roles and responsibilities can become blurred, leading to potential confusion of which professional is responsible for what and when.

Seabury et al. (2011) identified three steps that social workers often use to clarify roles within practice, and they can be applied to interprofessional collaboration as well: explicating various expectations, comparing and identifying discrepancies in expectations, and negotiating agreements on expectations. The first step requires collaborators to identify what they expect from each member of the interprofessional team, including their own responsibilities. In the second step, collaborators compare and examine the different expectations. Conflict and ambiguity that exist are identified. Finally, collaborators come to an agreement on the conflicting perspectives and reinforce areas of agreement. As stated earlier, conflict is to be expected in collaboration, and as such, differences should be viewed as constructive and informative. Done early in the process, role clarification saves time, resources, and potential emotional stress.

Field Reflection Questions

What can you achieve in your field placement by working across systems? What systems can you identify as interconnecting with your field agency?

From your experience in field, how does the system you are in and the systems you work across impact service delivery to clients?

As a social worker, you will hold multiple accountabilities and responsibilities. You are accountable to the clients you work with, to your licensure board, to the NASW (2021) *Code of Ethics*, to your employer, to your colleagues, and to the other professionals with whom you work with. Responsibility and accountability are inextricably linked to trust, discussed earlier in the chapter, and they also require integrity, self-awareness, and a clear sense of responsibility. Interprofessional collaboration can make the lines of accountability difficult to distinguish, and it is your responsibility to make clear your multiple accountability levels to those you are collaborating with.

WORKING ON A TEAM

Ambrose-Miller and Ashcroft (2016) discuss social workers' perspectives on interprofessional collaboration, including what you can expect while working in a team environment. Some of the perspectives reported include:

- Get comfortable in a leadership capacity.

- Attract team members who are seeking out collaboration.

- Be prepared to nurture the collaborative process.

- Advocate for an organization culture that supports collaboration over time saving.

- Be prepared to advocate for social work's contribution to the team.

- Embrace the flexibility of your role as a social worker as a strength.

- Know that your role as client advocate can create tension within the collaborative team.

Social workers identified leadership qualities as important, as those qualities help the social worker to collaborate and speak up within the team environment. They also help to reinforce collaborative ideas. Additionally, it was suggested that individuals who gravitate toward collaboration and egalitarian work environments thrive in the interprofessional process. As such, identifying potential team members who have the skill and mindset for that process and encouraging them to join in is useful. Those interviewed explained that the collaborative process requires nurturance in the form of intentional planning and carving out time for the process. This is easier to do when the overall organization also supports and values interprofessional collaboration. The attitudes of both leadership and employees about interprofessional collaboration seemed to greatly influence the nurturance, of lack thereof, of a collaborative culture. Because so many organizations are overly concerned about efficiencies, you may need to advocate for an intentional push toward collaborative models.

In some settings, your contribution as a social worker will be clear to all members of the collaborative team. However, in other settings, for example, a healthcare setting, the

Field Reflection Questions

How does professional supervision allow you to evaluate your own practice?

How does this process prepare you for interprofessional social work practice?

social worker must utilize their expertise to ensure a humanizing, broad perspective is being taken by the interprofessional team. This takes confidence and speaks to the necessity to have confidence in your role and competence, as discussed earlier in the chapter.

Also identified as a strength was social workers' ability to be flexible in their role and fill a variety of service gaps when necessary. Finally, recognize that the social worker is, at times, the interprofessional team member who is filling the role as client advocate, and this can create tension between team members as there are instances when all other members have a different, often more expedient, plan in mind.

COLLABORATION CHALLENGES

While there are many benefits to interprofessional collaboration, discussed in detail in the next section, there are also potential challenges. Ambrose-Miller and Ashcroft (2016) reported that in-place decision-making procedures at times caused a barrier for a more collaborative decision-making process to exist within the interprofessional team. Typically, interprofessional team members called for a collaborative decision-making process; however, there may be differences across professions regarding the most appropriate decision-making process, especially for team members who often had the final call on decisions in their everyday work life.

Additionally, due to ethical and legal mandates regarding confidentiality, fears around information sharing can be another potential barrier to interprofessional collaboration. Radford (2010) acknowledges the efficient sharing of information is vital to intervention and risk reduction, so a clear delineation of what information is truly confidential and what is appropriate to be shared with the interprofessional team is necessary for the team to operate in the most beneficial way. O'Sullivan (2011) highlights the dire need for effective information sharing strategies in that lack of communication between social service agencies has resulted in cases of children and vulnerable adults being involved in significant tragedies. Clear protocols shared with the interprofessional team early in the process will allow for fewer delays as team members try to establish the confidentiality of specific, vital information.

Power imbalances within the interprofessional team can also cause barriers (Crawford, 2011). Lymbery (2006, as cited in Crawford, 2011) identified three types of interprofessional rivalries that can be a result of power imbalances: Professional identity and territory; relative status and power of professions; different patterns of discretion and accountability between professions. This underlines the importance of a shared purpose, as well as an atmosphere of teamwork. Sharing differing opinions with the same goal looks very different than personal feuds or in-fighting. A constant focus on the goal of the interprofessional team—the outcome for the clients—helps interprofessional collaborators refocus their energies within disagreements.

BENEFITS

Interprofessional collaboration allows professionals from different fields to come together, develop proficiency as a group, share information and knowledge, and see circumstances from a variety of perspectives. Research on the topic of interprofessional collaboration has found multiple benefits (Darlington & Feeney, 2008), including lower anxiety levels of team members, faster access to services for clients, and lower instance of separation in child welfare cases.

In the healthcare area, research has shown the interprofessional collaboration has resulted in improved client experiences, improved health outcomes, and reduction of costs (Vega & Bernard, 2016). This is due to a reduction of errors as a result of the client being switched to a different provider. The interprofessional collaboration approach supports the sharing of essential information to all team members, reducing the risk of errors association with transitions. Additionally, interprofessional collaboration requires a client-centered approach, as discussed earlier. This requires a shift of all team members, including those in the healthcare setting, to move away from the physician-centered system, which has also been found to improve outcomes (Vega & Bernard, 2016). Finally, research indicates that clients and patients who receive interprofessional care are more satisfied and have better health outcomes, including a 30% reduction in ED visits. Finally, healthcare professionals also report being more satisfied with interprofessional collaboration than traditional approaches—with over 95% of professionals stating that it was an improvement (Vega & Bernard, 2016).

While interprofessional collaboration has also been found to be an effective practice model in multiple settings (Darlington & Feeney, 2008; Vega & Bernard, 2016), it is also becoming the expectation for social service and medical providers through policy or organization mandates in some cases. A shift toward interprofessional collaboration has been documented in the United States, the United Kingdom, other parts of Europe, and Australia (Darlington & Feeney, 2008). Perhaps this mandate is justified, as O'Sullivan (2011) points out that information sharing between agencies may have provided social workers the information they needed to intervene and potentially avoid tragic outcomes for vulnerable individuals.

CASE SUMMARY: "NOT SURE WE WILL EVER CLICK"

PRACTICE SETTING DESCRIPTION

My name is Brianna and I am a first-year MSW student completing an internship at a family service agency in a medium-size city on the East Coast. The agency provides individual and family counseling services on a sliding fee scale. The agency also accepts mandated clients referred to fulfil counseling requirements often tied to sentencing related to nonviolent felonies. I was assigned to work with R., who was sentenced to counseling after being charged with possession of illegal prescription medications.

IDENTIFYING DATA

R. is 16 years old and has been in legal trouble once before related to marijuana posses-sion. R. lives with his mother and two younger siblings. R. attends an alternative high school and was working part-time but lost his employment due to missing work after his arrest. The judge in R.'s case decided that R. might benefit from counseling due to his defi-ant attitude over the course of the proceedings. The judge believes R. may have some anger issues and required counseling as a part of a deal to avoid jail time.

PRESENTING PROBLEM

R. is resistant to counseling and has shown little interest in forming a helping rela-tionship. He has indicated that he does not think he needs to be there and has noth-ing to benefit from. He has come in for three sessions and has only spoken about four sentences.

ASSESSMENT

While R. has not shared much information, I do know a little about him from the records we received upon accepting him as a client. I know that R.'s mother is a single-parent who is employed in two part-time jobs, that he has two younger siblings ages 8 and 6, and that R. utilized a public defender for his trial. R.'s mother was supportive of R. receiving counseling.

While R. is obviously extremely reluctant to actually share anything with me during his sessions, I have identified some obvious strengths. First, R.'s mother is supportive of R.'s receipt of counseling. Second, R. has made mention of wanting to fulfil the obligations of his probation, including continuing with the counseling, so he can "move on with his life." When pressed, he shared he wanted to complete high school and obtain training to become an auto mechanic because it pays well, and he believes he would be able to help out his family with that decent income.

CASE PROCESS SUMMARY

I will admit that I am feeling frustrated with the lack of progress that we have made so far. While three sessions over 3 weeks is not a significant amount of time, I am much more used to working with voluntary clients. So, this slow speed is challenging. My typical conversation starters result in one-word answers from R. I know that R. is resistant to the idea of counseling in general, but I also have to wonder if the fact that I am a fairly young White woman, and he is a teenage Latino male may be impacting his ability to see me as someone capable of helping him in any way. I wonder if I should transfer R. to one of the two male social workers who work in the agency, even though there would be a bit of a wait. I am just not sure if we will ever "click."

Brianna, MSW Student Intern

CASE DISCUSSION QUESTIONS

1. *If you were Brianna's supervisor, what questions might you ask Brianna to gauge how she is attempting to build trust with R.?*

2. *If R. was your client, what ways would you attempt to engage him beyond simply asking him questions? What are some of the potential pitfalls to your suggested approaches?*

3. *Thinking back to what you read in this chapter, why might Brianna believe that referral to another social worker makes the most sense in this case? Do you believe it is solely due to their inability to "click" or may there be some other potential barrier for Brianna?*

4. *Imagine Brianna needed to build an interprofessional team to ensure R.'s successful completion of his sentence. Who should Brianna consult to be a part of that interprofessional team? How might this team be able to help R. be successful?*

END-OF-CHAPTER RESOURCES

A robust set of instructor resources designed to supplement this text is located at http://connect.springerpub.com/content/book/978-0-8261-3753-1. Qualifying instructors may request access by emailing textbook@springerpub.com.

CRITICAL THINKING QUESTIONS

1. Earlier in the chapter, we discussed the trust-building process. How might the trust-building process vary for a mandated client in comparison to a voluntary client?

2. In thinking about interprofessional collaboration, how do the necessary skills discussed in the chapter also apply to the competency of demonstrating ethical and professional behavior?

3. Similar to engaging diversity and difference in practice, interprofessional collaboration, and collaboration with groups and organizations, involves humility, curiosity, and ongoing self-reflection. Can you identify a time when you found yourself making an assumption about a professional in another field (e.g., a doctor, a teacher)? In reflecting upon your experience working interprofessionally, how might these assumptions impact your ability to be a fully engaged member of an interprofessional team?

4. Earlier in the chapter, the trust-building process is described as a two-way street. The client must trust your intentions and competence as the helping

professional, but you must also trust the client has the capacity to make positive changes. Reflect on your experience in your field placement. Have you ever worked with a client in which you were unsure of their capacity or desire to make positive changes? Or perhaps you were convinced otherwise? Identify how this may have impacted your practice with that client? Do you agree that, in order to be effective, both parties must trust that a positive outcome is possible?

LEARNING ACTIVITIES

1. Identify a time during your field placement that you worked on a team or participated in interpersonal collaboration. What did you find helpful in this experience? What was more challenging? What engagement skills did you utilize? What skills might have made the process better?

2. Consider the different skills listed in the chapter relating to engagement and the helping relationship. Which do you think comes easiest to you? Why? Which is the most challenging for you? Identify one or two strategies to grow in this skill and take it to your next supervision.

3. If in your field placement, you provide services in person, what barriers would exist if forced to move to a telehealth, online delivery system? How would you mitigate those barriers? If you already provide services in a telehealth delivery system, identify what would be easier in an in-person setting. What would be more challenging?

ELECTRONIC RESOURCES

WEBSITE LINKS

Inter-Professional Collaboration: A Social Work Ethic—Shelley Cohen Konrad: www.slideshare.net/CEIPE/social-work-leadership-in-ethics

VIDEO LINKS

Communication Skills in the Client-Social Worker Relationship—Rebecca Davis: https://www.youtube.com/watch?v=mJoZG7jfolk

Social Work & Models of Interprofessional Education—CHAS
UChicago: www.youtube.com/watch?v=HDvd9_sgdOg

REFERENCES

Ambrose-Miller, W., & Ashcroft, R. (2016). Challenges faced by social workers as members of interprofessional collaborative health care teams. *Health and Social Work, 41*(2), 101–109. http://doi.org/10.1093/hsw/hlw006

Barker, R. L. (2014*). The social work dictionary* (6th ed.). NASW Press.

Behnia, B. (2008). Trust development: A discussion of three approaches and a proposed alternative. *British Journal of Social Work, 38*(7), 1425–1441. https://doi.org/10.1093/bjsw/bcm053

Chang, V., Decker, C., & Scott, S. (2018). *Developing helping skills: A step-by-step approach to competency* (3rd ed). Cengage Learning.

Council on Social Work Education. (2022). *Educational policy and accreditation standards for baccalaureate and master's social work programs.* https://www.cswe.org/getmedia/94471c42-13b8-493b-9041-b30f48533d64/2022-EPAS.pdf

Cournoyer, B. (2017). *The social work skills workbook* (8th ed). Cengage Learning.

Craig, S. L., Iacono, G., Pascoe, R., & Austin, A. (2021). Adapting clinical skills to telehealth: Applications of affirmative cognitive-behavioral therapy with LGBTQ+ youth. *Clinical Social Work Journal, 49*(4), 471–483. https://doi.org/10.1007/s10615-021-00796-x

Craven, M., & Bland, R. (2013). Depression in primary care: Current and future challenges. *Canadian Journal of Psychiatry, 58*(8), 442–448. https://doi.org/10.1177/070674371305800802

Crawford, K. (2011). *Interprofessional collaboration in social work practice.* SAGE Publications.

Darlington, Y., & Feeney, J. A. (2008). Collaboration between mental health and child protection services: Professionals' perceptions of best practice. *Children and Youth Services Review, 30*(2), 187–198. https://doi.org/10.1016/j.childyouth.2007.09.005

Ferguson, J. (2010). *Serious case review under chapter VIII. Working together to safeguard children' in respect of the death of a child: Case reference - BSCB/2009-10/1.* Birmingham Safeguarding Children Board. https://cscp.org.uk/wp-content/uploads/2019/06/Birmingham-SCR-BSCB2009101-2010.pdf

Gamble, V. N. (2006). Trust, medical care, and racial and ethnic minorities. In D. Satcher, & R. J. Pamie (Eds.), *Multicultural medicine and health disparities* (pp. 437–448). McGraw-Hill.

Glicken, M. D. (2009). *Evidence-based practice with emotionally troubled children and adolescents.* Academic Press.

Hammick, M., Freeth, D., Copperman, J., & Goodsman, D. (2009). *Being interprofessional.* Polity Press.

Hepworth, D., Rooney, R., Rooney, G. D., & Strom-Gottfried, J. (2017). *Direct social work practice: Theory and skills* (10th ed.). Cengage Learning.

Kvarnström, S. (2008). Difficulties in collaboration: A critical incident of interprofessional healthcare teamwork. *Journal of Interprofessional Care, 22*(2), 191–203. https://doi.org/10.1080/13561820701760600

Levin, D. Z., Whitener, E. M., & Cross, R. (2006). Received trustworthiness of knowledge sources: The moderating impact of relationship length. *Journal of Applied Psychology, 91*(5), 1163–1171. https://doi.org/10.1037/0021-9010.91.5.1163

Lymbery, M. (2006). United we stand? Partnership working in health and social care and the role of social work in services for older people. *The British Journal of Social Work, 36*(7). https://doi.org/10.1093/bjsw/bch348

National Association of Social Workers. (2021). *Code of ethics.* https://www.socialworkers.org/About/Ethics/Code-of-Ethics/Code-of-Ethics-English

Norcross, J. C. (Ed.). (2011). *Psychotherapy relationships that work: Evidence-based responsiveness* (2nd ed.). Oxford University Press.

O'Sullivan, T. (2011). *Decision making in social work* (2nd ed.). Palgrave Macmillan.

Saleebey, D. (2008). The strengths perspective: Putting possibility and hope to work in our practice. In K. M. Sowers, & C. N. Dulmus (Eds.), *Comprehensive handbook of social work and social welfare* (pp. 123–142). John Wiley and Sons.

Seabury, B. A., Seabury, B., & Garvin, C. (2011). *Foundations of interpersonal practice in social work: Promoting competence in generalist practice* (3rd ed). SAGE.

Shulman, L. (2009). *The skills of helping individuals, families, groups and organizations* (6th ed.). Cengage Learning.

Sinai-Glazer, H. (2020). The essentials of the helping relationship between social workers and clients. *Social Work, 65*(3), 245–256. https://doi.org/10.1093/sw/swaa028

Vega, C. P., & Bernard, A. (2016). Interprofessional collaboration to improve health care: An introduction. *Medscape.* https://www.medscape.org/viewarticle/857823

Warren, C. S. (2001). Book review: Negotiating the therapeutic alliance: A relational treatment guide. *Psychotherapy Research, 11*(3), 357–359.

Weigel, G., Ramaswamy, A., Sobel, L., Salganicoff, A., Cubanski, J., & Freed, M. (2020, May 11). *Opportunities and barriers for telemedicine in the U.S. during the COVID-19 emergency and beyond.* Kaiser Family Foundation. https://www.kff.org/womens-health-policy/issue-brief/opportunities-and-barriers-for-telemedicine-in-the-u-s-during-the-covid-19-emergency-and-beyond

Whittington, C. (2003). Collaboration and partnership in context. In J. Weinstein, C. Whittington, & T. Leiba (Eds.), *Collaboration in social work practice* (pp. 13–38). Jessica Kingsley Publishers.

Micro Assessment: Individuals, Families, and Groups

CASE VIGNETTE

Julie is a first-year MSW student placed in a unit of a drug and alcohol center. She is assigned to the intake unit. Typically, Julie has two interviews with her clients prior to admission into the outpatient recovery program. The first interview focuses on conducting a biopsychosocial assessment and the second focuses on developing the client's treatment goals.

Before she entered the MSW program, Julie worked for 2 years in a foster care agency that served children who were in long-term placement. She spent a lot of time with her clients, and she felt that she got to know them and developed strong helping relationships with them. In contrast, her work at the rehabilitation center is fast paced and short-term. She has to complete the assessment and treatment goals after two brief client contacts.

By the end of her third week of placement, Julie was concerned about the effectiveness of her work. She felt that her approach was too task focused and that she was not truly understanding her clients' strengths and challenges. She felt that she did not really understand who they were. Instead, she was getting information as quickly as possible, filling out a form, and telling the clients about their treatment goals and the outpatient program. It felt rote and dehumanizing to her. She wondered what she could do to make the experience more positive for her clients and for herself. Julie felt that she needed a better understanding of her clients to develop realistic and appropriate treatment goals. How can she complete her biopsychosocial assessments and get the information the agency requires while gaining a beginning understanding of her clients' strengths, challenges, and life experiences in order to develop meaningful treatment goals?

COMPETENCY 7: ASSESS INDIVIDUALS, FAMILIES, GROUPS, ORGANIZATIONS, AND COMMUNITIES

Social workers understand that assessment is an ongoing component of the dynamic and interactive process of social work practice. Social workers understand theories of human behavior and person-in-environment, as well as interprofessional conceptual frameworks, and they critically evaluate and apply this knowledge in culturally responsive assessment with clients and constituencies, including individuals, families, groups, organizations, and communities. Assessment involves a collaborative process of defining presenting challenges and identifying strengths with individuals, families, groups, organizations, and communities to develop a mutually agreed-upon plan. Social workers recognize the implications of the larger practice context in the assessment process and use interprofessional collaboration in this process. Social workers are self-reflective and understand how bias, power, privilege, and their personal values and experiences may affect their assessment and decision-making.

Social workers

- apply theories of human behavior and person-in-environment, as well as other culturally responsive and interprofessional conceptual frameworks, when assessing clients and constituencies; and
- demonstrate respect for client self-determination during the assessment process by collaborating with clients and constituencies in developing a mutually agreed-upon plan. (Council on Social Work Education, 2022, p. 11)

LEARNING OBJECTIVES

By the end of this chapter, you will be able to:

- Apply critical thinking skills in conducting assessments with individuals, families, and groups.
- Describe the strengths perspective and its six key principles.
- Conduct individual and family client system assessments.
- Conduct assessments of individual group members and the group as a whole.
- Use a range of micro system assessment tools.

CRITICAL THINKING

Critical thinking is more than a rational step-by-step problem-solving process (Gibbons & Gray, 2004). It involves an intuitive process as well as disciplined evaluation and analysis. Thinking critically includes the synthesis, comparison, and evaluation of ideas from a variety of sources, such as texts, direct observation and experience, and social dialogue (Gibbons & Gray, 2004). A critically thinking social worker attempts to understand the client systems' perception of their reality and how their perceptions inform their work together. Critical thinking in social work assessment is the process of figuring out what is going on with your client, including what to believe or not about a situation. Social work is by definition a process in which there is no definitive answer. There are often multiple pathways to address a situation or reach a targeted goal. Effective social work assessment requires critical thinking. A key component of the assessment process is formulating hypotheses and critically assessing them to better understand the client system. Practice interventions and/or strategies flow out of our understanding of the client's perception of their situation and social reality. Critical thinking is the open-minded search for understanding.

Associated with critical thinking is the process of considering evidence when making decisions (Gambrill, 2013). Walker et al. (2007) point out that there are two kinds of evidence that social workers must balance in making informed decisions about their work with clients. The first is "empirically based knowledge generated through the scientific method" (p. 361). The second is "knowledge that is acquired through relationships with unique individuals (or unique groups like families, communities and organizations)" (pp. 361–362). Balancing empirical knowledge and practice wisdom allows social workers to move forward and make assessments with "reasonable confidence while also acknowledging uncertainty" (Walker et al., 2007, p. 362).

> **Field Reflection Questions**
>
> In your field placement, what do you need to do to strengthen your critical thinking skills in relation to your cognitive processing, affective reactions, and professional judgments?
>
> What clues can you give yourself to remember to self-reflect upon your affective reactions while in the moment with your clients at your field placement?

STRENGTHS PERSPECTIVE

The idea of building on clients' strengths has received a lot of attention in social work. Most social work agencies now claim adherence to "the strengths perspective." A strengths-based assessment is very different from approaches that focus on client problems and history taking (Hepworth et al., 2017). Social work has a long history of helping disadvantaged clients overcome individual problems and problem situations. Clients come to us with problems, and there is a natural tendency to attempt to resolve the problems and to view the clients from a deficit perspective. Often social workers' perceptions are different from their clients' self-perceptions. The clients viewed themselves as proactive, autonomous human beings who were using counseling services to enhance their functioning and competence. Unfortunately, in contrast, social workers tended to underestimate clients' strengths, focusing on their problems, underlying weaknesses, and limited potential.

When social workers focus on problems, they tend to perceive clients in essentially negative terms, as a collection of problems and diagnostic labels. This negative perception may lower expectations for positive change. More likely than not, clients are seen as diagnostic categories or their presenting problems, or both. These labels may create distance between clients and helpers (Saleebey, 2013). They also create pessimism in both parties. Negative labels and expectations obscure the unique capabilities of clients. The social worker's ability to recognize and promote a client's potential for change is markedly reduced. The focus is on what is wrong and the client's inability to cope with their life situation. Saleebey (2013) suggests that instead of focusing on problems, we should focus on possibilities.

The pathologic problem approach searches the past for causes. How did the client get into this situation? Why is the client experiencing these difficulties? The search for causes and rational explanations assumes a direct link between cause, disease, and cure (Saleebey, 2013). Human experience is rarely that simple. More often than not, it is uncertain and tremendously complex. In addition, looking to the past diverts attention away from exploring the present. The shift from problems to strengths moves the focus from the past to the present and future. Strengths-oriented social workers seek to discover the resources clients currently have that can be used to change their futures. The past cannot be completely dismissed, because it provides a context for the present. However, in strengths-based practice the focus is on the present and the future. Rather than focusing on why clients are having problems, social workers who have adopted a strengths perspective focus on what clients want, what they need, and how they have managed to survive (Saleebey, 2013). These and similar questions will help you and your clients identify, use, build, and reinforce clients' strengths, resources, and abilities. Saleebey (2013) identified six principles of strengths-based assessments:

1. Every individual, group, family, and community has strengths.

2. Trauma, abuse, illness, and struggle may be injurious, but they may also be sources of challenge and opportunity.

3. Assume that you do not know the upper limits of the capacity to grow and change, and take individual, group, and community aspirations seriously.

4. We best serve clients by collaborating with them.

5. Every environment is full of resources.

6. Caring, caretaking, and context are important.

Field Reflection Questions

After reviewing the six strengths principles, which principle do you feel you have the most difficulty applying in your field placement work?

Which principle is the easiest for you to apply? What makes one harder to incorporate into your practice than the other?

ASSESSING INDIVIDUAL AND FAMILY CLIENT STRENGTHS

Strengths-based assessments enhance the individualization of clients. The focus is on what is unique about each client in terms of interests, abilities, and how they have coped with their problem situation. The work should focus on what the client has achieved and what resources are currently available to the client. Give pre-eminence to the client's understanding of the facts and figure out what the client wants. Above all, avoid blame and blaming. Join with your clients in a collaborative effort to understand their reality and their strengths.

Adherence to these concepts will help ensure that your assessment interviews are collaborative and that the process will identify client strengths. The tendency to focus on pathologic symptoms and dysfunction will be minimized. Identifying client strengths is not always easy. Clients are often unable to name specific strengths they have used in coping with a problem situation. They often indicate that they do not have any strengths, or they respond in very general terms. The challenge is to help clients recognize how they have taken steps, summoned up resources, and coped (Saleebey, 2013).

Using a strengths perspective does not negate the very real problems clients face. The problems that cause clients to seek professional help cannot be disregarded or ignored. The assessment process must attend to both the obstacles and the strengths that potentially affect the resolution of the problem and the helping process. Much of the assessment that takes place in social work is focused on client problems and deficits (Saleebey, 2013). The strengths approach seeks to provide a balance between client obstacles and strengths.

Cowger (1997) proposed an assessment axis to help attain this balance. It has two coordinates: the environmental–personal continuum and the strengths–obstacles continuum. There are four quadrants: environmental strengths, personal strengths, environmental obstacles, and personal obstacles. The quadrants for personal strengths and obstacles include both psychological and physiologic components. Attention to all four quadrants helps ensure a comprehensive assessment that is balanced in terms of individual and environmental strengths and obstacles.

Creating an empowering assessment process with families is similar to doing strengths-based assessment with individuals. The main difference, and the biggest challenge, is to focus your attention and efforts on the family as a whole as well as on each individual member. To be able to effectively help families, you need to develop a shared understanding of their concerns, their strengths, potential resources, and the challenges they face. The assessment process provides an opportunity for families to tell their stories. It is more about listening than asking questions. Strengths-based assessments focus on clients' perceptions of their situation and their goals, rather than on diagnostic labels. Ideally, the process should lead to increased family empowerment and create a sense of hopefulness. Focusing on strengths rather than deficits helps create expectations about the possibilities of change.

The key to conducting an assessment in which you begin to truly understand your client is to use your social work interviewing skills. Your agency will have an assessment form with many questions they need answered. Asking the questions on the form is not enough. You need to be able to get the whole story in order to understand your client's unique situation. This requires your ability to engage your clients in a helping relationship in which trust is built and sensitive information shared, and your clients are willing to expose their vulnerability. This is not easy to accomplish. You must use your social work interviewing skills to make this happen. More than anything, we believe, that clients need to feel heard and understood. Active listening, empathic responding, reaching for feelings, elaboration skills, and summarizing are all key skills in conducting assessments. Remember, your task is to understand your client and provide a professional assessment. This requires skill and compassion. It is not just about filling out the form.

ASSESSING GROUPS

As with the assessment of families, assessing small groups is similar to assessing individuals. Again, the main difference is to focus your attention and efforts on the group as well as on each individual member. The use of groups in generalist social work practice is very prevalent in almost all fields of practice. The chances of you being asked to facilitate or co-facilitate a group in your field placement are very high. Facilitating a group can be very scary, especially for those without prior experiences in group work. When groups are working well together it can be a very powerful and rewarding experience for both the participants and the facilitator. When groups are not working well the opposite is true.

Facilitating or co-facilitating a group requires you to monitor the functioning of each member of the group. You must be sensitive to each group member's participation, nonverbal communication, emotional responses, and behaviors. Your assessment of the individual members is done primarily by observation. Your observations and your knowledge of the client are the data you will use to assess the individual members in your group. This combined with your critical thinking skills will provide you with hypotheses about what might be going on with individual members in terms of their functioning in the group. You then must make a professional judgment as to whether you should address the possible concern in the group or handle it individually with the group member. This is never an easy decision, especially when you have limited experience in facilitating groups. Adding to the difficulty is the fact that you have to make the decision in the moment and while you are also attending to the needs of the group as a whole. Nevertheless, your ongoing assessment of each participant in the group is a critical component of effective group facilitation.

Concerns about group functioning may arise from the group, or you may raise them. In this respect, group assessment is different from individual and family system assessment. Individuals and families usually seek professional help for a problem they are aware of and want to correct. Problems in group functioning, however, are not always apparent to individual members or to the group as a whole, and groups usually do not seek professional help. An important part of your job as the group leader is to identify potential issues and concerns and to bring them to the attention of the group. Following is an example of a group not functioning well and another of one that is more successful.

CASE EXAMPLE 12.1: A GROUP THAT IS NOT FUNCTIONING WELL TOGETHER

Gwen has been involved on a team to address the quality concerns in her agency. There are 10 people on the team. They are positive and productive supervisors and administrators across the agency. Their goal is to review a policy or a procedure each time they meet. Most of the time they "wordsmith" it and set up a new deadline for project completion. Work assignments are given to group members between meetings. However, members rarely complete the assignments. The meetings are often interrupted as members step out to answer cell phone calls, come in late, or leave early. Members jump at any excuse not to attend meetings, citing work obligations that Gwen knows are not so urgent that they could not be addressed after the meeting time. In addition, no matter how far in advance the meetings are scheduled, members plan their compensatory day and vacation days for the days the meetings are scheduled. Gwen is under the impression that members of the team would rather be anywhere else than in this group. She feels that trying to manage the team is like "herding cats." It has become a waste of time for everyone, including Gwen.

Gwen dislikes attending these meetings. They ruin her day. She feels like a failure with respect to this project. She is worried that her reputation as a competent worker is at stake. She has tried being more strict and authoritative around attendance and compliance with assignments, but the harder she works, the less the group members cooperate. It seems that they expect her to do all of the work so that they can just criticize and shoot-down her efforts (Barol, 2010).

CASE EXAMPLE 12.2: A GROUP THAT IS WORKING WELL TOGETHER

Andrea is responsible for a team in her agency whose mission is to address quality within the agency. She is excited by the assignment. She enjoys working with this group of focused, productive, and positive supervisors from across the agency. The time that they meet together seems to fly by. They are usually on the same wavelength with what they are doing, and they have healthy discussions and occasional friendly arguments when they work on issues that represent their different vantage points. However, even when there is a disagreement with some tension attached to it, they are issue focused rather than person focused. After working through the tension and issues, they always seem to find common ground. Members know and respect each other and are not worried that a disagreement within the meeting will have a negative effect on their relationships on the team and their reputation outside the meeting time. Team members are creative and excited in this work and strive to include all members of the agency in parallel processes. In fact, people think that it is an honor to be on this team and are excited when they are chosen to participate (Barol, 2010).

GROUP SUBSYSTEMS

As shown in Exhibit 12.1, there are five major subsystems within the group-in-environment system that have potential relevance for the assessment process: purpose, structure, life-cycle stage, culture, and alliances. Like family subsystems, group subsystems are highly interrelated. Taken as a whole, they provide a comprehensive picture of the internal structure and functioning of a group system. A strengths-based assessment requires the social worker and the group to mutually and continually assess the effect the various subsystems have on one another and on the functioning of the group.

EXHIBIT 12.1

GROUP SUBSYSTEMS

Purpose (type)	Life-cycle stage
Therapy	Developmental stage
Support	
Education	**Culture**
Growth	Traditions
Project	Values
Administrative	Norms
Professional	
Citizen	**Alliances**
	Communication patterns
Structure	Interpersonal attraction
Membership composition	Power
Size	Leadership
Duration	
Open/closed	

Purpose

Every formed group has a purpose. The purpose varies according to the type of group. Because in many respects, the type defines a group's purpose, assessment of purpose is an excellent first step in assessing group functioning. The group's purpose should be clearly stated and agreed on by group members. It is from the purpose that all other aspects of a group evolve. Is the identified problem or concern related to confusion or disagreement about the purpose of the group? Is the purpose clear and unambiguous? Is there agreement about the purpose of the group? Does the group have more than one purpose? If so, are the different purposes in conflict?

Structure

Structure is the composition of the group, its size, whether the group is time limited or ongoing, and whether the group is open to new members or closed. Problems in group functioning can often be traced back to structural issues. Examination of a group's structure and the effect that the four structural dimensions are having on the area of concern is an important aspect of group assessment. The four dimensions are group composition, size of the group, how long the group stays together, and open versus closed group membership. All of these factors can influence group functioning and need to be considered in conducting an assessment of the group.

Life-Cycle Stages

This aspect of group functioning deals with group development. Groups go through a number of developmental stages. They change and evolve as they mature. Like humans, groups have a pattern of development. There are the various typologies of group development, ranging from three stages (Schwartz, 1986) to nine (Beck, 1983) and there is considerable overlap in the labels applied to the stages and in their conceptualization. One widely used conceptualization is Tuckman's (1965) four-stage model of group development: forming, storming, norming, and performing. Magen (1995) added a fifth stage, adjourning, to Tuckman's model.

Forming

The initial stage of the group, forming, occurs when members come together for the first time. In most groups, especially client groups, this is an exciting and anxious time for both the members and the leader. The participants are anxious about what will happen, what their experience in the group will be, and how they will perform. At this point, the group is a collection of individuals with individual concerns. Dependency on the worker is common in the early stages (Barol, 2010). Group members look to the leader for answers and direction. Interactions among members are superficial and guarded. Members do not have a strong commitment to the group and have not developed an identification with the group as a whole.

Storming

The second developmental stage is characterized by conflict among the members and with the leader. The emotional climate is characterized by tension. Members exhibit hostility toward one another and frustration with the group. The worker's leadership is challenged, and the purpose, structure, and operation of the group may often be questioned. Conflict is an expression of the group's emerging identity and group members' efforts to obtain power and control of the group. Group members challenge, attack, or withdraw. Through this process, the group begins to develop a collective identity and a sense of togetherness. Although this stage of group development is difficult for the worker, it presents an opportunity to model behavior for the group. In the face of often unpleasant challenges, members need to stay calm, nondefensive, and open to criticism, and they should demonstrate a willingness to share power and control with the group.

Norming

The third stage is the period during which group identity is solidified and the various roles, norms, and boundaries of the group emerge. Guidelines for group functioning are agreed on during this stage of development; they are the product of the group's coming together and developing a sense of itself. Guidelines are not just the leader's vision of what the group should do and how they should do it; they are the group's guidelines. At this point, the group has established ownership, and a collective sense of purpose and expected behavior has emerged.

Performing

The action phase of the group's life cycle, performing, is the time when the group has worked out its leadership issues, structural concerns, and behavioral expectations. The performing stage is characterized by solidarity, cohesion, and commitment. Patterns of communication have become more predictable, and the members are more comfortable with one another. Exchanges are open and honest, and differences are less likely to lead to conflict. The group has worked out mechanisms for managing and resolving conflict. There is a sense of cohesiveness among the members. They are now a group, and they are ready to work on and accomplish the tasks at hand.

Adjourning

This is the ending phase or termination stage of the group's development. A wide range of feelings among the members often characterizes it. If the group has developed a sense of closeness characteristic of the performing stage, the adjourning phase can be difficult for group members and the leader. Feelings of loss and abandonment are common. There is often regression on the part of some members. They revert to earlier stages in an attempt to keep the group going. Reasons for continuing are put forth. Groups may go through a grieving process similar to that seen in individuals: denial, rage and anger, bargaining, depression, and acceptance. Group members have a range of feelings and emotions about ending. The worker needs to help each member examine their responses to ending.

Assessment of the group's stage of development is an important aspect of understanding group functioning. Groups develop at different rates and progress in their development differently. What might seem like a problem in group functioning may be a normal stage of the group's development. To what extent is the behavior being exhibited by group members related to the group's developmental stage? How far has the group progressed developmentally?

Culture

The traditions, beliefs, and norms developed by the group constitute the cultural components of group functioning. Traditions, beliefs, and norms are highly interrelated. An examination of a group's culture and the effect it has on an identified area of concern is an important aspect of group assessment. All groups develop *traditions*, which are ritualized activities, such as ceremonies, prayers, and songs, that are incorporated into group meetings. A group's traditions are influenced by members' ethnic, racial, and cultural backgrounds (Seabury et al., 2011). They are important symbols for group members, strengthening group identification and helping members feel closer to the group. They also help define the uniqueness of a group. Members who violate group traditions are not viewed favorably by fellow members. Violations can lead to reprimand and rejection by the group. To avoid this, you should learn their traditions as quickly as possible (Seabury et al., 2011).

Group *norms* are the understandings group members have about behaviors. They define what members should and should not do within the group (Hepworth et al., 2017; Seabury et al., 2011). All groups develop unwritten rules that govern the behavior of the members. Norms may have a positive or negative influence on group functioning. Regular attendance at meetings, treating one another with respect, and communicating concerns directly to the group are examples of norms that have a positive effect on groups. Norms that have a negative or dysfunctional effect on the group include encouraging discussion of topics not related to the purpose of the meeting, letting a few members dominate the group, and avoiding talking about group problems. Group norms are not explicitly expressed. They are implicit rules of behavior. Norms are discerned by observing the behavior of members and reactions to it. Sanctions and social disapproval are given for violating a norm; praise and social approval are given for compliance (Toseland & Rivas, 2012).

Groups also develop *values* or beliefs that are held in common by all or most group members. Values are what group members believe to be true. They are the shared belief system of the members. The values held by a group can have a positive or negative influence on group functioning. As with norms, values can only be inferred through observation. They are not written down, nor are they usually stated explicitly.

Assessment of a group's culture is an important function of the group leader. Cultural influences can have positive or negative effects on a concern or problem. To be able to effectively assess a group's culture you need to be aware of the traditions, values, and norms that have developed. This is an ongoing process. How does group culture affect the target problem? What are its positive influences? What are its negative influences?

Alliances

There are four dimensions of alliance: communication patterns, interpersonal attractions, power, and leadership. These four dimensions are highly interrelated. Taken together, they provide a comprehensive overview of the alliance component of group functioning.

Communication Patterns

Communication patterns involve who talks to whom and about what (Seabury et al., 2011). It is the structure of the interactions among members. An analysis of communication patterns indicates who dominates group discussions, whether some members are isolated, and who the informal leaders are. It also provides insight into subgroup formation and the effect of the various subgroups on the functioning of the group. Subgroups do not necessarily adversely affect a group. In fact, the formation of subgroups helps members form closer attachments to other members and to the group as a whole. Subgroups negatively affect the group when they become exclusive or when power struggles between subgroups interfere with member support for the larger group (Hepworth et al., 2017).

Interpersonal Attraction

Closely associated with communication patterns and subgroup formation is *interpersonal attraction* of members. As members get better acquainted, some members are attracted to others and some are not. Interpersonal attraction is influenced by race, culture, and gender as well as physical appearance, personality, and interests, among other factors (Seabury et al., 2011). Members with similar backgrounds and interests are more likely to be attracted to each other than those who are very different from one another.

Power

Power is the ability of one individual to influence another in a specific way. There are five types of power:

1. *Reward power* is the ability to influence others by providing them with something that they value. A group member may offer friendship, support, praise, or other goods and services.

2. *Coercive power* is the ability to influence others using punishment. A group member may use coercive power by criticizing, insulting, or physically threatening another group member.

3. *Legitimate power* is the ability to influence others by virtue of one's position in the group. The social work leader may exercise legitimate power based upon their assigned role.

4. *Referent power* is the ability to influence others by being liked or respected. A group member may have referent power based upon their personality or attractiveness.

5. *Expert power* is the ability to influence others because of specialized knowledge or skills. A member may exercise expert power by virtue of their special training. (Seabury et al., 2011)

Both the sources of power and the locus of power within the group may vary. Power does not itself negatively affect group functioning. Problems arise when there are power struggles within the group. Groups, in fact, sometimes fall apart because of unresolved power issues (Hepworth et al., 2017). The issue in group assessment is not so much who has the power but rather the group's ability to share power and to find resolutions to power conflicts that do not result in some members feeling that they have been forced to give up too much.

Leadership

In simple terms, leadership it is the capacity to mobilize group members into action. Leadership as a process that grows out of interactions among group members related to the attainment of goals (Seabury et al., 2011). *Task leadership* occurs when the individual helps the group move toward defining and achieving group goals. *Social-emotional leadership* occurs when the member positively affects the interaction among group members by such things as reducing conflicts and facilitating the expression of positive feelings (Seabury et al., 2011).

The alliance component has powerful influences on group functioning. A comprehensive assessment needs to carefully evaluate the effect of these processes on an identified problem area or concern. As the social worker involved with the group, part of your leadership task is to become aware of the alliance structure of the group. This requires ongoing observation of group behavior. Before you can assess the impact the processes have on the group, you need to understand how the group functions. Once you have a clear understanding of communication patterns, interpersonal alliances, power, and leadership within the group, you can assess their effect on a specific area of concern.

STRENGTHS-BASED GROUP ASSESSMENT

Group assessment is a collaborative process that the leader and members of the group undertake to change conditions that impede the group from achieving its purpose or improving its functioning. An empowering approach to group assessment involves the members in the analysis of group functioning and the problem situation. You may raise an issue or concern, but the entire group explores it and its effect on the group. The group decides whether it is a problem, what contributes to the concern, and what should be done to help correct the situation. The group and its members are the experts. Your starting point is their perceptions of the problem situation. Do not force your analysis and assessment of the group's problems, interpersonal relationships, or individual dysfunctions on the group. Engage in a collaborative exchange with the group, share your insights and perceptions, and explore the perceptions of the members. You guide the assessment process, but the group members conduct the assessment. Ensure that each member's perception of the situation is acknowledged and validated. There is no single correct view. There are always multiple perceptions of reality. Each member's perception of the situation is accurate from their perspective. Seek consensus about the target problem. If that is not possible, seek agreement about the need to address the concern. The group has the power to set the agenda. It has ownership of the problem as well as the potential solutions.

A strengths-based assessment emphasizes the identification of group strengths as well as strengths of each individual member. Group members have individual and collective power to bring about positive change. Incorporating a strengths perspective in the assessment process, however, is the professional leader's responsibility. Regardless of the type of group, emphasizing strengths requires a conscious effort on your part. All groups, regardless of the level of functioning of individual members, have strengths. Do not expect group members to recognize or be aware of their individual and collective strengths. Adopt the attitude that strengths exist and that they can be used to help the group resolve the problem situation.

CASE EXAMPLE 12.3: WHAT IS GOING ON WITH THE GROUP

Alex's field instructor suggested that she conduct a preliminary assessment of their treatment group for male sex offenders. During the last session Alex felt that the group probably did not feel like a safe space for some of the members including Juan with whom she is also assigned to work with individually. Prior to the next weekly group meeting Alex reviewed the five dimensions and subdimensions of group functioning—purpose, structure, life-cycle stage, culture, and alliances. Alex and her field instructor agreed that during the next group session her field instructor would be the lead facilitator and she would observe the group functioning and prepare an assessment for review in supervision.

At the group meeting Alex noticed a couple of factors that might be hindering the life-cycle development of the group. Her first observation was that the group was still in the forming stage. They appeared to be a collection of individuals with individual concerns. The group members all look to either her or her field instructor for answers and direction. The communication patterns tend to be back and forth between the facilitator and a group member and then the same thing with another group member. During these exchanges the other group members appear bored and distracted. They are not engaged. This communication pattern and member behavior suggested that the purpose of the group was probably not clear to the members and the clear norms for participating in the group had not been established.

Alex also observed that some of the group members appeared to be in denial about the sex offenses and their need for treatment. These members tended to make jokes on the side when others were talking, pointing again to the need to establish norms of behavior for the group. The side joking appeared to be a significant contributor to Alex's feeling that the group probably did not feel like a safe space to share sensitive information.

In supervision Alex and her field instructor reviewed her assessment and identified some interventions. They agreed that the first step was to go back and review the purpose of the group and to have the group members identify rules for the group. They felt that it was important for the members to come up with the rules and that they would write them down on poster paper and always bring the rules to future group meetings. The also decided to do their best to change the communication patterns so that there would be less facilitator/individual member interactions and more facilitator/group interactions.

MICRO SYSTEM ASSESSMENT TOOLS

Generalist social workers practice in a multitude of settings. The types of assessment tools they use are as varied as the settings. Agencies adopt or develop assessment procedures based on the kinds of information they need and the types of services they provide. Most assessment tools are variations of the generic biopsychosocial assessment that has been taught in schools of social work for many years. Typically, these instruments are used to collect information on client problems and past behaviors and experiences. Little or no attention is given to client strengths. Tools that focus on client strengths are now emerging, and strengths-based assessments are beginning to be incorporated into agency-based practice.

STRENGTHS-BASED ASSESSMENT WORKSHEET

An Individual and Family Strengths and Obstacles Worksheet is available by accessing Springer Publishing Connect™ via the instructions on the opening page of this book, and clicking on the drop down Show Supplementary, Student Materials, Individual and Family Strengths and Obstacles Worksheet. The strengths-based worksheet was developed to help social workers and clients identify clients' strengths as well as the obstacles they face in resolving problem situations. It can help you and your clients summarize areas of concern and priorities, identify strengths and obstacles, and help assess the effects of the obstacles and strengths on the target problem.

You should try to complete as much of the worksheet as possible between your first and second meetings with the client. During the second meeting, review your initial assessment findings and then, with the client, revise and finish the worksheet. Be sure to review the completed worksheet with your client and make any needed adjustments. Ensuring your clients have a clear picture of their strengths and obstacles is as important as you having an understanding of the client's situation.

ECOMAPS

Ecomaps graphically display the person-in-environment perspective and can help you identify strengths and challenges in your client's life. They focus on the relationships between the client and the major systems in the client's environment. The major systems vary by client. Typically, they include kin and friendship relationships; work, school, community, and neighborhood organizations; and the social worker, agency, and other social service and healthcare organizations. An ecomap shows the relevant systems, whether the relationships are positive or negative and strong or weak, and the direction or flow of energy and resources between the client and the systems. A dashed arrow indicates a weak relationship, a solid arrow indicates a strong relationship, and a dashed line indicates the absence of a relationship between the client and the subsystem. A plus sign (+) or minus sign (–) indicates whether the relationship is positive or negative. The direction of the arrowhead indicates the direction of the energy or resource flow (Hepworth et al., 2017).

Ecomaps are constructed in collaboration with the client. The worker begins by placing the client in the middle of the ecomap, and then identifies the various personal and environmental systems with which the client interacts. The social worker reviews the relationships with the client using open-ended questions and elaboration techniques. Together, the worker and client complete the ecomap. The worker and client review and analyze the completed ecomap. This process encourages collaboration in the worker–client relationship. Ecomaps can be very useful tools in helping clients understand their person-in-environment systems and the effects the various relationships or absence of relationships have on the presenting problem. They also help the worker and client identify areas of strength and resources.

Figure 12.1 is a completed ecomap for an individual client. The client is a 55-year-old African American male named Harry M. He is divorced, has two adult children, lives alone, and is currently working as a school janitor. He attends a partial hospitalization program for adults with mental health problems.

The ecomap indicates that Mr. M. has strong, mutually supportive relationships with the partial program, the social worker, his mother, and his next-door neighbor. He also receives support from his church and his belief in God, and from his job. Mr. M. has a weak but supportive relationship with his son and weak stressful relationships with his sister and daughter. His relationship with his ex-wife is completely dissolved. He does not have any romantic or friendship relationships or other connections with neighbors or the community.

Overall, Mr. M.'s person-in-environment assessment reveals a number of strengths and sources of support. He receives a great deal of support from formal associations, such as the partial program, his social worker, and his church.

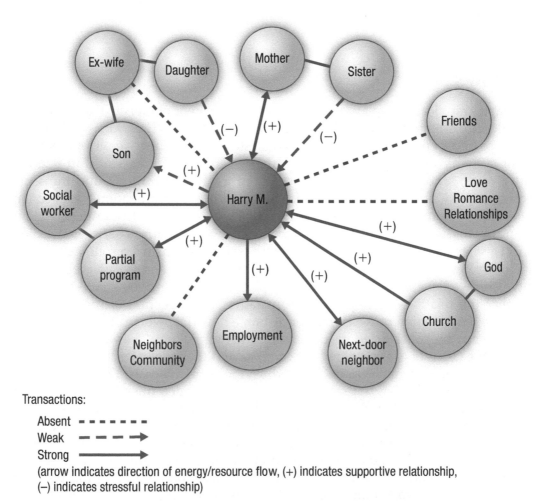

Transactions:

Absent ‑ ‑ ‑ ‑ ‑ ‑ ‑
Weak ‑ ‑ ‑ ‑ →
Strong ⟶
(arrow indicates direction of energy/resource flow, (+) indicates supportive relationship,
(–) indicates stressful relationship)

FIGURE 12.1 **Ecomap for individual client.**

His informal support network appears to be limited to his mother and a next-door neighbor. His relationship with his ex-wife, children, sister, friends, and lovers are either weak or nonexistent.

Figure 12.2 is a completed ecomap for a family client system. The family consists of a single mother and her two daughters, ages 11 and 15. The mother has requested help from a family service agency for problems she is having with the 11-year-old daughter. She reports that the younger daughter is having problems in school and is acting out at home by not obeying her. She is disrespectful and defiant.

The ecomap shows that the mother has a stressful relationship with her younger daughter and a positive relationship with her older daughter, and that the two girls have a conflicted relationship. The father does not live with the family. He and the mother have no contact or ongoing relationship. The older daughter has a stressful relationship with her father, and the younger daughter feels close to him.

The identified patient is the 11-year-old daughter. She is having problems in school and in her relationships with her mother and sister. Her mother is also concerned about the girl's friends. She feels that they are a negative influence on her

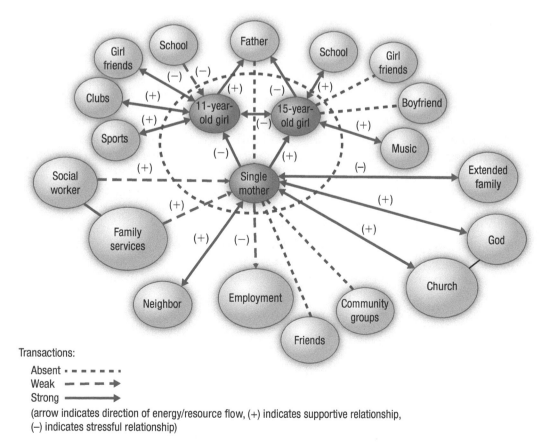

Transactions:

Absent · · — · · — · ·
Weak — — — →
Strong ——————→
(arrow indicates direction of energy/resource flow, (+) indicates supportive relationship, (–) indicates stressful relationship)

FIGURE 12.2 **Ecomap for family client.**

daughter. On the positive side, the daughter is active in clubs and sports. She has a supportive relationship with her father.

The older sister is close to her mother, does well in school, and gets a great deal of satisfaction from her musical pursuits. On the negative side, she does not have any close friends, and her relationships with her father and sister are strained.

The mother has a supportive extended family network and derives a great deal of support from church-related activities. She also has a neighbor who is a source of support. Other than her neighbor, she does not have close friends, nor is she involved in the community beyond her church activities. Her relationship with the social worker and the family service agency at the time of the interview was weak but supportive, while her job was viewed as moderately stressful.

SOCIOGRAMS

Field Reflection Questions

In what ways could you use any of the micro assessment tools in your field placement? What would you need to do to incorporate any into your field placement practice?

What do you see as a benefit of using an assessment tool? What are the challenges for you in using assessment tools in your field placement?

A group sociogram is similar to an ecomap. The ecomap describes a person-in-environment system; the sociogram describes the relationships among members of the group. Hartford's (1971) approach to sociogram construction examines attraction and repulsion between members of the group. It is a graphic representation of the alliances within a group and can help identify strengths and challenges facing the group. Usually, a worker constructs a sociogram based on observations of the group interactions. You include yourself in the sociogram. Doing so recognizes that you are part of the group-in-environment system and forces you to try to objectively analyze your relationships with each member of the group. Seabury et al. (2011) point out that discussion of alliances within groups creates anxiety and concerns about rejection. Therefore, sharing a sociogram with the group should be approached with caution. However, a sociogram can be an effective tool for helping group members understand the dynamics of the group and the effect of group alliances on a problem area or concern.

The sociogram shown in Figure 12.3 consists of six members, three males and three females, and the social worker. The sociogram shows that the social worker has strong positive relationships with members 3 and 5, weak positive relationships with members 1, 4 and 6, and a strong negative relationship with member 2. Members 3 and 6 are somewhat isolated. Each only has a strong relationship with one other member. Member 2 appears to be the informal leader of the group. She has strong positive relationships with members 1, 5, 3, and 4. She also appears to be in competition for leadership with the social worker with whom she has a strong negative relationship.

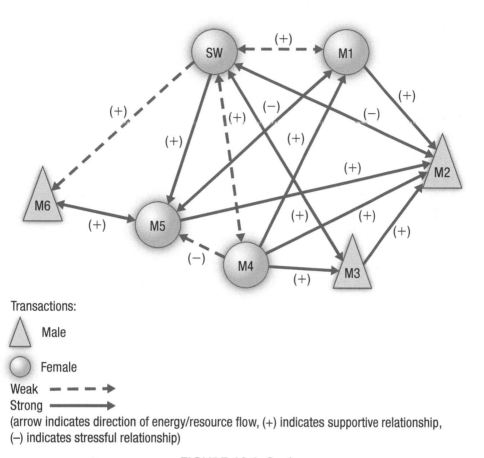

Transactions:

△ Male

○ Female

Weak ‑ ‑ ‑ ‑ →
Strong ———→
(arrow indicates direction of energy/resource flow, (+) indicates supportive relationship,
(–) indicates stressful relationship)

FIGURE 12.3 **Sociogram.**

CASE SUMMARY: "ADJUSTING TO LIFE WITHOUT MOM"

PRACTICE SETTING DESCRIPTION

My name is Janson and I am a first-year MSW student completing an internship at a family service agency in a medium-size city in the Midwest. The agency provides individual and family counseling services on a sliding fee scale. The agency also runs a number of educational and treatment groups. My field instructor assigned me to work with the K. family, who are seeking help in dealing with the accidental death of the wife and mother in a car crash.

IDENTIFYING DATA

The K. family consists of the father, Bob, and three children, Sharon, Chad, and Jason. Ellen, Bob's wife and the children's mother, passed away 8 months ago as a result of injuries she sustained in an automobile accident. Bob is 45 years of age, Caucasian, and works in the banking industry. Sharon is 18 years old and a senior in high school. Chad is 17 years of age and is currently a junior in high school. Jason is 15 years of age and in the ninth grade. Bob has steady employment as a salesman with adequate income to support his family. Ellen worked part-time in retail sales and her income was used primarily for family vacations and family outings.

PRESENTING PROBLEM

Chad has taken the death of his mother especially hard. This past year, he has been receiving failing grades in school and has been involved in numerous fights. He also has begun to experiment with drugs and alcohol. Ellen had been a constant source of support for Chad and the other children. However, the children describe Bob as not being supportive of them, and as having an especially stressful relationship with Chad.

In addition to the preceding problems, the family seems to not have allowed outsiders, even extended family members, to help them deal with their grief and loss. Family traditions ended with Ellen's death, as did involvement with the church and other organizations. The family's emotional climate has become tense, and the family's communication patterns have been greatly altered since Ellen's death.

ASSESSMENT

The greatest obstacle facing the K. family is Ellen's absence. It is clear that she maintained the closest relationships with the children, led family traditions, was the mediator between Bob and the children, kept communication open, and allowed family boundaries to remain open to the outside world. Ellen was involved with the schools her children attended, the church she and the rest of the family attended weekly, and numerous community-wide events. Ellen also kept the lines of communication open between extended family members, including Bob's mother, siblings, and cousins.

Upon Ellen's death, the K. family seemed to completely "shut down." While Sharon's and Jason's performance at school has not changed as drastically as Chad's, the two children reported not feeling as good about themselves as they once did and also reported not wanting to continue participating in extracurricular activities.

Chad's sudden change in behavior and school performance is directly related to the death of his mother. His recent experimentation with drugs and alcohol is related to his mother's death and to the fact that alcoholism is prevalent in Ellen's family history. Ellen's father and brother are both recovering alcoholics. Chad, like the rest of his family, is dealing with Ellen's death in an unhealthy manner.

The weak relationships between Bob and his children had an effect before Ellen's death and now greatly affects the family's identified problem situation. Another obstacle the family faces is the fact that Bob never learned effective coping or parenting skills.

However, the K. family does have several strengths. All family members realize that there are definite obstacles and that no one has been dealing with Ellen's death in a healthy fashion. Chad appears to want to stop using drugs and alcohol and to change his recent behavior patterns at school. The children have expressed interest in maintaining strong and supportive relationships with their father. Bob has admitted that he never had a strong relationship with any of his children or with his own father.

Another major strength is that the family wants to return to family traditions, change their emotional climate, open communication patterns, reset the family's boundaries, and utilize family resources. In addition, the children seem to have strong and supportive relationships among themselves, and extended family members have expressed an interest in being active participants in the lives of Bob, Sharon, Chad, and Jason. External strengths include a sincere desire by all family members to again become a part of their church, the community, and other associations.

CASE PROCESS SUMMARY

Bob and the children all recognize that, first and foremost, they need to deal with the sudden death of Ellen. They also acknowledge the need to deal with the strained relationship between Chad and his father and to strengthen Sharon's and Jason's relationships with their father. Chad has also agreed to receive help for his academic and behavioral problems at school. I feel that I have made excellent progress in assessing the families' strengths and challenges. After discussing my family assessment with my field instructor, we decided that the next step would be for me to share my preliminary assessment with the family and to engage the family in completing a family ecomap to help identify supports and areas that need work.

Janson, MSW Student Intern

CASE DISCUSSION QUESTIONS

1. *Critique the family assessment on the K. family. What are the strengths of the assessment? What areas need to be strengthened? What additional information is needed to better understand the functioning of this family?*

2. *Based upon the information provided in the case summary, identify at least three individual and/or family issues that you think need to be addressed and discuss why and how the issues impact family functioning.*

3. *Jason's case summary did not include any of his affective reactions to the family's situation or their interactions together. If this family was assigned to you, reflect upon what your emotional response to the family and its members would be. How would their circumstances affect you emotionally? Is there anyone in the family you probably would feel a close identification with? Anyone who might bring up negative feelings for you? What are some possible counter-transference feelings you should watch out for?*

END-OF-CHAPTER RESOURCES

A robust set of instructor resources designed to supplement this text is located at http://connect.springerpub.com/content/book/978-0-8261-3753-1. Qualifying instructors may request access by emailing textbook@springerpub.com.

CRITICAL THINKING QUESTIONS

1. In Example 12.3, Alex completed, with her field instructor, an initial assessment of their treatment group's functioning as a group. They identified some issues that might be interfering with the functioning of the group. A major issue of concern is that a couple of the group members seem to dislike another member and that person is getting scapegoated by the group. It appears that the other group members are joining in on the scapegoating. Alex is unsure how to approach this sensitive topic with the group and how to engage the group in the assessment process. Identify at least three possible pitfalls that could occur when broaching this topic with the group. Describe how you would minimize the pitfalls. Discuss how you would conduct your group as a whole assessment around this potential issue. Describe your affective reaction to your proposed plan.

2. In the case summary example, what engagement skills would you employ to conduct in your group assessment? What engagement skills are you most confident using? What skills are you less sure about? What would you do to prepare and strengthen your engagement skills to conduce a more effective assessment?

3. Assessment involves critical thinking, self-reflection on your affective reactions, and the rendering of your professional judgment. It also involves your ability to engage your clients in a helping relationship. In reflecting upon your work with clients in your field placement, describe an experience in which your engagement skills were in conflict with your ability to conduct a strengths-based client assessment. What was the conflict? In reflection, how could you have more effectively dealt with the conflict?

LEARNING ACTIVITIES

1. Consider the kind of practice you are doing in your field agency. Identify as many ways as you can to monitor progress toward client goals, which will look vastly different depending on the types of clients you are working with.

2. Observe an assessment and document what you noticed. Utilize what you learned from your observation in a role-play with your supervisor or a peer.

ELECTRONIC RESOURCES

WEBSITE LINKS

 Strengths-Based Assessment—Social Care Institute for Excellence: https://www.scie.org.uk/strengths-based-approaches/guidance

Family Assessment Tools Slideshow—Aileen Pascual: www
.slideshare.net/abpascual?; www.slideshare.net/abpascual/
tools-in-family-assessment

VIDEO LINKS

Assessment Process Video—ORGovDHS: www.youtube.com/
watch?v=kagGIylgAnw

Social Work Assessment Video—Rebecca French: https://www
.youtube.com/watch?v=LklCLVHgt5E

Family Assessment Video—Austen Riggs: www.youtube.com/
watch?v=khWzUzfvtLg

REFERENCES

Barol, B. (2010). Generalist practice with groups. In J. Poulin (Ed.), *Strengths-based generalist practice: A collaborative approach* (pp. 219–253). Cengage.

Beck, A. (1983). A process analysis of group development. *Group, 7*(1), 19–28. https://doi.org/10.1007/BF01456476

Council on Social Work Education. (2022). *Educational policy and accreditation standards for baccalaureate and master's social work programs.* https://www.cswe.org/getmedia/94471c42-13b8-493b-9041-b30f48533d64/2022-EPAS.pdf

Cowger, C. (1997). Assessing client strengths: Assessment for client empowerment. In D. Saleebey (Ed.), *The strengths perspective in social work practice* (2nd ed., pp. 59–73). Longman.

Gambrill, E. (2013). *Social work practice: A critical thinker's guide* (3rd ed.). Oxford University Press.

Gibbons, J., & Gray, M. (2004). Critical thinking as integral to social work practice. *Journal of Teaching in Social Work, 24*, 19–38. https://doi.org/10.1300/J067v24n01_02

Hartford, M. (1971). *Groups in social work.* Columbia University Press.

Hepworth, D. H., Rooney, R., Rooney, G. D., & Strom-Gottfried, K. (2017). *Direct social work practice: Theory and skills* (10th ed.). Cengage.

Magen, R. (1995). Practice with groups. In C. Meyer, & M. Mattaini (Eds.), *The foundations of social work practice* (pp. 156–175). NASW Press.

Saleebey, D. (2013). *The strengths perspective in social work practice* (6th ed.). Pearson.

Schwartz, W. (1986). The group work tradition and social work practice. *Social Work with Groups, 8*(4), 7–28. https://doi.org/10.1300/J009v08n04_03

Seabury, B., Seabury, B., & Garvin, C. (2011). *Interpersonal practice in social work: Promoting competence and social justice* (3rd ed.). SAGE Publications.

Toseland, R., & Rivas, R. (2012). *An introduction to group work practice* (7th ed.). Allyn & Bacon.

Tuckman, B. (1965). Developmental sequence in small groups. *Psychological Bulletin, 63*(6), 384–399. https://doi.org/10.1037/h0022100

Walker, J., Briggs, H., Koroloff, N., & Friesen, B. (2007). Implementing and sustaining evidence-based practice in social work. *Journal of Social Work Education, 43*(3), 361–375. https://doi.org/10.5175/JSWE.2007.334832007

Assessing Organizations and Communities

Aysha's foundation MSW field placement is with a large nonprofit agency providing residential placement and foster care services to abused and neglected children and their families. The agency has a professional staff of about 200 social workers providing a wide range of services. During her first month Aysha worked closely with her field instructor to learn the agency operating procedures and begin her work with a caseload of foster children, biological parents, and foster families. She liked her field instructor, their team, and the work.

Over the next few months Aysha noticed some concerning organizational issues. The first was that staff morale was very low. Most of the social workers were unhappy, and many were looking for other jobs. The staff members were distrustful of the administration, and several of the social workers advised Aysha to never admit any mistake and to be very careful in what she said to supervisors and administrators. Aysha also began to realize that many of the social workers made disparaging comments and jokes about their clients. They seemed to view them as failures incapable of change and with almost no compassion or empathy.

Aysha discussed her observations with her field instructor, who understood her concerns. Together they decided that Aysha would interview a sample of the professional social work staff to come up with recommendations to improve staff morale and retention.

COMPETENCY 7: ASSESS INDIVIDUALS, FAMILIES, GROUPS, ORGANIZATIONS, AND COMMUNITIES

Social workers understand that assessment is an ongoing component of the dynamic and interactive process of social work practice. Social workers understand theories of human behavior and person-in-environment, as well as interprofessional conceptual frameworks, and they critically evaluate and apply this knowledge in culturally responsive assessment with clients and constituencies, including individuals, families, groups, organizations, and communities. Assessment involves a collaborative process of defining presenting issues and identifying strengths with individuals, families, groups, organizations, and communities to develop a mutually agreed-upon plan. Social workers recognize the implications of the larger practice context in the assessment process and use interprofessional collaboration in this process. Social workers are self-reflective and understand how bias, power, privilege, and their personal values and experiences may affect their assessment and decision-making.

Social workers

- apply theories of human behavior and person-in-environment, as well as other culturally responsive and interprofessional conceptual frameworks, when assessing clients and constituencies; and
- demonstrate respect for client self-determination during the assessment process by collaborating with clients and constituencies in developing a mutually agreed-upon plan. (Council on Social Work Education, 2022, p. 9)

LEARNING OBJECTIVES

By the end of this chapter, you will be able to:

- Discuss purposes of organizational assessment.
- Summarize five organizational theories.
- Describe five methods used in organizational assessments.
- Conduct a organizational assessment of your field placement agency.
- Design a community needs assessment for your field placement agency.
- Conduct a community asset assessment of your field placement agency's local community.

ASSESSING ORGANIZATIONS

The key to a good assessment is knowing what represents optimal functioning of the organization. Yet, at the same time, there is no "one best way" to construct an organization to meet all desired ends. Organizations may be structured in any one of several ways, each of which may be effective at achieving the goals of the organization under some conditions, but may be problematic at other times. Various groups or "constituencies" make up an organization. These may variously include line staff, supervisors, support staff, administration, clients, and external collaborators. Each typically has their own set of needs and perceptions about the organization, and thus each will have something valuable to contribute to the assessment (Kauffman, 2010).

Exhibit 13.1 shows the organizational components that are covered by five organizational theories. Taken together the five organizational theories cover almost all functions of an organization. A review of the five theories can be found in Poulin and Matis (2020). When designing an organizational assessment, the dimensions shown here provide a beginning list of organizational components to include in the assessment.

Organizational assessment allows an agency to evaluate whether it is meeting its mission and its goals. This is a planned systematic review of an organization's processes, work environment, and organizational structure within the constantly changing work environment; there is a periodic need to review how jobs are defined, departments organized, processes structured, and problems managed. Awareness of the variables that affect the agency, its workers, services, and climate is only part of the process of assessment.

Because organizations are complex entities, determining the questions in variables you hope to examine is a critical first step. Capacity assessments can examine the organization broadly, hoping to learn about all the various aspects, or narrowly (Poulin et al., 2022).

Nevertheless, whether broad or narrow, a good capacity assessment should begin with questions that allow the thorough description of the organization. Exhibit 13.2 shows examples of organizational assessment questions.

EXHIBIT 13.1

ORGANIZATIONAL THEORIES AND ORGANIZATIONAL ASSESSMENT

Theory	Organizational Dimension
Scientific Management	Worker Tasks and Functions Worker/Task Fit
Administrative Theory	Manager Effectiveness Administrative Functioning
Bureaucratic Theory	Task Specialization Hierarchical of Authority Formal Selection Rules and Requirements Impersonal Career Orientation
Rational Decision-Making Theory	Decision-Making Process
Organizational Development	Organizational Climate Organizational Culture Organizational Strategies

EXHIBIT 13.2

CAPACITY ASSESSMENT QUESTIONS

Overall Organizational Description

- What is the name of the organization?
- What are the mission and vision of the organization?
- What are the goals and objectives of the organization?
- What are the organization's legal auspices?
- Does the organization have a strategic plan? What are the organization's program goals for the future?

Existing Structure and Services

- What client population or populations does the organization serve?
- What services or programs does the organization provide?
- What is the administrative structure of the organization? (Provide an organizational chart.)
- How many staff members work at the organization?
- How are the programs funded?

Community and Environment

- What niche does the organization or program fill in the community (what needs does the agency address)?
- Are there other organizations in the area that also provide these same services? (Note—be brief here!)
- What is the demographic composition (# or percentage by age, race, income, gender) of the clients at the organization?
- What is the demographic composition (# or percentage by age, race, income, gender) of the staff at the organization?
- With which collaborating organizations or agencies does the organization work to provide services?

Performance and Change

- How well does the agency serve the identified goals and objectives?
- Does the agency meet its mission?
- What are the primary strengths of the organization?
- What are the current challenges facing the organization?

Source: Poulin, J., Kauffman, S., & Ingersoll, T. S. (2022). *Social work capstone projects: Demonstrating professional competencies through applied research* (pp. 109–110). Springer Publishing Company.

ORGANIZATIONAL ASSESSMENT TOOLS

Deciding how to assess and what tools to use is also very important. The first consideration is often the methodology, and almost any research methodology can be used. Following are a few of the more common organizational assessment methods.

FOCUS GROUPS

Focus groups are a wonderfully flexible method that may be used to obtain a large amount of data quickly under almost any set of conditions—except in case of a constituency that is unable to carry on a conversation. At its most general, a focus group is a group of 6 to 15 (usually) similar persons who are led through discussion of a series of open-ended questions with the purpose of finding consensus answers. Focus groups are very helpful in understanding the *why* question. A major limitation of this method is the lack of representativeness of the findings. Another limitation is the inability to provide descriptive data about the magnitude and scope of the issue being assessed.

SECONDARY ANALYSIS

For many assessment questions of need, secondary data and analysis of existing data are both desirable and reasonably simple. Agency records, both qualitative and quantitative, may contain large amounts of usable data. Qualitative data in the form of agency reports, legal documents, and other descriptive information can take you a long way to developing a rich description of the agency, its goals and purposes, and how it is organized. Similarly, for most issues of service provision, agencies can provide extensive records. These can include everything from case notes to sign-in sheets and even billing data. In many cases, quick transitions from spreadsheet to data analysis software are possible.

Of similar importance are the vast datasets that exist in the larger world. Many of the social problems we are interested in examining have entire organizations that are dedicated to doing little else but collecting relevant data. Crime, poverty, education, many health variables, many environmental variables, and occupation data at many geographic levels are quite easy to locate. However, two issues must be considered. First, if the data that you are accessing are used for comparative purposes, you must be certain that you have an appropriate justification for the comparison. If your organization is embedded in a larger geographic unit generally, you have a good justification. If you are looking to compare your data to a similar community, however, you need to be very careful about the criteria you use for comparison (Poulin et al., 2022).

SURVEYS AND INTERVIEWS

Surveys and interviews are indispensable tools for organizational assessments, most particularly if you are interested in getting descriptive data about experiences and opinions. The central issue here, however, is who to ask. Throughout an organization will be found a variety of different opinions about any number of things. Different opinions are good. However, different opinions that come from sources that are dramatically unlike one another can be a problem. Differences need to be considered in the analysis and interpretation of the data. Hopefully, you can survey or interview enough people with the same characteristics that you can obtain reasonably consistent results (Poulin et al., 2022).

OBSERVATIONAL PERFORMANCE RATINGS

> **Field Reflection Questions**
>
> What aspects of your field placement agency's organizational functioning need to be strengthened?
>
> How would you assess that component of your field placement agency's organizational functioning?

Another approach involves observation of the functioning of the organization, and then rating what is seen. Many organizational assessment tools can be used for this purpose. Many of them either are in the public domain or may be used with the

permission of the persons who hold the copyright. A sample organizational assessment tool can be found in the Student Mateirals at www .springerpub.com/fieldwrk.

ASSESSING COMMUNITIES

An empowerment approach to assessing community needs focuses on building relationships with community members. With this approach, the community is known to be capable of identifying and addressing its own issues. As a social worker, you are a partner in the assessment process. You provide technical assistance and support to the community members and constituent groups. Conducting a community needs assessment entails the same processes as any other research. You need to (1) define the purpose of the assessment, (2) identify your research questions, (3) identify your data sources, (4) design your research and data collection plan, (5) design your data collection instruments, (6) collect the data, (7) analyze the data, (8) interpret and disseminate your findings.

COMMUNITY ASSESSMENT APPROACHES

There are many ways to collect the data that you need for your community assessment. Observation, surveys, and focus groups provide three options.

Observation

This approach focuses on documenting behavior as it occurs. The observation may be conducted independently from the group being observed or as a participant. Observation includes going out into the community, walking the streets, interacting with community members, or attending meetings. It allows you to get to know the people and the environment. The key here is to systematically record your observations using journal entries, observational rating forms, and so forth.

Surveys

Survey data are collected using questionnaires and/or interview schedules. Both tools are excellent ways of "collecting information that you hope represents the views of the whole community or group in which you are interested" (Center for Community Health and Development at the University of Kansas, n.d., What Are Surveys? section). When developing a community survey, it is important to consult with community partners to understand the purpose for conducting the survey and reaffirm the need or problem that they seek to address. The three most common types of community assessment surveys are key informant surveys, community surveys, client satisfaction surveys, and focus groups.

Key Informant Surveys

This approach collects data from those who are informed about a given problem because of training or work experience—usually because they are involved in some sort of service with that population (Royse et al., 2005). Typically, they are the community residents, block captains, organizational leaders, local politicians, ward leaders, local business owners, law enforcement officers, school officials, and human services professionals who work with the client population whose need is being assessed.

Snowball sampling techniques are often used to generate a list of key informants. The person developing the survey begins with a few key informants and asks them to identify other persons knowledgeable about the problem or population being studied. Depending on the size of the key informant list, the key informants can be interviewed by telephone, in person, or by a mailed questionnaire. Key informant surveys are a relatively inexpensive and convenient way to obtain subjective (expert opinion) needs assessment data.

Community Surveys

Collecting data from households or community residents is another approach for assessing community needs. Typically, these types of surveys are more expensive and require a high level of survey research expertise to carry out. Community surveys can provide information about residents' perceptions of their needs and community conditions as well as empirical data that can be extrapolated to the community or population being investigated. The benefit of a well-executed community survey is that the findings are representative and can be generalized with a specified degree of confidence to the community or population being studied. The downside is cost and difficulties in carrying them out.

Client Satisfaction Surveys

This approach is like community surveys except that current or past recipients of a service or program are queried instead of community residents in general. Obtaining a sample of former or current clients tends to be easier than conducting a community survey because the study population is known, defined, and more limited. Client satisfaction studies can provide useful information for needs assessments. Clients are in a unique position to provide feedback on how well the service or program is meeting their needs, additional unmet needs, and the operation of the service or program.

Focus Groups

Another approach to documenting community needs is to conduct focus groups with key informants, community members, or clients. As described earlier, the social worker facilitating the focus group uses open-ended questioning and elaboration skills to obtain in-depth information about the topic under investigation. Focus group participants are selected based on their knowledge of the problem as well as how representative they are of the population group.

Field Reflection Questions

What are some of the needs of the community that your field placement agency serves? In what ways could your field placement agency better serve the community in addressing those needs?

How would you determine what the community thinks about its needs? How might the perceptions between the professionals and community members differ?

ASSET ASSESSMENT

Asset assessment is the process of determining the amount of social capital within the community. The solutions to community challenges are seen as residing within the community residents themselves. Community assets, as defined by Kretzmann et al. (2005), refer to those strengths that exist in a community. They include individual, economic, institutional, and organizational resources that are available to community residents. Components of an asset assessment may include the following:

- local residents, their skills, experiences, passions, capacities, and willingness to contribute to the project (special attention is paid to residents who are sometimes "marginalized")

- local voluntary associations, clubs, and networks—for example, all the athletic, cultural, social, and faith-based groups powered by volunteer members—that might contribute to the project

- local institutions—for example, public institutions such as schools, libraries, parks, and police stations, along with local businesses and nonprofit organizations—that might contribute to the project

- physical assets—for example, land, buildings, infrastructure, and transportation—that might contribute to the project

- economic assets—for example, what people produce and consume, businesses, informal economic exchanges, and barter relationships

An excellent resource for organizers seeking to understand Asset-Based Community Development (ABCD) is the ABCD Institute at DePaul University (https://resources.depaul.edu/abcd-institute/Pages/default.aspx). The three basic steps of ABCD are the following: (a) discovering the strengths in the community, (b) connecting with each other and with the community, and (c) coming together to build on knowledge and skills. The ABCD website provides a detailed description of ABCD, tools, and instruments for conducting assessments, and case examples of the use of ABCD.

ASSET MAPPING

A useful community assessment tool is the development of an asset map. Asset maps are visual representations of a community's resources. Organizers use capacity assessment instruments to determine the strengths and skills of individual residents (individual capacity assessment) and the opportunities and resources available to residents through the provision of social services programs offered by agencies or organizations (organizational capacity assessment). Once information is collected regarding community resources, community social workers use geographic information system (GIS) mapping to depict the special relationships between the existing resources and the community residents. Simple asset maps can be created by conducting a community resources assessment and plotting the addresses of the resources found on a map. The community resources assessment allows the social worker to identify potential assets and resources that are available to the client.

Although some resources can be found by conducting a simple internet search, many resources in low-income communities may not be documented. To uncover hidden assets, walk the neighborhood in which your agency resides. Often services exist in faith-based organizations, in hospitals, within fraternal and sorority organizations, or even in recreation centers. Social workers can develop a helpful resource for their agencies and their clients by collecting this information and geographically plotting it on a map. These asset maps allow clients to see where resources exist and how far they are from their homes, as well as identify gaps or underresourced areas.

Programs that use GIS software are available at ESRI.com. Mapping for 200 or fewer addresses can be plotted using free programs such as Batchgeo.com. Both programs interface with Excel spreadsheets. Be sure to read licensing agreements to determine the charges for your organization or personal use of such software.

COMMUNITY MEMBERS CAPACITY ASSESSMENT

This type of assessment is designed to measure the skills of individual residents in the community and to determine what resources they have available to address a particular social problem. Community members respond to questions that assess their vocational, interpersonal, and associational capacities. The goal is not only to ascertain the individual's personal assets, but also to determine the amount of interaction that a person has in the community. Often community members belong to or have connections with organizations or associations that can be helpful in addressing a problem. The inventory also asks residents to identify skills they would like to learn or that they could teach.

RESOURCE MAPPING

Resource mapping is a visual representation of the data that allows you to see where the resources in a community are in relation to your client population. Data can be mapped using a variety of tools that are available either through purchase or by using free resources on the internet. Programs such as Microsoft MapPoint are relatively inexpensive and are easy to learn. It is necessary to develop a database of information to categorize your resource findings prior to mapping.

CASE SUMMARY: "PRESCRIPTION DRUG COVERAGE?"

PRACTICE SETTING DESCRIPTION

My name is Rachel and I am a graduate social work student doing my first-year field placement at county services for the aging (COSA). COSA provides a wide range of free and low-cost services to seniors in the county. I am assigned to the Towers, a residential facility for seniors and disabled community members run by the local housing authority. My assignment is to provide case management services to the residents.

Sandra, my field instructor, is the director of communication and community services at the agency. One of her tasks is to conduct information sessions with seniors and assist them in signing up for the prescription drug plan that best meets their needs. I was asked to assist Sandra in developing and implementing a plan for informing residents about their options and to answer any questions that they had about their coverage and participation. As part of the planning process, I was asked to conduct a community assessment of the residents' information needs and participation in prescription drug plans. In supervision, Sandra and I discussed possible ways I could conduct the community assessment.

IDENTIFYING DATA

There are 125 residents living in the Towers. Ninety-eight are seniors age 65 or older, and 27 are disabled adults. All the residents are low-income individuals. Almost all the residents receive Supplemental Security Income (SSI) and either Medicare or Medicaid for their health insurance coverage. Approximately 90% of the residents are African Americans, and all are single, divorced, or widowed. Only about 15% of the residents have completed high school and none attended college. In terms of health status, it appears that almost all have some health issues and very few would be characterized as being in good to excellent health. In sum, the Towers residents are for the most part, African American older adults or disabled persons with very low incomes, limited education, and poor health who live alone.

PRESENTING PROBLEM

The presenting problem is that the social work staff serving the Towers residents do not know if the community members have prescription drug coverage and, if they do, whether it is the best option available. Because all the residents have very low incomes and numerous health issues, it is quite possible that they are spending more for their medications than they can afford or need to. This is a community-wide problem, not just a problem for individual residents.

ASSESSMENT

I was charged with conducting a community assessment of the Towers residents to gather data about their prescription drug coverage and information needs regarding their prescription drug coverage options. After conferring with Sandra, my field instructor, I decided to conduct a series of focus groups with the community members. We eliminated a pen-and-paper survey approach because of the overall low educational level of the residents. We also eliminated conducting personal interviews because of the large number of residents and time constraints. We both felt that the focus group approach would work best with the Towers population. The focus group approach would be manageable in terms of the time constraint, and it would be a comfortable format for the residents, who enjoy talking with one another. We decided that holding the focus groups with between 8 and 10 participants would give us enough information about the community residents to plan for informational and advocacy sessions. We decided to randomly invite 36 residents to participate in one of three focus groups. We also decided that I would personally invite each person selected to explain the purpose of the focus group, answer questions, and obtain informed consent. As an incentive to participate, each focus group participant would be entered into a drawing for a food basket.

CASE PROCESS SUMMARY

I conducted three focus groups. One group had 10 participants, one had eight, and the other group had five participants. I used open-ended questions to obtain information about the participants' prescription drug plans, how much they were spending on medications, and their knowledge of the different coverage options. Conducting the focus groups was challenging. The community residents were much more interested in talking with one another and had a hard time staying on the topic of prescription drugs. They seemed to really enjoy socializing and being in a group. In each group, someone asked if they could meet again to talk about something else or just get together.

I compiled the findings and presented them to Sandra. I concluded that most of the residents are not sure what prescription drug plan they are using and that almost all felt that they spend too much of their limited incomes on medications. Their knowledge of different options was very limited to nonexistent. I also concluded that thinking about the complicated topics such as drug insurance and co-pays appeared to be too difficult for many of the residents.

Rachel, MSW Student Intern

CASE DISCUSSION QUESTIONS

1. *Based on this case summary, discuss whether the decision to use focus groups for the community assessment was appropriate. If you were tasked with conducting the community assessment, what would you have done differently?*

2. *Given Rachel's findings from her focus groups, describe how you would approach Sandra's task of implementing a plan for informing residents about their prescription drug plan options. Describe the intervention you would use to provide the information and help the residents enroll in insurance plans that work best for them.*

3. *In thinking about Rachel's experience in conducting the focus groups, what types of services or programs would you propose to your field instructor to better serve the needs of the Towers residents? Describe the reasons for your proposed programs.*

4. *Rachel conducted an assessment of a 125-person residential community of low-income older and disabled adults. Describe at least one macro implication of her findings. What macro-policy changes do you think need to be addressed?*

END-OF-CHAPTER RESOURCES

 SPRINGER PUBLISHING CONNECT™

A robust set of instructor resources designed to supplement this text is located at http://connect.springerpub.com/content/book/978-0-8261-3753-1. Qualifying instructors may request access by emailing textbook@springerpub.com.

CRITICAL THINKING QUESTIONS

1. All organizations have function-related issues that could be improved. What is an organizational issue that you have noticed in your field placement? How would you assess this issue to obtain data to present to the administration and/or board?

2. How does the communication pattern between the administration and professional staff in your field placement affect client services and/or staff morale?

How would you go about assessing communication and its impact on clients and staff? What are the strengths of your proposed assessment? What are some of its limitations?

3. Describe the local physical and professional communities of which your field placement agency is a member. How does your agency impact those communities, and how is your agency impacted by them? What could your agency do to strengthen its impact on its local community? What could your agency do to strengthen its impact on its professional community?

LEARNING ACTIVITIES

ORGANIZATIONAL ASSESSMENT ACTIVITIES

1. *Conduct an organizational assessment.* In collaboration with your field instructor identify an area of organizational functioning that is challenging for the social work staff. Develop a list of questions that you would like to address. Identify the data collection method you would like to use in your assessment. Prepare a brief proposal that describes the problem area and a rationale, your research questions, data collection and analysis methods, and proposed time frame. Obtain agency permission to conduct your organizational assessment. Carry out your organizational assessment. Prepare a summary of your findings and your recommendations. Submit your assessment to your field instructor.

2. *Use supervision to analyze agency functioning.* Each week identify some aspect of agency functioning to include on your supervision agenda. Come to your supervision meeting prepared to share your observations on the identified topic.

3. *Service delivery assessment.* In collaboration with your field instructor identify a service delivery issue that is challenging for clients. Develop a list of questions that you would like to address. Identify the data collection method you would like to use in your assessment. Prepare a brief proposal that describes the problem area and a rationale, your research questions, data collection and analysis methods, and proposed time frame. Obtain agency permission to conduct your service delivery assessment. Carry out the assessment. Prepare a summary of your findings and your recommendations. Submit your assessment to your field instructor.

COMMUNITY ASSESSMENT ACTIVITIES

1. *Community needs assessment.* In collaboration with your field instructor identify a community issue that impacts your field placement clients or population. Develop a list of questions that you would like to address. Identify the data collection method you would like to use in your community needs assessment.

Prepare a brief proposal that describes the problem area and a rationale, your research questions, data collection and analysis methods, and proposed time frame. Obtain agency permission to conduct your community needs assessment. Carry out the assessment. Prepare a summary of your findings and your recommendations. Submit your needs assessment to your field instructor.

2. *Asset mapping.* Identify an asset map of the resources in the community that are available for your clients. Plot the community resources on a map of the community. If you have access to a GIS program, we recommend you use it to automate the mapping process. If you do not, there are free GIS programs available on the internet. One is QGIS which can be accessed at https://www .qgis.org/en/site. Analyze your GIS map and prepare a map summary to be discussed with your field instructor. Discuss with your field instructor ways that your asset map can be disseminated and how gaps in services can be addressed.

3. *Resource mapping.* Resource mapping is similar to asset mapping. The difference is that resource mapping allows you to see where community resources are located in relation to the client population. Prepare a resource map for your field placement agency's geographic community. If your agency serves a large number of clients select a random sample and plot the subjects' residential locations on the map. If it serves a small number of clients select a time frame and plot the residential locations for all the clients served within the time period. Analyze your results and prepare brief report for your field instructor.

ELECTRONIC RESOURCES

WEBSITE LINKS

 Organizational Assessment Tool: http://nonprofit.adelphi.edu/ resources/organizational-assessment/

 Community Needs Assessments: www.childwelfare.gov/topics/ systemwide/assessment/community

 Asset Mapping: www.vistacampus.gov/what-asset-mapping

Resource Mapping: www.ncset.org/publications/essentialtools/
mapping/overview.asp

VIDEO LINKS

Organizational Assessment: www.youtube.com/
watch?v=SfSiYDID888

Organizational Culture: www.youtube.com/
watch?v=Rd0kf3wd120

Creating Cultures: www.youtube.com/watch?v=BlhM7vALtUM

Community Needs Assessments: www.youtube.com/watch?v=
624PSllFWsA

Conducting a Community Needs Assessment: www.youtube
.com/watch?v=CziB8X_4T7U

Asset Mapping: www.youtube.com/watch?v=mJ7pSoJ25Hc

REFERENCES

Center for Community Health and Development at the University of Kansas. (n.d.). *Chapter 3. Assessing community needs and resources: Section 13. Conducting surveys*. Community Tool Box. https://ctb.ku.edu/en/table-of-contents/assessment/assessing-community-needs-and-resources/conduct-surveys/main

Council on Social Work Education. (2022). *Educational policy and accreditation standards for baccalaureate and master's social work programs*. https://www.cswe.org/getmedia/94471c42-13b8-493b-9041-b30f48533d64/2022-EPAS.pdf

Kauffman, S. (2010). Generalist practice with organizations. In J. Poulin (Ed.), *Strengths-based generalist practice: A collaborative approach* (3rd ed., pp. 254–321). Cengage.

Kretzmann, J. P., McKnight, J. L., Dobrowolski, S., & Puntenney, D. (2005). *Discovering community power: A guide to mobilizing local assets and your organization's capacity*. Asset-Based Community Development Institute. https://wlcvs.org/wp-content/uploads/2015/07/ABCD_and_organisations.pdf

Poulin, J., Kauffman, S., & Ingersoll, T. S. (2022). *Social work capstone projects: Demonstrating professional competencies through applied research*. Springer Publishing Company.

Poulin, J., & Matis, S. (2020). *Social work practice: A competency-based approach*. Springer Publishing Company.

Royse, D., Thyer, B. A., Padgett, D. K., & Logan, T. K. (2005). *Program evaluation: An introduction* (4th ed.). Brooks Cole.

Intervening With Individuals, Families, and Groups

Chelsea is an MSW student completing her first-year internship at a public child welfare agency. She had worked at the same agency for 4 years as a child protective services worker conducting investigations and assessments of reports of abuse and neglect. Although Chelsea had learned a great deal while doing her job, she was very happy to have been selected by her agency to pursue her MSW degree under the agency's education leave program.

In the 4 years that Chelsea had been a child welfare caseworker, she had felt both challenged and gratified by her job. She felt challenged by the extraordinary unmet needs of the children and families with whom she worked, but also gratified by the many opportunities she found to make a big difference in their lives by helping them to access resources and making sure that children were safe. Chelsea was aware that she had relied on her "gut feelings" and innate empathy to guide her in her work. With MSW education, Chelsea looked forward to learning the theories, techniques, and skills to make more informed assessments and decisions. She was also eager to learn about new methods that might provide more effective services for the children and families she had encountered.

When Chelsea arrived at her internship on Monday morning, she could feel the tension in the air. She soon learned from coworkers that over the weekend, 14-year-old Daniella Patrick had died as a result of dehydration and malnutrition. Although the girl was living with her mother and three younger siblings at the time of her death, the family had been known to the agency for over 3 years as a result of repeated reports from family and friends alleging neglect and abuse of Daniella and her siblings. A protective services worker, assigned to the family when the initial reports were received, was responsible for assessing the safety of the Patrick children and making recommendations regarding needed services.

The family had also been referred for services from a private provider agency under contract with Chelsea's agency. The role of the provider agency was to deliver intensive supervision and supportive services for the Patrick family in their home. It was routine practice to assign a public agency caseworker to monitor the provision of services by private provider agencies to make sure that appropriate support was available to the family.

Accordingly, a second caseworker from Chelsea's agency was responsible for visiting the family monthly to evaluate the situation and to review the reports of the provider agency regarding the family's status.

Chelsea was horrified, and the mood among the staff at the agency was one of depression and anxiety. The media and the public already viewed child welfare workers negatively. This would just make that perception worse. Two agencies—one public and one private—were responsible for ensuring the welfare and safety of Daniella. Three caseworkers had been involved in and charged with the responsibility of making sure that Daniella was safe. Yet she was found dead in her home, a victim of extreme neglect. How could this happen?

Chelsea already knew that her job required her to make decisions about the safety of vulnerable children in potentially high-risk situations. She was working with several families who could be considered "high risk." Could one of the children on her caseload die? Was she assessing safety and risk accurately? Was she using effective interventions in working with the parents or caregivers of the children for whom she was responsible? Were the current policies in place sufficient for protecting children from maltreatment and supporting families? If not, what changes in policies should be considered to prevent something like this from happening again? Should she reconsider the field of practice in which she had chosen to specialize?

COMPETENCY 8: INTERVENE WITH INDIVIDUALS, FAMILIES, GROUPS, ORGANIZATIONS, AND COMMUNITIES

Social workers understand that intervention is an ongoing component of the dynamic and interactive process of social work practice. Social workers understand theories of human behavior, person-in-environment, and other interprofessional conceptual frameworks, and they critically evaluate and apply this knowledge in selecting culturally responsive interventions with clients and constituencies, including individuals, families, groups, organizations, and communities. Social workers understand methods of identifying, analyzing, and implementing evidence-informed interventions and participate in interprofessional collaboration to achieve client and constituency goals. Social workers facilitate effective transitions and endings.

Social workers

- engage with clients and constituencies to critically choose and implement culturally responsive, evidence-informed interventions to achieve client and constituency goals; and

- incorporate culturally responsive methods to negotiate, mediate, and advocate, with and on behalf of clients and constituencies. (Council on Social Work Education, 2022, p. 9)

LEARNING OBJECTIVES

By the end of this chapter, you will be able to:

- Define generalist social work practice.

- Understand the difference between micro, mezzo, and macro social work practice.

- Describe the role that goals play in an intervention plan.

- Identify micro social work practice interventions.

- Describe different case management interventions.

GENERALIST SOCIAL WORK INTERVENTIONS

Generalist social work practitioners work with individuals, families, groups, communities, and organizations in a variety of social work and host settings. A classification of generalist social work practice interventions is shown in Exhibit 14.1. In this conceptualization, intervention tasks are categorized by practice level (micro, mezzo, and macro) and system level (individual, family, group, organization, or community). Generalist practice often requires simultaneous interventions on multiple levels. In any case situation or practice setting, you might be involved in several interventions on different practice and systems levels.

Generalist social work practice entails change activities at the micro, mezzo, and macro levels. *Micro social work practice* is interventions with individuals, couples, and families (Hepworth et al., 2017). Regardless of the client system, the purpose of micro-level practice is to enhance functioning and empower the client. *Mezzo-level practice* involves interventions with organizations and communities or neighborhoods. The purpose of mezzo-level practice is to improve organizational functioning and service delivery and community well-being for vulnerable populations. *Macro-level practice* involves change efforts at the municipality, county, state, national, or international level, and the purpose of macro-level practice is to help vulnerable populations indirectly through policy change, program development, and advocacy.

Micro interventions commonly used by generalist social workers are divided into two broad groups: counseling and case management (Exhibit 14.1). Counseling interventions include supportive counseling as well as education and training. Case management includes service linkage, service coordination, service negotiation, resource mobilization, and client advocacy.

Field Reflection Questions

In your field placement, what practice level will be the primary focus of your work?

What levels of practice will need special efforts to ensure learning opportunities?

EXHIBIT 14.1

GENERALIST PRACTICE INTERVENTIONS

System Level	Client System	Generalist Interventions
Micro Individual Family Group	Individuals Families/couples Small groups	Counseling Assessment Supportive counseling Education and training Case management Service linkage Service coordination Service negotiation Resource mobilization Client advocacy
Mezzo Organization Community/neighborhood	Administrators Task forces Committees Advisory boards Community groups Professional task forces Community coalitions Neighborhood groups	Education and training Strategic planning Program development and grant writing Program evaluation Needs assessments Policy analysis Community organizing Community development Cause advocacy Resource coordination
Macro Municipality County State National International	Governmental bodies Advocacy groups Professional organizations Policy think tanks Foundations Research institutes Intergovernmental organizations	Policy analysis Policy proposals Advocacy Basic research Program evaluation Needs assessments

Mezzo-level interventions focus on organizational and community change. Typical client systems at the organizational level are organizational leaders, task forces, and committees. The system level is the organization, and the client systems that the social worker engages are the decision-makers and decision-making structures of the organization. The worker usually participates in formally organized work groups, such as agency task forces or committees, often to develop new services or improve existing services. The client system might also be the organization's decision-makers—that is, administrators and supervisors. Thus, a generalist social worker seeking to change an organization may view the decision-makers or the decision-making structures as the client system when trying to improve how decisions are made or how the organization communicates about decisions, activities, or services. An organization that does not function well may not serve its clients or even the very staff who work within those organizations. Thus, at the organizational level, the purpose of macro-level practice is to improve the functioning of the organization, improve services and service delivery, or develop new services through program development and/or grant writing. All three purposes involve change of the organization or agency.

Typical client systems at the community level are professional task forces, community coalitions, and neighborhood or community citizens' groups. Often, the purpose of community practice is to improve community or neighborhood conditions, empower residents, develop resources, increase community awareness of social and economic problems, and mobilize people to advocate for needed resources and changes. Generalist social workers engaged in community change usually work with professional or community groups. Some groups have both professional and citizen members. Social workers engaged in community practice may view the group they are working with as the client system. In other words, the client system may be the professional task force, neighborhood group, or community coalition that is seeking to change or improve the community. Alternatively, the client system may be the residents of the community.

Macro-level generalist social work practice focuses on larger system change. Macro-level client systems typically include governmental bodies, advocacy groups, intergovernmental organizations, professional organizations, and other entities focused on larger system change to improve the well-being of individuals, families, and communities. Macro interventions include policy analysis, development of policy proposals, cause advocacy, basic research, program evaluations, and needs assessments. There are even roles for international collaboration. In recent years, more and more social problems have begun to cross borders. Such issues as globalization, immigration, and climate change often require social workers to dialogue and work with international partners.

Importantly, all the micro-level skills generalist social workers develop may well be needed when working with mezzo- and macro-level client systems. Effective communication, goal setting, and sensitivity to the needs of individuals in some ways become even more important when working with the (often) large and complex client systems that are found at the organizational, community, and national levels. Case Example 14.1 illustrates the variety of roles played by generalist social workers.

CASE EXAMPLE 14.1: PROFILE OF A GENERALIST SOCIAL WORK INTERN

Gina had her first-year MSW field placement at Social Work Consultation Services (SWCS), an innovative agency developed by her graduate school of social work and a community-based agency. SWCS provided generalist social work learning experiences for social work students and capacity-building services for the residents and organizations of an economically disadvantaged community.

At SWCS, Gina undertook a range of generalist social work tasks and activities. As a member of the senior services team, she provided micro-level counseling and case management services for older residents of a senior housing facility. Gina met with her senior clients weekly. For some, she provided supportive counseling addressing a variety of concerns, such as family relationships, isolation, depression, and a host of loss issues. For other clients, she served as a case manager. She referred clients to other service providers (service linkage), negotiated on their behalf with other service providers (service negotiation), obtained resources for them (resource mobilization), and advocated for them in any way she could (client advocacy).

Gina's work on the senior team also entailed a number of mezzo-level practice activities. Gina and two of the senior team interns established a 1-day-a-week drop-in center at the senior housing facility (program planning) and began holding monthly meetings with local providers who served older clients to share information, reduce service duplication, and increase coordination (resource coordination). Gina helped develop programs and monthly group activities for residents and organized two ongoing support groups (program planning). In addition, Gina and her team organized a community service day that targeted older community residents (community development). The student volunteers provided cleaning and chore services for 125 older adults. Gina also wrote a grant proposal (program planning) for additional funding for the SWCS program, helped conduct a program evaluation (program planning), and conducted a series of training workshops for another agency's case managers (education and training).

Gina engaged in mezzo-level practice by organizing a 3-day community event designed to promote community awareness of violence against women (education and advocacy). Gina and two other student interns planned, organized, obtained funding for, and implemented the city-wide event. Approximately 200 community residents, students, faculty, and staff participated in the program.

SMART GOALS

Client goals are derived directly from client problems and concerns. The assessment process focuses on identifying the areas of concern that clients want to address in the helping process. It also identifies client system strengths and resources. The contracting process follows up on this work by focusing on what the client system hopes to accomplish. Problems are negative statements about the client's current situation, whereas goals are positive statements about what the client's situation will be after the identified problem has been resolved or ameliorated.

One of the major purposes of goals is to set the direction for the work. When writing goals, we encourage you to use the SMART acronym. SMART stands for specific, measurable, achievable, relevant, and time-bound (see Exhibit 14.2). Specifying goals ensures that you and your client agree about what is expected. Without specific

EXHIBIT 14.2

SMART GOALS

	Definition	Poor Example	Rationale and Improvement
Specific	You are clearly articulating what exactly you expect. Anyone who reads this goal would be able to easily understand the exact criteria. Create operational definitions whenever necessary for clarity.	The client will learn to cope with their anxiety.	It is not clear how the client will be coping—we could specifically list the coping strategies we expect the client to utilize to help assist in managing their anxiety.
Measurable	You clearly state the quantity or quality that is required for the goal to be accomplished.	The client will practice using positive self-talk statements.	It is not clear how often this will occur—we could add a quantifiable number to the goal and say that the client will practice this strategy one time per day.
Achievable	Your goal is attainable by the client.	The client will eliminate all depressive thoughts.	Though ideally, we would love to help rid our clients of all depressive thoughts, it is not realistic that we will accomplish this as an initial goal. Rather aiming for a specific symptom reduction is a more achievable goal that could give the client a greater chance of success at meeting the goal. Remember, we can always update our treatment plan and develop new goals if a client meets their goals!
Relevant	Your goal relates to the problems and issues shared by the client.	To deal with feelings of loneliness, the client will practice deep breathing.	For this goal we need to make sure that the subject of our goal relates to the problem being targeted. In our example, we are trying to illustrate that disconnect between loneliness and the intervention. Maybe a more appropriate goal would be "To deal with feelings of loneliness, the client will attend one social activity in the next 2 weeks."
Time-bound	There is a clearly stated window of time by which the goal is to be achieved.	The client will attend a peer recovery support group.	As it is written the current goal does not reflect any time. We can make it time bound by saying, "Within the next month the client will attend a peer recovery support group."

Field Reflection Questions

In your field placement, how do you set goals with your clients?

How do you incorporate client goals into your practice?

goals, you may have different expectations about what needs to be accomplished. Goals also help facilitate the development of your intervention plan by identifying tasks and activities that will be undertaken to address the identified target problems and concerns. Finally, goals provide benchmarks for monitoring client progress. Without clear and specific goals, it is impossible for you or your client to determine whether progress is being made and whether a desired end has been attained. Goals provide direction for the helping process, ensure agreement between you and your client about what you hope to achieve, facilitate the development of your intervention plan, and provide a benchmark for judging progress.

INTERVENTION PLAN

The intervention plan specifies what will be done by whom to achieve the identified goals. It is the plan of action for the helping relationship. This action plan is essentially a contract between you and your client about how you will collaboratively work toward the identified goals.

Several considerations are involved in developing the intervention plan. The contract is an evolving entity and continues throughout the entire course of the helping process (Hepworth et al., 2017). The intervention plan should not be viewed as fixed once it is developed. The nature of social work practice is such that priorities, goals, and plans change and are modified as the helping process unfolds. Consequently, the contract evolves and is modified to reflect the changing nature of the work.

The intervention plan developed by you and your client is a collaborative undertaking. Your task is to provide guidance and technical support. Your client's task is to create the substance of the plan. Regardless of the client's level of functioning, it is imperative that the client participate in creating the action plan. The plan should belong to the client, not to you or anyone else. It should specify who will do what within what time frame to achieve each of the identified goals. For each goal, specify the tasks and activities that will be undertaken. The time frame for accomplishing each task also should be specified in the plan.

INDIVIDUAL AND FAMILY INTERVENTIONS

Most interventions are usually done in collaboration with your client. Sometimes you provide an intervention on behalf of your client. The two micro interventions usually undertaken by generalist social workers are supportive counseling and case management. Within each of these broad categories, there are a variety of more specific intervention tasks and activities. This section describes several micro interventions used by generalist social workers. The ones selected for inclusion here are the most common generalist interventions; they do not represent the full range of intervention strategies and approaches.

COUNSELING

Supportive counseling and education and training are two traditional direct service interventions that are frequently used by generalist social workers. Both are counseling-type interventions.

CASE EXAMPLE 14.2: SUPPORTIVE COUNSELING INTERVENTION

Jim is a 15-year-old sophomore previously diagnosed as having a moderate learning disability. He takes regular college preparation courses and has managed to maintain a B grade average. He receives tutoring in math and science and uses the writing center at the school to help him write all his papers. Although he struggles academically, he has been relatively successful in school.

Jim has no close friends and very few friendly acquaintances. His peers view him as odd and as a "loser." His attempts to fit in and make friends have met with rejection and ridicule, and he has withdrawn socially and makes no attempt to interact with classmates. Jim spends all his free time at home watching television and playing computer games.

While at home, Jim appears to take out his frustration on his family. He is very demanding of his parents and causes many disturbances within the family. He gets angry quickly and lashes out at his parents over little things. He constantly picks on his younger sister, puts her down in front of her friends, criticizes her looks and abilities, and treats her with general disrespect. When Jim gets into "one of his moods" or is "on the warpath," the tension in the family gets very high. During these times, everyone seems to be mad at everyone else. His parents start fighting, and the general mood in the family is tense and hostile.

Jim's parents are concerned about his lack of peer relationships and his behavior at home. They contacted the school social worker to inquire about help for their son. To his family's surprise, Jim agreed to meet regularly with the school social worker, and together they developed an intervention plan.

SUPPORTIVE COUNSELING

In supportive counseling, the social worker takes the enabler role in the helping relationship (Hepworth et al., 2017). The social worker and the client agree to meet for a specified time and engage in a collaborative therapeutic or counseling process. The purpose of the intervention is to help the client resolve concerns and challenges, enhance coping, and improve functioning.

Case Example 14.2 illustrates a supportive counseling intervention. In this case example, supportive counseling was one of the agreed-upon interventions.

Jim recognized his difficulties with peer and family relationships, and he wanted to do something to improve the situation. Jim and the school social worker met once a week to help him improve his relationships. The social worker provided supportive counseling to help Jim gain insight into the problem and to help him develop coping strategies that would increase his effectiveness with peers and family members. Jim also used the counseling sessions to deal with his feelings of low self-worth and the hurt and anger he felt toward his classmates.

Within the supportive counseling framework, the social worker and the client can engage in a variety of therapeutic modalities. The choice of a specific modality is determined, in part, by the focus of the work and the identified concerns. Walsh (2015) provides an excellent review of the theories behind many specialized interventions. It is beyond the scope of this book to review the various specialized individual and family interventions that might be used in your field placements. Exhibit 14.3 provides a brief description of some of the more widely used individual and family interventions and website links to obtain more detailed descriptions for each. All the interventions listed in the following text are evidence-based programs that have been researched, tested empirically, and shown to be effective interventions.

EDUCATION AND TRAINING

Education and training is a micro intervention that involves helping individuals, families, and groups learn new concepts and skills. Generalist social workers empower clients through an exchange of information in this form of intervention. This kind of information exchange occurs as a normal part of most social work interventions. However, when it is a primary goal of the interaction, it becomes an intervention.

When functioning as an educator or trainer with any client, especially with a disadvantaged and oppressed client, it is important to be mindful of power differences between you and your client. You have the knowledge and power, and it is easy to assume the role of expert. You can minimize this power differential by taking an empowering strengths-based approach and beginning with the capacities of your clients. Have them share their knowledge of the topic. An educational intervention may involve helping clients learn new skills, such as parenting, disciplining children, life care, budgeting, time management, and/or shopping. Case Example 14.3 illustrates an educational intervention.

CASE EXAMPLE 14.3: EDUCATIONAL INTERVENTION

Time Out for Tots is a parenting program for teenage mothers. The program consists of 15 two-hour sessions. The young mothers attend a weekly mother-only group session, during which information about child development and parenting is presented by the social worker. Group members also share their personal experiences and challenges. The second component of the program involves both the mothers and the children in a weekly group play session. During these sessions, the social worker models appropriate parent–child interactions and supports the mothers' use of the concepts and techniques covered in the group sessions.

EXHIBIT 14.3

SPECIALIZED INTERVENTIONS FOR INDIVIDUALS AND FAMILIES

Name	Brief Description	Website Links
Individual Interventions		
CBT	CBT is a time-sensitive, structured, present-oriented psychotherapy directed toward solving current problems and teaching clients skills to modify dysfunctional thinking and behavior.	Beck Institute for Cognitive Behavioral Therapy https://beckinstitute.org/about/understanding-cbt/
SFBT	SFBT is future focused, goal directed, and oriented toward solutions, rather than the problems that brought clients to seek therapy. With SFBT, the conversation is directed toward developing and achieving the client's vision of solutions by exploring previous solutions, exceptions, the present and future, and the miracle question.	Institute for Solution-Focused Therapy (2022) https://solutionfocused.net/what-is-solution-focused-therapy
MI	MI is a clinical approach that helps people with mental health and substance use disorders and other chronic conditions such as diabetes, cardiovascular conditions, and asthma make positive behavioral changes. The approach focuses on the following: expressing empathy and avoiding arguing, developing discrepancy, rolling with resistance, and supporting self-efficacy (the client's belief that they can successfully make a change).	SAMHSA-HRSA Center for Integrated Health Solutions https://www.samhsa.gov/sites/default/files/programs_campaigns/homelessness_programs_resources/path-spotlight-motivational-interviewing.pdf
NT	NT is an empowering and collaborative approach that recognizes people possess natural competencies, skills, and expertise that can help guide change in their lives. People are viewed as separate from their problems; in this way, a therapist can help externalize sensitive issues. This helps clients be more open to change or a new, healthier narrative.	Dulwich Center (2022) dulwichcentre.com.au

(continued)

EXHIBIT 14.3

SPECIALIZED INTERVENTIONS FOR INDIVIDUALS AND FAMILIES (*continued*)

Name	Brief Description	Website Links
TCP	TCP involves a four-step process to establish distinct and achievable goals on the basis of an agreed-upon presenting problem, usually called the target problem. The social worker and the client cocreate a contract that contains the target problem, tasks to be implemented by both client and practitioner to address the target problem, and overall goals of the treatment. The client's priorities and strengths are interwoven into the entire TCP process. Most TCP involves working briefly with clients, typically in 8 to 12 sessions over the course of a 6-month period.	*Encyclopedia of Social Work* (Kelly & Colindres, 2020) http://socialwork .oxfordre.com/view/10.1093/ acrefore/9780199975839.001 .0001/acrefore-978019997 5839-e-38
Family Interventions		
FFT	FFT is a short-term, intervention program that involves an average of 12 to 14 sessions over 3 to 5 months. It works primarily with 11- to 18-year-old youths who have been referred for behavioral or emotional problems. FFT uses a strengths-based model built on a foundation of acceptance and respect. The focus is on assessment and intervention to address risk and protective factors within and outside the family. FFT consists of five major components: engagement, motivation, relational assessment, behavior change, and generalization.	Functional Family Therapy (2022) https://www.fftllc.com
MST	MST is an intensive family- and community-based treatment that addresses the multiple causes of serious antisocial behavior across key settings, or systems within which youth are embedded (family, peers, school, and neighborhood). Because MST emphasizes promoting behavior change in the youth's natural environment, the program aims to empower parents with the skills and resources needed to independently address the behavioral problems. Initial therapy sessions identify the strengths and weaknesses of the adolescent, the family, and their transactions with extrafamilial systems (e.g., peers, friends, school, parental workplace). Problems identified by both family members and the therapist are explicitly targeted for change by using the strengths in each system to facilitate such change.	Blueprints for Healthy Youth Development https://www .blueprintsprograms.org/ programs/32999999/ multisystemic-therapy-mst/

(continued)

EXHIBIT 14.3

SPECIALIZED INTERVENTIONS FOR INDIVIDUALS AND FAMILIES (*continued*)

Name	Brief Description	Website Links
BSFT	BSFT is a short-term, problem-focused therapeutic intervention, targeting children and adolescents 6 to 17 years old, that improves youth behavior by eliminating or reducing drug use and its associated behavior problems, and that changes family members' behaviors that are linked to both risk and protective factors related to substance abuse. The therapeutic process uses techniques such as the following: • Joining: forming a therapeutic alliance with all family members • Diagnosis: identifying interactional patterns that allow or encourage problematic youth behavior • Restructuring: changing family interactions that are directly related to problem behaviors	Cherry (2021) https://www.verywellmind.com/what-is-structural-family-therapy-5193068
FAST	FAST is an 8-week program that brings multiple families together once a week after school. In each 2.5-hour session, the trained FAST team guides families through a scientifically structured agenda of evidence-based activities that enhance parenting skills and reduce family stress while encouraging family bonding. Each FAST session includes group activities as well as one-on-one parent–child interaction and parent group time.	Families and School Together (2022) https://www.familiesandschools.org/what-we-do/fast-program/

BSFT, brief structural family therapy; CBT, cognitive behavioral therapy; FAST, Families and Schools Together; FFT, functional family therapy; HRSA, Health Resources and Services Administration; MI, motivational interviewing; MST, multisystemic therapy; NT, narrative therapy; SAMHSA, Substance Abuse and Mental Health Services Administration; SFBT, solution-focused brief therapy; TCP, task-centered practice.

CASE MANAGEMENT

Many micro generalist interventions fall within the broad category of case management. Typically, a social worker provides one or more of the following case management interventions: service linkage, service coordination, service negotiation, resource mobilization, and advocacy (Poulin & Matis, 2021).

Service Linkage

Social workers have longed been rooted in the intervention of service linkage, which is another form of direct service. The social worker takes the broker role in the helping relationship (Hepworth et al., 2017), referring a client to another agency for service. The process is more than just making a referral, though: Service linkage creates a new link between the client system and an existing service. This is a major function of generalist social workers, especially because many clients who are referred to agencies for service do not follow through on the referral or, if they do, are not accepted for service.

It is important that social workers build and maintain collaborative relationships within the communities they serve. Having relationships with key contact people throughout the professional community will help you get your client accepted for service. Often, the client does not exactly fit the eligibility criteria, or there may be a limited number of service slots available. In these situations, your relationship with the agency contact person can help smooth the way so that the client is accepted for service. The importance of knowing someone in the system cannot be overstated. Becoming familiar with existing services within the community as well as developing relationships with professional colleagues is an important aspect of the broker role in generalist social work practice.

Service Coordination

Many clients have multiple problems and often need more than one service. In service coordination, you as the social worker coordinate the various services and professionals to ensure that they are integrated and working toward common goals.

In Case Example 14.2 a service coordination intervention was not used. Although the social worker stayed in contact with the social worker providing family therapy and the worker at the teen center, she did not coordinate the unrelated services. No effort was made to ensure that the services were integrated. If Jim's social worker and the family therapist had developed an integrated treatment plan for Jim and the family, and if Jim's social worker had assumed responsibility for coordinating their efforts, a service coordination type of intervention would have taken place.

Service Negotiation

Service negotiation involves helping individuals and families overcome difficulties they have encountered with service delivery systems. Service negotiation focuses on helping the client resolve problems and difficulties with existing service linkages. As a social worker, you take a position between your client and the service provider to improve linkage and resolve conflicts. You help your client negotiate with system providers to address duplication of services, ineligibility, and poor service quality. Your primary task is to facilitate communication between your client and service representatives so that they can reach an agreement (Poulin & Matis, 2021).

Service negotiation was not used in Jim's case (Case Example 14.2). However, later in her work with Jim, the social worker helped the family negotiate with the school system. Jim's parents asked the school to run a full battery of psychological and diagnostic tests to assess Jim's learning difficulties. The school system's first response was that he could not be tested until the start of the following school year, a delay of more than 9 months. Jim's parents asked the school social worker to intervene. She helped the family negotiate a much earlier testing date by assisting them in presenting relevant information about Jim's functioning at home and his social isolation at school at a meeting she set up with the school psychologist. Thus, the school social worker provided a service negotiation intervention for the family by facilitating better communication between the school psychologist and the family.

Resource Mobilization

Resource mobilization involves helping the client obtain needed resources, such as housing, clothing, food, furniture, financial support, or healthcare (Hepworth et al., 2017). The distinction between resource mobilization and service linkage is a very small. Resource mobilization is the acquisition of needed services, whereas service linkage is helping clients obtain such services. Both are concerned with helping the client system gain access to needed services, both require knowledge of service networks, and both involve a referral process. The difference lies in the type of service: Resource mobilization focuses on helping clients obtain resources needed to meet basic human needs, whereas service linkage helps them obtain social, psychological, and healthcare services.

CLIENT ADVOCACY

Social workers have a long tradition of advocating on behalf of issues and client systems. Our National Association of Social Workers (NASW) *Code of Ethics* (2021) calls upon us to actively advocate and empower the clients we serve to advocate on their own behalf as well. There are two types of client advocacy: case advocacy and class advocacy. In case advocacy, the social worker is advocating for a specific client system (possibly a person or family system). In class advocacy, the client system is a large collective or group of people defined by some demographic characteristic.

> **Field Reflection Questions**
>
> What micro interventions are used in your field placement agency?
>
> What micro interventions are you most comfortable performing? What micro interventions are you least comfortable using?

GROUP INTERVENTIONS

Generalist social workers are involved with many different types of groups. There are a variety of types of micro-level practice groups (see Exhibit 14.4). The primary purposes of treatment groups are to increase members' coping abilities and help them resolve sociopsychological needs. The primary purposes of task groups, by

EXHIBIT 14.4

TYPES OF MICRO-LEVEL PRACTICE GROUPS

Client Groups	Description
Therapy	Groups that focus on the remediation or rehabilitation of members' intrapsychic or interpersonal problems, such as groups for depression, anger management, and substance abuse
Support	Groups established to provide support to members and help them cope with an issue that is common to all the members of the group, such as a parent bereavement group
Educational	Groups that have an educational objective and use educational techniques, such as parent training groups and teen leadership groups
Growth	Groups that focus on self-improvement and personal growth of the members, such as consciousness-raising groups and empowerment groups

comparison, are to accomplish a specific undertaking, produce a product, or carry out a mandate (Hepworth et al., 2017).

CASE SUMMARY: "BUT I AM NOT READY TO LEAVE"

PRACTICE SETTING DESCRIPTION

Leslie, a first-year MSW student intern, is placed with the Senior Care Center, a 16-week partial hospitalization program for individuals ages 65 and older who are experiencing a mental illness. Most clients are experiencing depression, often following the onset of a medical condition (e.g., Parkinson's disease, cancer, a stroke) and/or following the loss of a spouse or loved one. Some clients have a long history of mental illness, including major depression, bipolar disorder, schizophrenia, and so forth. Many of the clients of the center are either coming out of psychiatric hospitalization or placed in this program to prevent hospitalization. Others are referred by their outpatient psychiatrist or primary physician or make a self-referral.

The Senior Care Center provides individual and group therapy. The groups consist of psychoeducation, music and art therapy, discharge planning, relapse prevention, and more intense psychotherapy groups. Clients also meet weekly with their social worker for supportive counseling. In addition, the social worker oversees the treatment plan and is responsible for developing the discharge plan.

IDENTIFYING DATA

Mrs. K. is a 77-year-old White woman with a 43-year history of depressive episodes. She and been diagnosed with both major depressive disorder and bipolar disorder. In late 1994, Mrs. K. was diagnosed with Parkinson's disease. Shortly after that, she was admitted to the hospital's inpatient psychiatric ward where she received electroconvulsive therapy (ECT). Following her discharge from the hospital, Mrs. K. was referred to the Senior Care Center for continued mental health treatment and therapy.

PRESENTING PROBLEM

After attending the Senior Care Center for more than 3 years, Mrs. K. was told several weeks ago that she is being discharged at the end of March. When she entered the program, there was no set time limit on how long a client could stay in the program. Recently, the center was informed by the managed care company that the maximum length of stay would be approximately 16 weeks per client.

Mrs. K.'s biggest obstacle is her physical health. Her Parkinson's disease has limited her ability to function independently, and it has also started to impair her cognitive abilities, including her memory. In addition, she is suffering from depression. With her medication and the benefits of the Senior Care Center, Mrs. K. has been coping with her depression very well. The concern is that she will fall back into her depression once she is no longer attending the center.

ASSESSMENT

Mrs. K. needs to improve her ability to be assertive regarding her needs and wishes. She acknowledges this in her individual sessions with her social worker and realizes that she especially needs to work on this around the time of her discharge.

Fortunately, Mrs. K. also has many strengths. She is a genuinely caring and optimistic person; she is intelligent and has a wonderful sense of humor. In addition, Mrs. K. is determined to stay active and fight the effects of Parkinson's disease. She rarely misses her scheduled days at the center and states that she cannot stand to sit around the house and do nothing. Mrs. K. has a caring, supportive husband and son.

CASE PROCESS SUMMARY

Given her current level of functioning, the treatment team does not feel that her continued participation in the program is justified given the new reimbursement guidelines and policies. Mrs. K., her husband, and their son are upset about her pending discharge. All of them feel that she benefits from the treatment she receives at the Senior Care Center and that after more than 3 years the center has become an important part of her life.

Leslie explored with Mrs. K. her feelings about termination. She was very clear that she did not want to stop coming to the center every day. She was very fearful of getting depressed again and also fearful about her health deteriorating. I acknowledged her feelings about the termination. Although I could not justify keeping Mrs. K. in the program based on the new guidelines, I felt that Mrs. K. needed the support and stability the program offered. Together we developed the following termination plan:

- *Mrs. K., in coordination with her case manager, will enroll in the aftercare group at the hospital and attend outpatient therapy at the center.*

- *Leslie will investigate the possibility of Mrs. K. receiving physical and/or occupational therapy for Parkinson's disease through the hospital.*

- *Mrs. K. will begin attending a Senior Activities Center once a week.*

- *Mrs. K. will continue to verbalize feelings about being discharged during individual counseling with Leslie and at home with her family members.*

- *Mrs. K. will verbalize her needs and wishes regarding her discharge to the Senior Care Center staff and her family members.*

CASE DISCUSSION QUESTIONS

1. *Discuss the ethics of discharging Mrs. K. and whether Leslie is facing an ethical dilemma. What benefits do you see in having Mrs. K. stay in the program? What are the benefits of termination? What are the negatives of staying and leaving? What would you do if you were Leslie?*

2. *Critique Mrs. K.'s discharge plan. What additional aftercare services need to be added to the plan?*

3. *List the types of activities you perform in your field placement. For each activity, identify the client system level and client systems. What client systems are relevant to this case?*

4. *What social work values appear to have a bearing on this case? Are there any ethical dilemmas that you would want to address? If so, how would you resolve them?*

END-OF-CHAPTER RESOURCES

A robust set of instructor resources designed to supplement this text is located at http://connect.springerpub.com/content/book/978-0-8261-3753-1. Qualifying instructors may request access by emailing textbook@springerpub.com.

CRITICAL THINKING QUESTIONS

1. In your field placement, what are the micro-level interventions that you use to intervene with your clients? How effective are those interventions? What makes them effective? What keeps them from being effective? How does diversity impact the effectiveness?

2. Describe the intersection between intervening with your individual and/or family clients and the diversity competency. How does your addressing diversity and difference affect how you intervene with your clients? What do you need to do to strengthen your cultural competence in your work with individual or family clients?

3. How have your field placement clients' life experiences with oppression, poverty, and/or marginalization informed your effort to provide micro-level social work services?

LEARNING ACTIVITIES

1. Reflect on writing SMART goals. Write five goals for yourself as a current social work student. What goals do you have for the next 3 months? Write out each goal and check that it is specific, measurable, achievable, relevant, and time bound.

2. Consider the specialized interventions for individuals and families shared in this chapter. Select one to learn more about. Find two research articles on the intervention you selected and summarize them to share with another social worker.

ELECTRONIC RESOURCES

WEBSITE LINKS

SMART Goals: How to Guide by University of California: https://www.ucop.edu/local-human-resources/_files/performance-appraisal/How%20to%20write%20SMART%20Goals%20v2.pdf

International Association for Social Work With Groups: www.iaswg.org

American Association for Marriage and Family Therapy: www.aamft.org/iMIS15/AAMFT

Clinical Social Work Association: www.clinicalsocialwork association.org

VIDEO LINKS

 Developing Treatment Plans—The Social Work Podcast: http://socialworkpodcast.blogspot.com/2007/03/developing-treatment -plans-basics.html

 Evidence-Based Practice—USC Suzanne Dworak-Peck School of Social Work: www.youtube.com/watch?v=BPqv9K-IZUI

 Solution-Focused Therapy—Ben Furman: www.youtube.com/ watch?v=OlGQDq2j6Gw

 Functional Family Therapy—George Kalarritis: www.youtube .com/watch?v=72YRyNlYNfw

REFERENCES

Cherry, K. (2021, July 31). *What is structural family therapy?* Verywell Mind. https://www.verywellmind.com /what-is-structural-family-therapy-5193068

Council on Social Work Education. (2022). *Educational policy and accreditation standards for baccalaureate and master's social work programs.* https://www.cswe.org/getmedia/94471c42-13b8-493b-9041 -b30f48533d64/2022-EPAS.pdf

Dulwich Center. (2022). *What is narrative therapy?* https://dulwichcentre.com.au/what-is-narrative-therapy

Families and Schools Together. (2022). *FAST program.* https://www.familiesandschools.org/what-we-do/ fast-program

Functional Family Therapy. (2022). *Evidence-based interventions for youth and families.* https://www.fftllc .com

Hepworth, D. H., Rooney, R. H., Rooney, G. D., & Strom-Gottfried, K. (2017). *Direct social work practice: Theory and skills* (10th ed.). Cengage.

Institute for Solution-Focused Therapy. (2022). *What is solution-focused therapy?* https://solutionfocused.net/what-is-solution-focused-therapy

Kelly, M. S., & Colindres, M. E. (2020). Task-centered practice. In *Encyclopedia of social work.* NASW Press and Oxford University Press. https://doi.org/10.1093/acrefore/9780199975839.013.388

National Association of Social Workers. (2021). *Code of ethics.* https://www.socialworkers.org/About/Ethics/Code-of-Ethics/Code-of-Ethics-English

Poulin, J., & Matis, S. (2021). *Social work practice: A competency-based approach.* Springer Publishing Company.

Walsh, J. (2015). *Theories for direct social work practice* (3rd ed.). Cengage.

15

Intervening With Organizations and Communities

CASE VIGNETTE

Kelly is a first-year MSW student placed in a community-based program that provides consultation services to grassroots human services programs in an economically disadvantaged community with numerous social problems. The agency's mission is to increase the number of services available to community residents as well as to strengthen the capacities of the local service organizations. Kelly is developing a collaborative program with the local legal aid clinic. The clinic provides legal services to the low-income residents, many of whom also need social work and case management services. The objective is to develop a program that will provide social work and case management services to the legal aid clients.

Kelly is excited but also feeling overwhelmed about helping develop a new service for the residents that would also strengthen an existing community agency. She knows that her first step is to learn all she can about the community and the experiences of the low-income residents who will use the new program. What is it like to be a member of a disadvantaged community? What is it like to be poor? What kinds of services and assistance do the potential clients need? How is working with disadvantaged communities and citizens different from working with other client populations? In what ways is it similar? What professional and community groups need to be involved in the planning process?

COMPETENCY 8: INTERVENE WITH INDIVIDUALS, FAMILIES, GROUPS, ORGANIZATIONS, AND COMMUNITIES

Social workers understand that intervention is an ongoing component of the dynamic and interactive process of social work practice. Social workers understand theories of human behavior, person-in-environment, and other interprofessional conceptual frameworks, and they critically evaluate and apply this knowledge in selecting culturally responsive interventions with clients and constituencies, including individuals, families, groups, organizations, and communities. Social workers understand methods of identifying, analyzing, and implementing evidence-informed interventions and participate in interprofessional collaboration to achieve client and constituency goals. Social workers facilitate effective transitions and endings.

Social workers

- engage with clients and constituencies to critically choose and implement culturally responsive, evidence-informed interventions to achieve client and constituency goals; and

- incorporate culturally responsive methods to negotiate, mediate, and advocate, with and on behalf of clients and constituencies. (Council on Social Work Education, 2022, p. 9)

LEARNING OBJECTIVES

By the end of this chapter, you will be able to:

- Understand the purposes of social work practice with organizations.

- Understand the purposes of social work practice with communities.

- Identify social work practice interventions with organizations.

- Identify social work practice interventions with communities.

ROLE OF ORGANIZATIONS AND COMMUNITIES IN GENERALIST PRACTICE

The National Association of Social Workers (NASW) *Code of Ethics* (2021) details important concepts and ideas affecting work with the mezzo systems of organizations and communities. Although many generalist practitioners find work with micro systems very important, it is often quickly found that many of the problems that clients experience are rooted in the larger systems of organizations, communities, national policy, and even global policy. Thus, it is not only individuals, families, and groups for which the social worker seeks to engage, assess, broker services, advocate, counsel, educate, or organize, but also the organizations and communities where micro systems exist. The context for the change process occurs at the organizational or community level. Furthermore, generalist practitioners will need to engage in community and organizational development, as well as to evaluate service outcomes to continually improve the provision and quality of services most appropriate to their clients' needs (Poulin, 2010).

MEZZO GENERALIST PRACTICE

Mezzo-level practice involves interventions with organizations and communities or neighborhoods. Exhibit 15.1 lists generalist social work practice interventions related

EXHIBIT 15.1

MEZZO GENERALIST PRACTICE INTERVENTIONS WITH ORGANIZATIONS AND COMMUNITIES

System Level	Client System	Generalist Interventions
Organization	• Administrators • Task forces • Committees • Advisory boards • Community groups	• Education and training • Strategic planning • Program development and grant writing • Program evaluation • Needs assessments • Policy analysis • Cause advocacy • Resource coordination
Community/neighborhood	• Professional task forces • Community coalitions • Neighborhood groups	• Policy analysis • Community organizing • Community development • Cause advocacy • Resource coordination

Field Reflection Questions

In your field placement, what practice level will be the primary focus of your work?

What levels of practice will need special efforts to ensure learning opportunities?

to organizations and communities. In this conceptualization, intervention tasks are categorized by practice mezzo-level systems (organizations and communities) and client systems. Mezzo-level interventions focus on organizational and community change (Poulin & Matis, 2021).

Typical client systems at the organizational level are organizational leaders, task forces, and committees. The system level is the organization, and the client systems that the social worker engages are the decision-makers and decision-making structures of the organization. The worker usually participates in formally organized work groups, such as agency task forces or committees, often to develop new services or improve existing services. The client system might also be the organization's decision-makers—that is, administrators and supervisors. Thus, a generalist social worker seeking to change an organization may view the decision-makers or the decision-making structures as the client system to improve how decisions are made or how the organization communicates about decisions, activities, or services. Addressing these client systems is often of the greatest importance because micro systems (individual clients) typically turn to organizations for help. An organization that does not function well may not serve its clients or even the very staff who work within those organizations. Thus, at the organizational level, the purpose of mezzo-level practice is to improve the functioning of the organization, improve services and service delivery, or develop new services through program development and/or grant writing. All three purposes involve changes within the organization or agency.

Typical client systems at the community level are professional task forces, community coalitions, and neighborhood or community citizens' groups. Often, the purpose of community practice is to improve community or neighborhood conditions, empower residents, develop resources, increase community awareness of social and economic problems, and mobilize people to advocate for needed resources and changes. Generalist social workers engaged in community change usually work with professional or community groups. Some groups have both professional and citizen members. Social workers engaged in community practice may view the group they are working with as the client system. In other words, the client system is the professional task force, neighborhood group, or community coalition that is seeking to change or improve the community. Alternatively, the client system may be the residents of the community as the client system.

Importantly, all the micro-level skills that generalist social workers develop may well be needed when working with mezzo-level client systems. Effective communication, goal setting, and sensitivity to the needs of individuals in some ways become even more important when working with the (often) large and complex client systems that are found at the organizational and community levels.

MEZZO INTERVENTIONS

It is beyond the scope of this book to review all the organization and community interventions listed in Exhibit 15.1. In this section, we review the mezzo interventions that social work field placement students are more likely to encounter in their internships.

AGENCY WORKSHOPS AND TRAININGS

The generalist social worker will often encounter situations wherein client systems will benefit from education and training. Education involves assisting the client system to develop or improve knowledge, skills, values, and/or ways of thinking (cognitive processes) about problems, clients, and the environmental contexts that affect people's lives. For the intervention to be effective, education must always be targeted to the specific audience, with literacy, preexisting knowledge, and cultural sensitivities being taken into consideration. One widely used application of education as a mezzo intervention is structured trainings, often conducted through workshops. In your field placement you should seek out opportunities to participate in various workshops and, even better, participate in delivering educational trainings.

CASE EXAMPLE 15.1: EARLY STEPS IN STAFF WORKSHOP DEVELOPMENT

Christiana, Laurie, and Pat all were graduate social work students doing their second-year field placements at Social Work Consultation Services (SWCS). SWCS provided generalist social work learning experiences for student interns and social work and capacity-building services for residents and organizations of an economically disadvantaged community. The Director of Adult Probation in the county contacted SWCS about conducting a staff development workshop for her probation officers. Christiana, Laurie, and Pat took on the project under the supervision of a school faculty member.

The training team scheduled a meeting with the Director of Adult Probation to get a better understanding of the agency's needs and her expectations about the purpose and objectives of the workshop. The director felt that her staff could benefit from a workshop on relationship-building skills and on how to engage reluctant, resistant, or hostile clients in a collaborative working relationship. She felt that many of the probation officers were showing signs of burnout and a lot of frustration with their clients and the legal system. Many seemed to have given up trying to make a difference in their clients' lives and were not making any efforts to connect with them. The team left the meeting with a clear understanding of what the director wanted. They felt it was something that they would be able to put together and deliver effectively.

With the approval of the director, the training team scheduled a preworkshop meeting with the probation officers who would be attending the workshop. The purpose of the meeting was to get an understanding of their training needs and interests. The meeting did not go as expected. The probation officers had absolutely no interest in learning "soft" relationship skills and were totally against the idea of having to attend a workshop on how to connect with reluctant or hostile clients. They felt that such training would be a total waste of time. They used the meeting to vent their feelings about the system and working with clients who lied and were manipulative.

The team struggled to find some common ground between the director's and staff's perceived needs. Because the probation officers were so clear about the frustrations of their job, Pat asked whether they would be interested in a workshop that focused on coping strategies and burnout prevention. This, too, was rejected as a waste of time. Most of the group members claimed not to have any problems in that area and said they could take care of themselves just fine.

Having struck out making suggestions to this group, Christiana asked them what would be helpful. After quite a bit of back-and-forth discussion among the probation officers, it was decided that a workshop on the link between mental health and substance abuse would be helpful. All of their clients were substance abusers, and the workers felt that for many, mental health issues compounded their difficulties with substance abuse and the law. The team agreed to the proposed focus, pending approval by the probation officers' director.

Case Example 15.1 illustrates the beginning steps in developing a staff workshop. This example illustrates the importance of getting input from members of the target group before implementing a training program. The probation officers' perceptions of what they were interested in were very different from their director's perceptions. The workshop turned out to be a success and was well received by the probation officers, even though it was not exactly what the director originally envisioned. If the training team had proceeded without any input from the participants, it would most likely have been less well received. The workshop would have been a trying experience for both the training team and the participants.

COMMUNITY EDUCATION

The value of education and training does not stop with small groups and organizations. Often, larger mezzo groups, such as communities, can benefit from education and training activities. In recent years, for example, generalist social workers have created or participated in community education programs to address issues as disparate as prevention of sexually transmitted infections (STIs), violence reduction, health education, cultural sensitivity, and environmental concerns.

Developing the appropriate education program is often complex. Issues as broad ranging as how to choose the best model and how to effectively communicate in a small group must be taken into consideration. Furthermore, social media provide useful tools for both identifying and contacting potential target groups, as well as distributing informational content.

Ideally, community education seeks to empower and build internal capacity among the members or residents. As with organizational training and education, it is important for the members of the target community to be involved in the definition of the problems and the structuring of interventions (Poulin & Matis, 2021).

PLANNING AND PROGRAM DEVELOPMENT

Generalist social workers may also find planning and program development to be a necessary mezzo-level intervention. Many of the problems identified by the target system may best be addressed by creating new programs and services. Sometimes an organization may choose to provide a new service, but communities may also benefit from programs that target the entire community. Planning, like education and training, has many dimensions and considerations. Nevertheless, two broad types can be distinguished: strategic planning and grant writing for program development.

Strategic Planning

Strategic planning focuses on giving the client system longer-term direction and identifies the steps to achieve the identified outcomes. Both organizations and communities may benefit from the development of strategic plans. Such plans can help identify concerns, assess, and identify group values, create and operationalize goals, articulate specific steps, and characterize challenges and opportunities.

One tool to assist in this process is called a SWOT analysis. SWOT stands for strengths, weaknesses, opportunities, and threats. The results of the data analysis are organized into a four-component framework, which is divided into two internal analysis components (strengths and weaknesses) and two external components (opportunities and threats). Strengths and opportunities are helpful to the organization, whereas weaknesses and threats are those things that may be harmful to the organization. SWOT analyses can help identify areas of strengths and those needing improvement to help inform the development of strategic plans. The components and related questions of a SWOT analysis are shown in Exhibit 15.2.

Grant Writing

One resource development skill set that all generalist social workers should develop is grant writing. Many organizations supplement or expand their resources through

EXHIBIT 15.2

SWOT ANALYSIS

Strengths	Weaknesses
• What do we do best? • What unique knowledge, talent, or resources do we have? • What advantages do we have? • What do other people say we do well? • What resources do we have available? • What is our greatest achievement?	• What could we improve? • What knowledge, talent, skills, and/or resources are we lacking? • What disadvantages do we have? • What do other people say we do not do well? • In what areas do we need more training? • What complaints have we had about our service?
Opportunities	**Threats**
• How can we turn our strengths into opportunities? • How can we turn our weaknesses into opportunities? • Is there a need in our agency that no one is meeting? • What could we do today that is not being done? • How is our field changing? How can we take advantage of those changes? • Whom could we support? How could we support them?	• What obstacles do we face? • Could any of our weaknesses prevent our unit from meeting our goals? • Who and/or what might cause us problems in the future? How? • Are there any standards, policies, and/or legislation changing that might negatively impact us? • Are we competing with others to provide service? • Are there changes in our field or in technology that could threaten our success?

Source: Louisiana Department of State Civil Service. (2015). *SWOT analysis: Questions for conducting an analysis with your team.* https://www.civilservice.louisiana.gov/files/divisions/Training/Job%20Aid/Supervisor%20Toolbox/Questions%20for%20 Professional%20SWOT.pdf

grant writing. The general steps for writing a grant are as follows: (a) develop a clear project or problem; (b) select the grant source; and (c) write the proposal. Each of these steps is described in detail in the following subsections.

Develop a Clear Project or Problem

This part of the process is not really very different from planning for any intervention, with perhaps two important differences. First, in many cases, the focus of the project may expand beyond the needs of a specific agency to possibly include other system client needs. Often, effective interventions will be strongest if many "partners" are a part of the process. A second difference that may apply here is that most successful grants depend on a grounding in the literature. An empirical basis for any project, as drawn from the literature of social work, sociology, psychology, or similar fields, will have a much greater chance of success than one that is based on anecdotes or practice wisdom alone. Funders, especially for larger grants, want to provide money to projects that are likely to succeed. And the empirical basis may provide the evidence needed to support that sense.

Overall, you can think about projects or problems as being one of several types. You will want to identify the type that is closest to your intent. Doing so will make searching for grants a bit easier and will improve the chances of being selected for funding. The various types of projects and problems include the following:

- *Research or planning projects/problems:* projects designed to help the agency examine a problem and/or plan for new services

- *Demonstration projects:* projects designed to implement new or untested services

- *Operating expenses and services support:* projects designed to raise funds for existing services

- *Endowment development:* projects designed to help build the endowment and long-term assets of the agency

- *Construction projects:* projects designed to help the agency build a new structure or renovate the existing physical plant

- *Capacity building:* projects designed to enhance the skills or knowledge of the staff, or to improve the agency's infrastructure

Select the Grant Source

To begin, you must find out who (what organization) is providing funding. This is, at least "on paper," easy, as organizations that give away money must notify the public that funds are available, although finding the right source might be more difficult. The notifications you will be seeking are variously known as an RFP (Request for Proposals), NOFA (Notice of Funding Availability), FOA (Funding Opportunity Announcement), or SUPER NOFA (groups of NOFAs).

Make sure you review these sections carefully. Many grant sources receive hundreds of applications, so you must prepare the right proposal for the right source. Although individuals may provide grant funds, most conceptualizations of grant funding sources focus on a government level (federal, state, local) or a foundation. There are advantages and disadvantages to the different grant sources. Government sources are often considered to be more prestigious and to offer high-dollar amounts, but their grants are very competitive, restrictive, and extremely complex to write. Foundations are more varied. With literally thousands of different sources, it is possible to find everything from large, high-dollar, complex grants to small, essentially noncompetitive microgrants.

Where does one find an RFP, or learn about grant sources? With the federal government, the *Catalog of Domestic Federal Assistance* was the standard source of such information until the internet arose and offered new opportunities. Now, almost every government agency provides information about sources on its website. And even easier access is available with www.grants.gov, which collects information across agencies.

Comprehensive information for foundations is harder to find simply because of the large number of foundations that exist. Yet again, several websites exist that can help, although they are often fee or subscription based. Some useful sites for government and foundational supports are given in Exhibit 15.3.

EXHIBIT 15.3

GRANT SEARCH ENGINE WEBSITES

www.grants.gov	Grants Learning Center: Your gateway to the federal grants. The Grants Learning Center is where you can learn more about the federal grants life cycle, policies on grants management, and profiles on grant making.
https://fconline.foundation center.org/?gclid=Cj0K CQiAvqGcBhCJARIsA FQ5ke6hv66pDF6wv kqoyjz5TxSRd7EOXfQ BwkK5MtmQI2dHm- oZca9Tq_0aAug2EALw_wcB	The Foundation Center is the leading source of information about philanthropy worldwide. It maintains a comprehensive database of U.S. and global grants.
www.grantwatch.com	This website provides information on international, Canadian, and U.S. federal, state, local, foundation, and corporation grants.

Write the Proposal

Writing the proposal may seem complex, but in many ways, it just involves pulling together information that may already exist, although that information must be put together in a clear, concise, and logical way. Although every proposal MUST be specific to the RFP, and MUST follow all the directions perfectly, it is also the case that the components of most proposals are similar. These components are shown in Exhibit 15.4 (Coley & Scheinberg, 2017).

Each of these sections should be logically connected to the others. This means that every section of the proposal builds on what has gone before and prepares for

EXHIBIT 15.4

TYPICAL GRANT PROPOSAL SECTIONS

Grant Section	Information Provided
Title or cover page	Often supplied by funder. Includes contact information for the submitting organization.
Abstract	Short overview of the proposal. Typically, 100 to 150 words.
Introduction/summary	One-to three-page summary of the project. Introduces the project and the agency to the funder. Includes the mission and vision of the agency.
Needs statement (problem statement)	Describes the problem/issue that the grant wants to address. Typically includes a problem definition, statistics describing the community setting, the size of the problem, and some evidence about the seriousness of the problem (such as statistics comparing the target group with other groups).
Project description	Identifies the project's goals and objectives and provides details about the implementation plan, including the timeline to complete project activities. This section often includes a scope of work grid of the project delivery plan.
Evaluation plan	Explains the measurement procedures that will be used to determine whether the goals and objectives have been met.
Budget request	Itemizes the expenditures of the project and includes a rationale or budget justification for the expenses.
Applicant capability	Demonstrates the applicant's past performance and ability to accomplish the proposed project. Often includes an organizational chart.
Organizational sustainability	Indicates the plan to continue the project beyond the requested funding period.
Letters of support	Letters reflecting support for the proposed project from program recipients, community leaders, partnering agencies, coalitions, religious organizations, universities, or political leaders.
Memoranda of understanding	A written agreement from each of the partners or co-applicant agencies on how they will cooperate to implement the grant.
Appendix materials	May include an audited financial statement, insurance documentation, or any other documentation required by the funder.

what comes after. Although this might seem evident and obvious, a lack of logical connections is a common flaw in many grant applications. One way to avoid this problem is to remember that the strongest proposals will have a clear relationship between indicators of need, your outcome objectives, and the degree of change in outcomes you seek to demonstrate in your evaluation. Do not identify and measure a need one way, while focusing your objectives and evaluation criteria somewhere else.

One tool that is commonly used as part of the grant development process is a logic model. The logic model serves several useful purposes, both for the organization that is submitting it and for the funders, who are increasingly requiring logic models with grant submissions. A logic model presents a picture of how your effort or initiative is supposed to work. Please see Chapter 16 for a detailed description of logic models.

COMMUNITY DEVELOPMENT

Community development involves the participation of community members in developing a capacity and consensus in identifying and solving their own problems (Fellin, 2001). Social work interventions are often aimed at improving community conditions and empowering residents to seek community change. Community development also has a social action component, which includes activities aimed at challenging inequalities, confronting decision-makers, and empowering people to change unjust conditions (Rubin & Rubin, 2008; Zastrow, 2013; Zastrow & Kirst-Ashman, 2016).

To achieve these purposes, the generalist social worker organizes constituent groups, builds community coalitions, conducts community needs assessments, lobbies political and government leaders, and advocates on behalf of constituent groups. Community development activities may also involve economic development projects, installation of public facilities, establishment of community centers, recruitment of new businesses, code enforcement, and developing homeowner assistance programs.

To achieve the varying ends of community development, almost every social work generalist skill is necessary. Social workers involved in organizing constituent groups often take responsibility for convening and facilitating meetings. They do the planning and the legwork to get participants to attend. This requires skill in managing groups and conducting meetings. An empowering approach to the process focuses on having community residents assume control and leadership of the development effort. The social worker helps get the process started, but ultimate responsibility for the ongoing effort rests with participants and indigenous leadership.

Coalition Building

Both an independent activity and a component of community development, coalition building occurs when representatives of diverse community groups join forces to influence external institutions on one or more issues affecting their constituencies (Mizrahi & Rosenthal, 2001). The process may be intended to be short or long term, but the idea is that there is strength in numbers. Often, the problems to be addressed are larger and more intractable than a single individual or group can effectively address. A coalition, then, has a goal to build a power base sufficient to influence decision-making and the allocation of resources (Gamble & Weil, 2009).

COMMUNITY EDUCATION AND TRAINING

Education and training at the community level tend to focus on increasing community awareness and understanding of social issues and community problems (DuBois & Miley, 2020). Generalist social workers make formal presentations at community meetings, serve as panelists at public forums, and conduct community workshops and seminars. Examples 1 and 2 in Case Example 15.2 illustrate how generalist social workers may use education and training as a mezzo-level practice intervention.

> **Field Reflection Questions**
>
> What mezzo interventions are used in your field placement agency?
>
> What mezzo intervention are you most comfortable performing? What mezzo intervention are you least comfortable using?

CASE EXAMPLE 15.2: EDUCATION AND TRAINING INTERVENTIONS

MARCUS

Marcus is the social worker with the Chester Community Improvement Project, a grant-funded agency that provides community residents with information to assist them in achieving homeownership. The project seeks to address the needs of families through its rehabilitation project, new housing construction project, mortgage counseling, and job training for youth. Marcus designed a series of workshops for the local residents that were designed to educate them about financial literacy, saving for a first home, and understanding mortgages. Marcus discussed the current condition of the local neighborhood and cited statistics showing that the neighborhood could be stabilized by increasing homeownership among the residents.

SHARON

Sharon is a second-year student placed with the local charter school. This past year, the school was in jeopardy of not making the Annual Yearly Progress benchmarks. Significant numbers of students scored below grade level in reading and math.

In consultation with parents, students, and staff, Sharon and a staff member from the school developed a homework after-school project for parents. The program is designed to tutor parents in upper-level math and science so that they will be able to help their children. In addition to the classes, Sharon has developed a monthly newsletter to communicate to parents about school events and provide tips on subjects such as time management and reducing stress.

CASE SUMMARY: "WE LOST EVERYTHING"

PRACTICE SETTING DESCRIPTION

My name is Shanna and I am a first-year MSW student completing an internship at a family services agency in a rural county near the Mississippi River. The agency provides individual and family counseling services as well as relief services and trauma services after emergencies and natural disasters. In the spring of my second semester of placement, the entire region was hit with a devastating flood during heavy rains. Everyone in the agency was dispatched to the surrounding communities to coordinate with Federal Emergency Management Agency (FEMA) officials and provide emergency relief services to flood victims as directed.

IDENTIFYING DATA

The W. family, Gloria and Henry, own 10 acres of land that they farm. They also have a small motel on their property and rent rooms to people who come during the hunting seasons every year. Gloria mentioned that Henry had just finished renovating the eight-room motel 3 weeks before the flood. Gloria and Henry have two grown children. Their son recently moved to New York City for a new job, and their daughter and her husband live in a nearby community in a small apartment with their two young children. Gloria also has a sister living in Georgia.

PRESENTING PROBLEM

The FEMA official assigned the W. family to our agency, and the case was assigned to my field instructor, Norman. Norman and I drove to the W. farm community and discovered that their home was surrounded by water. A community resident took us to the house by boat.

Gloria W. told us that she and her husband had not evacuated because her husband would not leave the home. He was staying in his room and refused to go to the city. In the 4 days since the flood began, Gloria and Henry had not left their house. Their daughter had brought some food by boat and registered her parents with FEMA. Gloria told me that the water covered their small motel next door and that most of the furniture had been destroyed. She indicated that her greatest concern was that the family would not receive compensation from FEMA because they did not have flood insurance.

Gloria indicated that she wanted to leave the house and move to the city shelter like everyone else, but she did not want to leave her husband alone. She was extremely worried about her husband. He was not sleeping or eating. She thought he might be suicidal. "I sometimes want to go and apply for loans or emergency assistance like everybody else, but I'm also afraid that if I leave him, he will hurt himself. I told him that we can't stay here by ourselves because we don't have a boat, and it does not seem that the water will go away soon." When I asked about her immediate need, she said, "I know we need food and stuff, but the most important thing is to leave and go where everybody is."

Gloria believed that her husband was traumatized by the experience. He had fought in Vietnam and still had dreams about the war. Since the flood, he had refused to take his blood pressure medicine, and she saw him crying the other day. She added, "We had a similar experience in the sixties, but the water didn't destroy everything. We helped each other, and the water receded 3 days after the flood." When we asked her what she thought would help her this time, she said, "I know we live in a floodplain area. We didn't buy insurance because the county decided to withdraw from the plan, but we have our will and many people are helping us. The thing that is difficult to accept is the flood. I try to work with the difficult circumstances, but my husband has a difficult time accepting that."

ASSESSMENT

Mr. and Mrs. W. had different perceptions of the situation. Henry was traumatized by the loss. Water covered their house, farm, and business. Henry felt isolated from his neighbors and immediate family. Gloria understood that living in a floodplain meant a high probability of flooding. She accepted the fact that the flood happened. Although she did not accept victimization, she struggled with their losses.

When we asked Gloria to assess the family's needs, she indicated that the most important thing was to move to temporary housing with the other survivors. She wanted to apply for assistance, communicate with people, and find out what resources were available. She also wanted to establish contact with her son, and with her sister in Georgia. She asked for help in convincing her husband to leave and in getting him medical and professional assistance to help him deal with his feelings of loss and depression. By the end of the first interview, Gloria and I agreed on the following needs:

- *Help Gloria convince her husband to move to a new place (she suggested asking Tom J., an old friend of her husband, to help convince Henry).*

- *Obtain information about possible places to move.*

- *Obtain copies of and review the application procedures of emergency relief programs and loans.*

- *Arrange for Henry to visit their family doctor.*

- *Make arrangements with someone who has a boat to take Gloria grocery shopping.*

CASE PROCESS SUMMARY

I visited the W. family the next day. Prior to the visit, I contacted FEMA and found out that the agency has an apartment available only 15 miles away from their farm. During my visit, I gave Gloria the application forms for compensation and emergency funds. I shared that many families from the community had withdrawn from the flood insurance plan and were also not eligible to receive compensation for their damaged homes. I told them that I would be meeting with a FEMA representative in 3 days to advocate on their behalf and I would share the results with them. Gloria was happy when I told her I had arranged a doctor's appointment for Henry and that Bob P., her neighbor, would take them to the appointment in his boat.

I talked about applications for emergency assistance and loans. By the end of the visit, Gloria had convinced Henry that they had to move. He agreed to begin working on the process. We agreed to meet on my next field placement day at the emergency center to fill out the forms and applications.

When I met the couple at the center, Henry looked better and engaged in conversation. I helped them fill out applications for small loans and for the apartment. I drove them to look at the apartment and visit with their daughter. Henry's spirit got a boost from visiting his daughter and seeing his grandchildren. The process of moving to the new place was easier than they thought it would be. Gloria was glad that the temporary apartment was close to her daughter's apartment.

Four days later, Gloria called me from their new apartment. She asked me to refer Henry to the community mental health center for help with his depression. I did so, and Henry had his first counseling session with a mental health therapist the following week. The W. family's support network began to take shape. Their son came from New York and spent 4 days with his parents. Neighbors and friends surrounded the family. They began to attend church services.

I worked with FEMA, the county administrator, state emergency officials, and a state representative to set up a community meeting at which residents expressed their anger and frustration with the local community leaders who had withdrawn from the National Flood Insurance Program 3 years before. Following a heated discussion, a FEMA representative announced that FEMA would meet with survivors to discuss their requests for assistance.

Some of the needs were for food and furniture. I contacted the local church and helped open a food pantry there. I also found a way to transport food and supplies that were donated by people in other states. I spent the rest of my field placement working with individuals, families, local organizations, and community groups involved in helping with the recovery efforts.

Shanna, MSW Student Intern

CASE DISCUSSION QUESTIONS

1. *How does social work practice in disaster relief differ from generalist practice with other client populations? How is it the same?*

2. *Describe the micro practice interventions used by Shanna in the case example. What mezzo practice interventions did she use? How are the micro and mezzo interventions used in the case example interrelated? In what ways are they separate?*

3. *This case example focused on the micro and mezzo interventions Shanna used in helping the W. family and their community. How does the social and economic justice competency impact the interventions provided by Shanna and her field instructor? What macro practice policies and interventions would help the community members and the community itself? Why?*

END-OF-CHAPTER RESOURCES

 A robust set of instructor resources designed to supplement this text is located at http://connect.springerpub.com/content/book/978-0-8261-3753-1. Qualifying instructors may request access by emailing textbook@springerpub.com.

CRITICAL THINKING QUESTIONS

1. In your field placement, what are the mezzo-level interventions you use? How effective are those interventions? What makes them effective? What keeps them from being effective?

2. How have your field placement clients' life experiences with oppression and poverty impacted your agency's efforts to provide mezzo-level social work services? What does your field placement agency do to address its client populations' life experiences with oppression, poverty, and/or marginalization?

LEARNING ACTIVITIES

ORGANIZATIONAL INTERVENTION ACTIVITIES

1. *Conduct a staff training.* In consultation with your field instructor identify a professional development topic that would be of interest and beneficial to the agency's staff or those in your unit/program. Research the topic and prepare a training workshop or a series of professional development seminars. Facilitate or co-facilitate the workshop or training.

2. *SWOT analysis.* Conduct a SWOT analysis of your field placement program. Review your SWOT analysis with your field instructor. Prepare a brief summary of your analysis with recommendations.

3. *Grant writing.* Explore with your field instructor the possibility to participating in any grant writing that is taking place in your agency. Volunteer to help with the various tasks that need to be completed. If no opportunity exists within your field placement agency, explore the possibility of participating in grant writing with another social service agency in the community.

COMMUNITY INTERVENTION ACTIVITIES

1. *Community task forces/coalitions.* Most communities have interagency task forces or community coalitions that are formed to collective address community needs and issues. Ask your field instructor about task forces or coalitions in which your field placement agency participates or those in the community that could use some agency representation. If opportunities are available, express an interest and willingness to attend and participate.

2. *Community education programs.* In collaboration with your field instructor identify a pressing community problem or issue that could benefit from some type of community education program. Together design a community education workshop or community education event. Plan, implement, and evaluate your community education project.

ELECTRONIC RESOURCES

WEBSITE LINKS

Association for Community Organization and Social Action: https://www.acosa.org/content.aspx?page_id=22& club_id=789392&module_id=335369

Network for Social Work Management: https://socialwork manager.org

VIDEO LINKS

Community Organizing for Social Change: www.youtube.com/ watch?v=-DtILpmsCcA

Logic Models for Planning and Evaluation: www.youtube.com/
watch?v=0Vfc2uX6ciI

How to Write a Grant Proposal: Step by Step: www.youtube.com/
watch?v=ByQRri_LTUE

REFERENCES

Coley, S. M., & Scheinberg, C. A. (2017). *Proposal writing: Effective grantsmanship for funding* (5th ed.). SAGE Publications.

Council on Social Work Education. (2022). *Educational policy and accreditation standards for baccalaureate and master's social work programs.* https://www.cswe.org/getmedia/94471c42-13b8-493b-9041 -b30f48533d64/2022-EPAS.pdf

DuBois, B., & Miley, K. K. (2020). *Social work: An empowering profession* (9th ed.). Allyn & Bacon.

Fellin, P. (2001). *The community and the social worker* (3rd ed.). Brooks/Cole.

Gamble, D., & Weil, M. (2009). *Community practice skills: Local to global perspectives.* Columbia University Press.

Mizrahi, T., & Rosenthal, B. B. (2001). Complexities of coalition building: Leaders' successes, strategies, struggles, and solutions. *Social Work, 46*(1), 63–78. https://doi.org/10.1093/sw/46.1.63

National Association of Social Workers. (2021). *Code of ethics.* https://www.socialworkers.org/About/ Ethics/Code-of-Ethics/Code-of-Ethics-English

Poulin, J. (2010). *Strengths-based generalist practice: A collaborative approach* (3rd ed.). Cengage.

Poulin, J., & Matis, S. (2021). *Social work practice: A competency-based approach.* Springer Publishing Company.

Rubin, H. J., & Rubin, I. S. (2008). *Community organizing and development* (4th ed.). Pearson/Allyn & Bacon.

Zastrow, C. (2013). *The practice of social work: A comprehensive worktext* (10th ed.). Cengage.

Zastrow, C., & Kirst-Ashman, K. K. (2016). *Understanding human behavior and the social environment* (10th ed.). Cengage.

Applied Research and Practice Evaluation in Your Field Placement

CASE VIGNETTE

Jeannette is a first-year MSW student doing her field placement at an after-school program serving disadvantaged elementary schoolchildren. The program provides academic support to the children and runs support groups for the parents. All the children are low-income and almost all are in single-parent families.

The after-school component is doing well, and Jeannette enjoys her work with the children. The parent support groups, however, are struggling with limited enrollment and poor attendance. The program director asked Jeannette and another MSW intern to evaluate the parent support group program to try to figure out why the program is struggling and to come up with recommendations for improvement. Jeannette, the other intern, and their field instructors embraced this challenge and set up a series of meetings to design a program evaluation. Jeannette's first task was to research the different types of program evaluations and to bring to the group suggestions for how they might proceed with their assigned task.

Where should she start? What resources at the school might be available? What questions should she ask herself? What questions should she ask others?

COMPETENCY 4: ENGAGE IN PRACTICE-INFORMED RESEARCH AND RESEARCH-INFORMED PRACTICE

Social workers use ethical, culturally informed, and anti-racist and anti-oppressive approaches in conducting research and building knowledge. Social workers use research to inform their practice decision-making and articulate how their practice experience informs research and evaluation decisions. Social workers critically evaluate and critique current, empirically sound research to inform decisions pertaining to practice, policy, and programs. Social workers understand the inherent bias in research and evaluate design, analysis, and interpretation using an anti-racist and anti-oppressive perspective. Social workers know how to access, critique, and synthesize the current literature to develop appropriate research questions and hypotheses. Social workers demonstrate knowledge and skills regarding qualitative and quantitative research methods and analysis, and they interpret data derived from these methods. Social workers demonstrate knowledge about methods to assess reliability and validity in social work research. Social workers can articulate and share research findings in ways that are usable to a variety of clients and constituencies. Social workers understand the value of evidence derived from interprofessional and diverse research methods, approaches, and sources.

Social workers

- apply research findings to inform and improve practice, policy, and programs; and
- identify ethical, culturally informed, anti-racist, and anti-oppressive strategies that address inherent biases for use in quantitative and qualitative research methods to advance the purposes of social work. (Council on Social Work Education [CSWE], 2022, p. 8)

COMPETENCY 9: EVALUATE PRACTICE WITH INDIVIDUALS, FAMILIES, GROUPS, ORGANIZATIONS, AND COMMUNITIES

Social workers understand that evaluation is an ongoing component of the dynamic and interactive process of social work practice with and on behalf of diverse individuals, families, groups, organizations, and communities. Social workers evaluate processes and outcomes to increase practice, policy, and service delivery effectiveness. Social workers apply anti-racist and anti-oppressive perspectives in evaluating outcomes. Social workers understand theories of human behavior and person-in-environment, as well as interprofessional conceptual frameworks, and critically evaluate and apply this knowledge in evaluating outcomes. Social workers use qualitative and quantitative methods for evaluating outcomes and practice effectiveness.

Social workers

- select and use culturally responsive methods for evaluation of outcomes; and
- critically analyze outcomes and apply evaluation findings to improve practice effectiveness with individuals, families, groups, organizations, and communities. (CSWE, 2022, p. 9)

LEARNING OBJECTIVES

By the end of this chapter, you will be able to:

- Describe ethical standards that social workers must abide by related to research and evaluation.

LEARNING OBJECTIVES

- Describe the differences between quantitative, qualitative, and mixed methods evaluations.
- Design a formative program evaluation.
- Design a summative program evaluation.
- Create a logic model.
- Carry out a single-subject design practice evaluation.
- Use supervision and client feedback to evaluate your practice effectiveness.
- Create client logs and behavioral observation instruments.
- Develop individualized and generalized rating scales.
- Retrieve standardized indices and scales.

RESEARCH AND THE NATIONAL ASSOCIATION OF SOCIAL WORKERS *CODE OF ETHICS*

The National Association of Social Workers (NASW) *Code of Ethics* (2021) sets forth ethical standards regarding research and evaluation for social workers. Social workers should aspire to contribute to the knowledge base of the profession (NASW, 2021). Professional social workers are called upon by this ethical principle to contribute to the knowledge base of the profession. Contributing to the knowledge base of the profession can take a variety of forms. It can be done formally by publishing findings in professional journals and by presenting at conferences. Contributions can also be done more informally by sharing your research findings with agency peers and administrators.

APPLIED RESEARCH

This chapter focuses on two types of applied research—program evaluation and practice evaluation. Applied research seeks solutions to organizational, community, and service delivery problems. Applied research addresses practical issues encountered in the provision of social work services to clients and constituents. Basic research, on the other hand, tends to focus on generalizations and theory development. The major difference between applied and basic research is in their purposes. The purpose of applied research is to solve problems while the purpose of basic research is to generate new knowledge or add to the existing body of knowledge (Poulin et al., 2022). Four widely used types of applied research are (1) organizational needs assessments, (2) community needs assessments, (3) program evaluations, and (4) practice evaluations. This chapter focuses on program and practice evaluation approaches. Organizational and community needs assessments are covered in Chapter 13. We have chosen to focus on these types of applied research because, in our view, they are the types of research social work students are most likely to encounter or conduct in their field placements.

Field Reflection Questions

At your placement, how are social work interventions evaluated?

How do you know whether what you are doing is effective?

All types of research methods can be used to conduct applied research studies. A common way to group research methods is quantitative versus qualitative approaches. Mixed method approaches combine both quantitative and qualitative data collection strategies.

Quantitative approaches involve collecting numerical data and using various statistical methods to analyze the collected data. A variety of data collection methods can be used with quantitative applied social work research, such as survey questionnaires and interview schedules.

Qualitative approaches, on the other hand, are subjective and descriptive. Data collection is based upon words or observations and the data analysis seeks to describe or interpret whatever is being researched. Instead of numbers, qualitative research collects information in the form of words. It relies on observation or participants' answers to open-ended questions.

PROGRAM EVALUATIONS

Here we will focus on two types of program evaluation. The first is formative or process evaluations, which examine the implementation of a program or service. The second is summative or outcome evaluations, which examine the extent to which the program/service has met its goals and objectives. Both formative and summative evaluations can be qualitative, quantitative, or mixed method evaluations.

As social workers committed to social justice you should design both formative and summative evaluations following anti-racist and anti-oppressive perspectives. This entails careful attention to the power relationships between you the researcher and the various stakeholders involved in the evaluation. Adopt a collaborative empowering approach in all aspects of the research process. Examine your research proposal in terms of power and how the proposed relationships will be structured. Reflect upon the value assumptions of your proposal and how equity, inclusion, and social justice are reflected in your proposed evaluation. Involve the service users in designing the evaluation, data collection, data analysis, interpretation, and dissemination of the results. Deconstruct your written and oral communication to avoid specialized language or jargon. Abandon the researcher as the expert role and adopt a collaborative partnership role (Rogers, 2012).

Formative Program Evaluations

Formative evaluations look at the implementation and operation of a program or service. These are useful for providing descriptions of what the program does and how it works. They are also used to observe the program in real time for the purposes of monitoring and improving the program. Formative evaluations can help determine why something worked, or why it did not work (Poulin et al., 2022).

Developing a Formative Program Evaluation

The first step in designing a formative evaluation is to specify your research questions. This is an important first step because the design of your evaluation will flow out of your research questions. Exactly what answers will help improve the program or service? What information will help your field placement agency staff better understand the functioning of the program or service? In collaboration with your field instructor and agency administrators create a list of the research questions that your evaluation will seek to answer.

Step two in developing your evaluation is identifying your data sources. Who or what will provide information on your research questions? Ask yourself: What are the best sources of information on the program or service I will be evaluating? Are there multiple sources of potential data? Will these data sources be accessible? This is a critical step in the evaluation process. You will need to identify data sources that are reliable or knowledgeable about your program.

Usually there are several potential data sources for a formative program evaluation. Possible sources of information include client records, agency policy manuals, program proposals, grant applications, clients, agency administrators, direct service workers, community members, and professionals in other community or human service organizations. Your task is to identify the data sources that have the strongest potential to provide information on your research questions. At a minimum you will need at least one source of data for your evaluation. It is usually preferable to have more than one data source for each research question. Having multiple sources of data helps reduce bias and increases the chances that your findings accurately reflect the implementation successes and challenges of the program/service being evaluated (Rubin & Babbie, 2017).

Once you have identified your research questions and potential data sources, the third step in this process is to decide upon your research methods. The basic choices here are to do a quantitative, qualitative, or mixed methods evaluation. All three are valid approaches and your choice is shaped primarily by your research questions. What is the best research approach to answer my research questions? If your research questions are descriptive and quantifiable, then a survey approach is often used. For example, you could survey the clients and/or the staff about their experiences in the program. On the other hand, if your research questions are more exploratory, then a qualitative approach is called for. For example, you could conduct focus groups with clients and/or staff to explore why or why not the program is working as anticipated. Often formative evaluations use a mixed methods approach with a combination of quantitative and qualitative data collection.

The choice of methods depends upon your research questions as well as your personal preferences, resources, and research skills.

The fifth step is identifying and/or creating your measures. The measures you use are dependent upon whether you are doing a quantitative, qualitative, or mixed methods evaluation. If you are doing a quantitative study, then we strongly recommend that you use standardized scales or indices if available. There are many that are publicly available. The trick is to find ones that measure the concepts you are trying to measure. You will also probably need to create rating scales and categorical variables for your survey instrument or questionnaire. After gathering and creating your survey measures you then create a survey instrument that the respondents complete or a questionnaire that is administered to the participants. If you are doing a qualitative evaluation, measurement usually entails creating a series of open-endeded broad questions that the participants answer in either a focus group or during individual interviews. In both settings the researcher asks probing follow-up questions to gain a deeper understanding of the topic in question. If you are doing a mixed method evaluation, you will do some sort of descriptive survey or data gathering as well as some type of exploratory investigation.

Steps five and six are data collection and data analysis. Data collection usually involves some sort of sampling. The different types of sampling methods will not be discussed here. Please review your research methods textbooks for detailed information on sampling. The same applies to data analysis methods. The topic is too broad for review here. There are numerous textbooks and online resources available on quantitative and qualitative data analyses. Exhibit 16.1 shows an example of a formative program evaluation proposal.

Summative Program Evaluations

Summative program evaluations are used to assess program outputs and program outcomes. Program outputs describe services delivered through program activities. Program outcomes describe the results of the services delivered. Outputs are usually measured quantitatively while outcomes can be measured quantitatively or qualitatively.

Logic models are often used to design summative program evaluations. Most logic models are presented in table form. The components of logic models often include inputs or resources, goals, services or activities, outputs, and outcomes. Program inputs are the resources used to operate the program. Program resources can include funding and staffing as well as community resources such as in-kind donations from other community organizations. Program services are the activities provided as part of the program such as individual counseling, support groups, and educational trainings. Outputs are the products of the activities such as number of clients served and number of group sessions. Program outcomes

EXHIBIT 16.1

BRIEF FORMATIVE EVALUATION PROPOSAL

The evaluator will conduct a formative evaluation of the new teen anti-bullying program. The evaluation data will provide feedback to the program staff regarding program fidelity as well as recommendations to improve the delivery of the program to the targeted client population. The formative evaluation will focus on two primary topics: (1) program implementation and (2) client feedback and perceptions. The program implementation evaluation will entail a mixed methods approach with quantitative and qualitative components. Client feedback will be obtained qualitatively using focus groups.

Program Implementation
The evaluator will closely monitor and document all aspects of program implementation. This component of the formative evaluation will address the following quantitative research questions. The data source for these questions will be the client's participation records.

- What services were provided?
- Who provided the services?
- Who received the program services?
- What was the level of service provided?
- What were the costs of the services provided?

The qualitative component of the program implementation evaluation will address the research questions shown below. The data source for these research questions will be in-person interviews with the program staff.

- How closely did the implementation match the proposed plan?
- What types of deviations from the plan occurred?
- What led to the deviations?
- What were the effects of the deviations?

Client Feedback and Perceptions
The second major topic of the process evaluation will focus on how clients perceive the program services and staff. This component will ascertain client feedback on all aspects of the program. The focus will be on documenting the clients' and caretakers' perceptions of what worked and what needs to be strengthened. These data will be collected from two focus groups, with approximately 10 former clients and 10 caretakers in each focus group. The evaluator will facilitate the focus groups and will ask several open-ended questions about the participants' experiences and perceptions of the program.

At the end of the program year, the evaluator will prepare a final process evaluation report that summarizes the findings from the ongoing implementation evaluation as well as participant feedback from the focus groups. The process evaluation report will also contain recommendations for changes to the anti-bullying program. The evaluator will schedule a meeting with the program director, program staff, and other interested stakeholders to review the process evaluation findings and recommendations.

are the measurable results for each program goal. The outcome objectives should specify a time frame, the outcome measure, and a benchmark level of success. Exhibit 16.2 is an example of a logic model.

EXHIBIT 16.2

SAMPLE LOGIC MODEL

Inputs (Resources)	Goals: Service or Activity, Output Objectives, and Outcome Objectives
Program Resources Budget ($300,000) Evaluation Budget ($3,000) Program Director (1 FTE) Clinical Director (1 FTE) Case Managers (1.5 FTE) Program Evaluator (.25 FTE) Research Assistant (.35 FTE) 3 Interviewers (225 hours each) Administrative Assistant (.5 FTE) **Community Resources** In-kind meeting space (Community Center)	**Goal 1: To decrease substance use among adolescents with histories of substance abuse.** **Activity 1.1.** Case management counseling services for substance-using adolescents. **Output Objective 1.1.** To provide 12-session case management services to 60 substance-using adolescents and their families during year 1. **Outcome Objective 1.1.** At least 50% of the adolescent alcohol users decrease the number of days of alcohol use during the past 30 days by 33% between intake and discharge from the 12-week case management program as measured by the GPRA Client Outcomes instrument. **Outcome Objective 1.2.** At least 50% of the adolescent drug users decrease the number of days of drug use during the past 30 days by 33% between intake and discharge from the 12-week case management program as measured by the GPRA Client Outcomes instrument. **Goal 2: To link adolescent substance users with appropriate community resources.** **Activity 2.1.** Case management referral/linkage services for substance-using adolescents. **Output Objective 2.1.** To assess the service needs of 75 adolescent substance users and link those needing additional services with appropriate community resources. **Output Objective 2.2.** To provide follow-up case management referral/linkage services to all adolescent substance users referred to community resources. **Outcome Objective 2.1.** 100% of the adolescent substance users with additional services needs will be linked with community resources as measured by the GAIN assessment instrument and client case records. **Outcome Objective 2.2.** At least 75% of the adolescent substance users referred to community resources will have followed up on the referral and contacted the community resource within 30 days of the referral as measured by the GPRA Client Outcomes instrument and client case records. **Goal 3: To strengthen adolescent substance user's family support systems.** **Activity 3.1.** Case management family intervention services for substance-using adolescents and their families. **Output Objective 3.1.** To provide at least two adolescent/family sessions to 60 substance-using adolescents. **Outcome Objective 3.1.** At least 50% of the adolescent substance user's scores on the Adolescent Family Support Scale will increase between initial assessment and discharge from the case management program.

FTE, full-time equivalent; GAIN, global appraisal of individual needs; GPRA, Government Performance and Results Act.

PRACTICE EVALUATION

This section focuses on informal and formal approaches to evaluating your practice effectiveness with clients and constituencies. As with program evaluation, you should adopt an anti-racist and anti-oppressive perspective in evaluating your practice effectiveness.

INFORMAL PRACTICE EVALUATION

One approach to evaluating the effectiveness of your social work practice with clients is through supervision. As noted in Chapter 4, social work supervision entails three components—administration, education, and support. The educational component can be used to evaluate your practice effectiveness.

An important part of the supervisory process is the willingness to share and be vulnerable. Sometimes we may not want to share certain things because they make us feel at risk. Vulnerability refers to a state of being open or exposed to criticism or judgment. This requires trust and it can be scary, especially within the context of your supervisory relationship (Poulin & Matis, 2021).

The critical element in developing trust is risk. The supervisor is an active partner in the search for understanding and insights. This cannot happen if the worker is unable to take a risk by being open and honest about their social work practice with clients. Social workers have to be willing to share their thoughts, insights, feelings, and questions about their practice to be able to use the supervisory relationship to access their practice effectiveness. Your field instructor's primary task is to facilitate your risk taking. Your task is to be self-reflective and to be willing to share information about your successes, mistakes, and ongoing challenges in order to evaluate your practice effectiveness (Poulin & Matis, 2021).

Ongoing Client Feedback

A second way to evaluate your practice effectiveness is through client feedback. This type of informal practice evaluation is based upon the subjective responses of the clients. It is a joint and collaborative effort. Both you and your client have roles in this type of practice evaluation.

In keeping with the principles of collaboration and empowerment, in which the client is the expert about their progress, subjective assessments play a prominent role in evaluating practice effectiveness. The critical factor is whether the issues or concerns for which they are seeking help have, in their view, improved. It also helps the social worker and client identify what is working and what is not.

The key to ongoing assessment of client progress and practice effectiveness is persistently and relentlessly following through on the intervention plan. It is checking in with your client between meetings. It is regularly monitoring progress and exploring why or why not progress is being made. In addition to providing feedback, seeking ongoing client feedback helps create expectations for success and for making the identified changes. It communicates that you care and that you are committed to helping your clients overcome the challenge they are facing.

FORMAL PRACTICE EVALUATION

At the micro level of practice, social workers can engage in evaluation to determine whether the intervention they are using is effective. The most common method of evaluation at the micro level is a very practical research design—single-subject design. In the simplest terms, single-subject designs compare baseline phases (referred to as the A phase) with treatment phases (referred to as the B phase). Several types of single-subject designs may be used (see Exhibit 16.3). For the sake of clarification, note that in single-subject design, the single subject refers to a single case that can be an individual person, a family unit, a group, an organization, or a community. For our purposes, we discuss single-subject design as a micro intervention with a single client.

The process of single-subject design involves collecting and recording data, analyzing data, and then making treatment decisions based on the findings. When completing a single-subject design, it is necessary to clearly identify the target problem and to operationally define that problem. An operational definition is a very specific definition that serves to clearly illustrate the behavior. For example, a vague target problem would be "aggression." An operational definition for this target behavior could be "throwing items at peers, pinching, poking, slapping, or hitting." Whenever possible, we should always try to define our targets in positive terms, rather than as the absence of something. When creating our operational definitions, we should also consider terminology related to measurement, including frequency, duration, interval, and intensity.

Once you have collected your single-subject design data, you can graph your data using a line graph. Simple line graphs are quite easy to make in a variety of computer programs. Exhibit 16.4 has a sample single-subject design graph. Notice that both the horizontal (y) axis and the vertical (x) axis are labeled. When creating a graph, it is very important that you label the axes. You should also give your chart a title so that the reader understands what they are looking at in the graph. When graphing single-subject design data, it is customary to point out the break in data between the baseline and treatment phases. In Exhibit 16.4, the break between the baseline and treatment phases is indicated in three ways. First, the line graph is not continuous, which shows the change in phases. Second, a vertical line in the graph marks the change in phases. Finally, we labeled each section as baseline or treatment.

Field Reflection Questions

At your current field placement, how might single-subject design be a useful evaluation strategy?

Which type of single-subject design would you be able to incorporate into your social work practice?

EXHIBIT 16.3

COMMON TYPES OF SINGLE-SUBJECT DESIGNS

Design Type	Description of Design
B	Measurement occurs during the intervention phase. There is no baseline data collection phase. Example: A client enters an inpatient drug and alcohol rehabilitation program. On entry into the program, he immediately begins receiving medication to treat his physical symptoms of withdrawal and begins individual cognitive behavioral therapy with a social worker. Because the social worker did not have a baseline period prior to starting her therapeutic work with this client, all of the data collected while providing the therapy would be considered the treatment phase (B).
AB	There is a period of baseline data collection when no intervention is given. Following the baseline phase, the intervention is administered, and data are collected. Example: A new student has recently transferred into an autism support classroom. The first week that the student is in the classroom, she is observed and evaluated to determine her current levels of functioning and behavioral needs. Data collected during this initial week would be considered baseline (A). Starting in her second week in the classroom, an applied behavior analysis intervention is implemented. Data collected during the intervention of applied behavior analysis would be considered the treatment phase (B).
ABA	There is a period of baseline data collection where no intervention is given. Following the baseline phase, the intervention is administered, and data are then collected. After a period of time, the intervention is withdrawn, and another period of baseline data collection occurs. Note that treatment carryover effects can interfere with the second baseline in this type of design. Example: A child with behavioral outbursts begins BHRS. During the intake process, the treatment team collects data in the forms of observations, interviews, and scales to determine current needs and establish goals. This is the baseline phase (A). After collecting the baseline data, the team implements a behavior modification plan that includes reinforcements and punishments in an attempt to increase positive behaviors and eliminate undesired behaviors. While the behavior modification plan is being implemented, data are collected (B). Once the child has met his treatment goals, before discharging him from services, the treatment team stops implementing the behavior modification plan and tracks rates of behaviors. The period in which data are being collected after the intervention has been removed is the second baseline phase (A).
BAB	Measurement occurs during the intervention phase. The intervention is then withdrawn to collect baseline data. Following collection of baseline data, the intervention is reintroduced. Example: A woman with anxiety comes to a community mental health clinic for support. During her first session, the treatment begins, with the social worker teaching her techniques to calm down, focus on her breath, and engage in mindfulness. The therapist asks the client to continue this intervention. Because there was no baseline period before the intervention was introduced, this case starts with the treatment phase (B). After several successful weeks using the intervention, the social worker stops the intervention and continues to collect data. Because there is no intervention being delivered, this is a baseline phase (A). The social worker eventually reintroduces the intervention and data are collected during the second treatment phase (B).

BHRS, behavioral health rehabilitation services.

EXHIBIT 16.4

SAMPLE SINGLE-SUBJECT DESIGN GRAPH

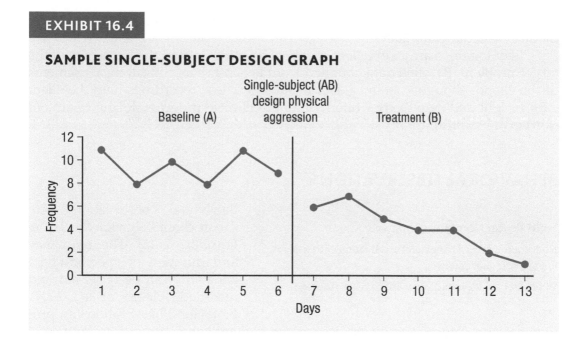

MEASUREMENT TOOLS

There are several measurement methods that involve clients, are easy to construct and implement, and are appropriate for informal and formal practice evaluations. The more frequently used methods are the following:

- client logs
- behavioral observations
- rating scales
- standardized measures

CLIENT LOGS

Having clients prepare narrative accounts of their activities, thoughts, and feelings is an effective method of monitoring progress. Client logs or journals help clarify the nature of client problems and the circumstances that contribute to the problem situation. Clients often find that keeping a log helps them increase their understanding and awareness of the factors that contribute to the identified problem situation. It enables them to "track the antecedents and consequences, or the feelings and thoughts, surrounding the occurrence of a specific event" (Berlin & Marsh, 1993, p. 99). Client logs allow a client to systematically take notes on the occurrence of a target problem and the events surrounding each occurrence. Doing so prevents distortions and misperceptions caused by faulty memory (Bloom et al., 2009).

Client logs also are an excellent source of baseline data on the frequency of the target problem. Baseline data obtained from logs serve as clinical measurements of the client's thoughts, feelings, and behaviors. These recordings help the client gain insight and help the practitioner monitor clinical progress during treatment (Jordan & Franklin, 2015).

BEHAVIORAL OBSERVATIONS

Field Reflection Questions

How could you use behavioral observation with a client in your field placement?

Which behaviors would you want to have observed?

Behavioral observations are direct client behavior (Jordan & Franklin, 2015). The frequency and duration of specific client behaviors can be observed and recorded (Bloom et al., 2009). Behavioral observation can provide detailed information on the occurrence of client behaviors and the context of those behaviors. It represents one of the most reliable and valid methods of measuring client change.

Behavioral observation requires a specification of the target behavior. An example would be specifying the types of disruptive behavior a child displays in the classroom, such as getting out of their seat or talking with classmates while the teacher is talking. The target problem must be clearly defined in behavioral terms and must be observable. Observation cannot be used to measure target problems that focus on feelings or thoughts. It is limited to measuring the frequency, duration, and context of behaviors.

Overall, direct observation is an excellent method for assessing client outcomes. It is one of the most effective tools we have for measuring behavior. When it is used with two or more observers, it can provide reliable and valid outcome data. It also has the potential to provide valuable clinical information on the context within which target problems occur. Direct observation should be seriously considered when a target problem is behavioral in nature, the situation allows for direct observation, and implementing direct observation is feasible.

RATING SCALES

Individualized rating scales are measures of client problems that are created by the client and the social worker together (Bloom et al., 2009). These types of measures are also referred to as self-anchored rating scales (Jordan & Franklin, 2015). The major advantage of an individualized rating scale is that it measures the specific problem or concern that you and your client have identified as the focus of intervention. Thus, a rating scale is directly linked to the feeling, thought, or event that is being addressed in the helping process.

Another advantage of individualized rating scales is that they are based on the client's unique experiences and perceptions. The anchor points of the scale are defined by the client. The low, middle, and high points of the scale are labeled with short, succinct terms. The labels (anchors) describe what the numbers represent (e.g., behaviors, thoughts, and feelings that the client would experience at various points along the scale). Having the client define the anchor points gives the measure great relevance for the client. It becomes a unique measure of the client's feelings, thoughts, or behaviors; it represents the client's perceptions and experiences. An example of an individualized rating scale is shown in Exhibit 16.5.

EXHIBIT 16.5

INDIVIDUALIZED RATING SCALES

Comfort in social situations						
1	2	3	4	5	6	7
Terrified, overwhelmed, completely unable to engage in conversation with strangers			Somewhat anxious, yet able to respond when spoken to		Relaxed, confident, able to initiate conversations with strangers	

Individualized rating scales are excellent tools for measuring client progress and change on identified target problems. They have a high level of face validity because they are derived directly from client problems or concerns. There is some evidence that the validity of single-item rating scales is comparable to that of standardized measures (Nugent, 1992). However, the validity and reliability of individualized rating scales cannot be readily established because they are designed for use with individual clients (Berlin & Marsh, 1993). Rating scales do, however, have a high level of clinical applicability and are excellent tools for measuring client target problems and assessing progress.

STANDARDIZED MEASURES

Standardized measures are instruments developed following empirical scale construction techniques with uniform administration and scoring procedures (Jordan & Franklin, 2015). Their reliability is known, and their validity has usually been empirically tested.

Standardized measures are available for a wide range of client behaviors, including marital satisfaction, self-esteem, anxiety, and family relations. Some standardized measures assess global behaviors, such as generalized contentment, whereas others assess specific behaviors and problems, such as fear, depression, or sexual satisfaction. Standardized measures are available in rapid assessment formats with up to 25 scale items, as well as in lengthy, comprehensive formats with hundreds of scale items. Rapid assessment instruments are easy to use and to incorporate into generalist social work practice.

"Standardized measures represent the most useful quantitative clinical measurement tools that are available to practitioners" (Jordan & Franklin, 2015, p. 53). There are numerous sources of standardized measures. *Measures for Clinical Practice* by Corcoran and Fischer (2013) is an excellent two-volume collection of rapid assessment instruments. Volume 1 contains measures for use with couples, families, and children, and Volume 2 contains instruments for individual adults. The two-volume set contains more than 300 different brief assessment instruments, with supporting information on each instrument's purpose, scoring, reliability, and validity. Another great source of rapid assessment instruments is *Measures of Personality and Social Psychological Attitudes* by Robinson et al. (1991). In this book, measures are organized by clinical topic (e.g., self-esteem, depression, anxiety). Another useful list of measures can be found in *Clinical Assessment for Social Workers* by Jordan and Franklin (2015).

Standardized measures, especially the rapid assessment variety, are well suited for use in evaluating your practice effectiveness. If you can locate one that closely corresponds to identified client problems or concerns, standardized measures offer several advantages. They have known psychometric properties—that is, their reliability and validity have been established. They are also efficient, do not require extensive training, and are easy to administer and score (Corcoran & Fischer, 2013).

CASE SUMMARY: "STOPPING MEDICATION"

PRACTICE SETTING DESCRIPTION

My name is Brantley, and I am an MSW field student. This semester, I have been placed at a long-term structured residence (LTSR). An LTSR is a therapeutic mental health treatment facility for adults. On the continuum of care, an LTSR is less restrictive than an inpatient hospitalization, but more intense than outpatient treatment. While participating in LTSR services, clients live at the facility and receive mental health treatment from a team of professionals including social workers, therapists, and medical staff. The staff work together to support the residents. We meet weekly to have interdisciplinary team meetings to discuss resident progress, concerns, and other treatment information. My primary responsibilities at the LTSR are to facilitate therapy, both group and individual, with the residents.

IDENTIFYING DATA

The first resident assigned to me was Joel, a 26-year-old male. Joel has been a resident at the LTSR for a little over 1 month. He has an extensive history of psychiatric hospitalizations that began when he was approximately 20. Joel has been diagnosed with schizophrenia. He experiences auditory hallucinations and delusions. Joel engages in ritualistic behavior and can at times be compulsive as well. Joel does not like to socialize with the other residents and has a hard time opening up to peers or staff as a result of a general distrust related to some of his delusions that are paranoid.

PRESENTING PROBLEM

Joel was admitted directly to the LTSR from his most recent inpatient psychiatric hospitalization. At the time of discharge, Joel's psychotropic medications had been adjusted to a level where he reported no positive symptoms related to his schizophrenia (hallucinations and delusions). Despite the reprieve from these symptoms, Joel does not like taking his medication because of the side effects he has been experiencing. Some of those side effects include weight gain, dizziness, muscle spasms, and nausea. Joel has shared with the doctor that he wants to try a different course of treatment because he reports being so miserable on the medication.

During an interdisciplinary team meeting, Joel's request to stop his psychotropic medications was discussed. My field supervisor, a licensed social worker, advocated for Joel's right to self-determination. She told the others on the team that Joel is coherent and capable of making his own treatment decisions, and that we should respect his wishes to try another course of treatment. A nurse at the meeting disagreed with my field supervisor. She shared that she felt strongly that because Joel's hallucinations and delusions have been virtually eliminated on the medication, stopping the medication should not be up for discussion. She added that research suggests medication and therapy together are the standard of treatment for individuals with this diagnosis. The group talked about the ethics related to this situation and in the end agreed that Joel was indeed competent to make the decision to attempt another course of treatment at this time. The psychiatrist plans to wean Joel off his current medications and try another family of medications that are known to have less harsh effects. Everyone agreed that it would be very important for Joel to continue to participate in therapy to continue to address his mental health needs. Everyone also agreed that Joel needed to be monitored quite closely during this transition of medications to evaluate whether the new course of treatment is beneficial for him.

After the meeting, I met with my field supervisor about the meeting and decision to allow Joel to try an alternative course of treatment. My supervisor asked me how I planned to evaluate Joel during this transition. At first, I was not sure what to do. I told my field instructor that I really was not sure. Together, we brainstormed ways to collect data. We also talked about the benefits of collecting data from various sources. After my conversation with my field instructor, I designed a data collection tool that I could use with Joel during my individual sessions. I also designed a self-reporting data tool for Joel to use as well so that he could share his experiences. I also created a general data collection tool that I put in Joel's chart where any staff member who needed to record an incident at the LTSR regarding Joel could make a notation of the event.

ASSESSMENT

Two weeks after the initial interdisciplinary team meeting where it was agreed to transition Joel to new medication, we came together to discuss Joel's case again. At the meeting the nurse who was initially resistant to the change of medication said that she thought Joel was decompensating since changing medications. Another therapist said that he thought Joel was doing better. Luckily, I had been collecting data for 2 weeks, from a variety of sources. I shared the data I had collected and analyzed; it illustrated that Joel was doing quite well with his new course of treatment. Based on my observations, client self-reports, and reports from other staff, it appeared that Joel was engaging with peers and staff more, still not experiencing any positive symptoms, and not experiencing any of the previously concerning side effects. My data were able to demonstrate that Joel's treatment is successful for him at this time.

CASE PROCESS SUMMARY

I have been learning so much at field placement, and with Joel's case especially, I feel like I am really learning how to be an effective social worker. With the help of my field supervisor, I was able to design data collection tools that allowed me to gather the data necessary to be able to share treatment progress. Because I had actual data, I was able to advocate for Joel's current treatment in the interdisciplinary team meeting. Without the data, I am not sure if Joel's current course of treatment would have been continued. With this experience, I learned that as a social worker I can use evaluation to improve the lives of my clients and at the end of the day that is why I want to be a social worker!

Brantley, MSW Student Intern

CASE DISCUSSION QUESTIONS

1. *Why do you think the field supervisor encouraged Brantley to collect actual data?*

2. *Why do you think Brantley decided to collect data from multiple sources (himself, Joel's self-reports, and notes from other staff)? What are the benefits from having multiple sources of data when conducting an evaluation?*

3. *If you were the social work student and needed to collect data on this case, how would you set up your data collection tool? What questions would be on your tool? How would your tools differ depending on who was using it (e.g., how would your data tool be different from the one for the resident and from the one for the other staff)?*

4. *In your field placement, if you needed to collect data on a client, how would you go about gathering those data? What sources would you use? What data would be important to collect?*

END-OF-CHAPTER RESOURCES

A robust set of instructor resources designed to supplement this text is located at http://connect.springerpub.com/content/book/978-0-8261-3753-1. Qualifying instructors may request access by emailing textbook@springerpub.com.

CRITICAL THINKING QUESTIONS

1. How are applied and basic research similar? In what ways do they differ from each other?

2. How can you ensure that you are following the standards set forth by the NASW *Code of Ethics* related to research and evaluation at your field placement? Provide three specific examples.

3. If you were asked to design a formative evaluation of your field placement program, what research questions do you think should be evaluated? What would be your data sources? What type of evaluation method would you choose? What type of measurement would you use?

4. Create a logic model for your field placement. What are the resources necessary for your program to run? What activities are required within your program? What are the outputs and outcomes of your program? How would you measure your outcomes?

LEARNING ACTIVITIES

1. In collaboration with your field instructor develop a plan for obtaining ongoing feedback from a client regarding their experiences working with you and their perceptions on their progress toward their goals. Discuss your feedback with your field instructor during your weekly supervision and make any needed changes in your work with the client.

2. In collaboration with your field instructor design a single-subject evaluation with one of your clients. Identify the client problem that you will measure and create or locate an appropriate measure. Role-play with your field instructor how you will introduce the single-subject design to your client. Review your findings with your field instructor and share them with your client.

3. Identify an aspect of your program that needs improvement. Design a program evaluation and share it with your field instructor. Create a proposal to evaluate the program and seek permission to conduct the evaluation.

4. Create a logic model for your program. Determine how your program is currently being evaluated and compare it to your logic model. Review your findings with your field instructor and make recommendations to your agency administrators on any needed improvements to their evaluation procedures.

ELECTRONIC RESOURCES

WEBSITE LINKS

 The Evolution of a Social Work Researcher: www.socialworker .com/feature-articles/practice/The_Evolution_of_a_Social _Work_Researcher

 Focus Groups: https://scientificinquiryinsocialwork.pressbooks .com/chapter/13-4-focus-groups

 Program Evaluation: https://omerad.msu.edu/meded/progeval/ step4.html

VIDEO LINKS

 How Do Focus Groups Work? www.youtube.com/watch ?v=3TwgVQIZPsw

 Mixed Methods: www.youtube.com/watch?v=PSVsD9fAx38

 Single-Subject Design: www.youtube.com/watch?v=A1idx6djJlY

REFERENCES

Berlin, S., & Marsh, J. (1993). *Informing practice decisions*. Macmillan.

Bloom, M., Fischer, J., & Orme, J. G. (2009). *Evaluating practice: Guidelines for the accountable professional* (6th ed.). Pearson.

Corcoran, K., & Fischer, J. (Eds.). (2013). *Measures for clinical practice: A sourcebook* (5th ed., Vols. 1–2). Oxford University Press.

Council on Social Work Education. (2022). *Educational policy and accreditation standards for baccalaureate and master's social work programs*. https://www.cswe.org/getmedia/94471c42-13b8-493b-9041-b30f48533d64/2022-EPAS.pdf

Jordan, C., & Franklin, C. (2015). *Clinical assessment for social workers: Quantitative and qualitative methods* (4th ed.). Oxford University Press.

National Association of Social Workers. (2021). *Code of ethics*. https://www.socialworkers.org/About/Ethics/Code-of-Ethics/Code-of-Ethics-English

Nugent, W. R. (1992). Psychometric characteristics of self-anchored scales in clinical application. *Journal of Social Service Research*, *15*, 137–152. https://doi.org/10.1300/J079v15n03_08

Poulin, J., Kauffman, S., & Ingersoll, T. S. (2022). *Social work capstone projects: Demonstrating professional competencies through applied research*. Springer Publishing Company.

Poulin, J., & Matis, S. (2021). *Social work practice. A competency-based approach*. Springer Publishing Company.

Robinson, J. P., Shaver, P. R., & Wrightsman, L. S. (1991). *Measures of personality and social psychological attitudes*. Academic Press.

Rogers, J. (2012). Anti-oppressive social work research: Reflections on power in the creation of knowledge. *Social Work Education*, *31*(7), 866–879. https://doi.org/10.1080/02615479.2011.602965

Rubin, A., & Babbie, E. R. (2017). *Empowerment series: Research methods for social work* (9th ed.). Cengage.

Index